KT-520-177

Musculoskeletal
Physiotherapy

in s are charged on overdue books at 10p per day. You can renew by:

phone: Sandwell Internal 3645,   City Internal 4491
Sandwell external 21 607 3551,   City external 0121 507 5245

REMOVED
FROM
STOCK

For Butterworth-Heinemann:

Senior Commissioning Editor: Heidi Allen
Project Development Editor: Robert Edwards
Project Manager: Jane Dingwall
Senior Designer: George Ajayi
Illustration Manager: Bruce Hogarth
Illustrations: David Gardner

Musculoskeletal Physiotherapy

Clinical Science and Evidence-Based Practice

SECOND EDITION

Edited by

Kathryn M. Refshauge
DipPhty, Grad Dip Manip Ther (Cumb), MBiomedE (NSW), PhD, MAPA, MPAA
Professor, School of Physiotherapy, The University of Sydney, Australia

and

Elizabeth M. Gass
DipPhty, BAppSc, MAppSc (Cumb), PhD, MPAA
Associate Professor, School of Physiotherapy and Exercise Science, Griffith University, Queensland, Australia

Foreword by

Lance Twomey AM
President and Vice-Chancellor, Curtin University of Technology, Perth, Australia

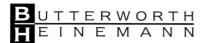

EDINBURGH   LONDON   NEW YORK   OXFORD   PHILADELPHIA   ST LOUIS   SYDNEY   TORONTO   2004

BUTTERWORTH-HEINEMANN
An imprint of Elsevier Limited

© Reed Educational and Professional Publishing Ltd 1995
© 2004, Elsevier Limited. All rights reserved.

The right of Kathryn M. Refshauge and Elizabeth M. Gass to be identified as
editors of this work have been asserted by them in accordance with the Copyright,
Designs and Patents Act 1988.

No part of this publication may be reproduced, stored in a retrieval system, or
transmitted in any form or by any means, electronic, mechanical, photocopying,
recording or otherwise, without either the prior permission of the publishers
or a icence permitting restricted copying in the United Kingdom issued by
the Copyright Licensing Agency, 90 Tottenham Court Road, London W1T 4LP.
Permissions may be sought directly from Elsevier's Health Sciences Rights
Department in Philadelphia, USA: phone: (+1) 215 238 7869, fax: (+1) 215 238 2239,
e-mail: healthpermissions@elsevier.com. You may also complete your request
on-line via the Elsevier homepage (http://www.elsevier.com), by selecting
'Customer Support' and then 'Obtaining Permissions'.

First edition 1995
Second edition 2004
  Reprinted 2005

ISBN 0 7506 5356 6

British Library Cataloguing in Publication Data
A catalogue record for this book is available from the British Library

Library of Congress Cataloging in Publication Data
A catalog record for this book is available from the Library of Congress

Note
Knowledge and best practice in this field are constantly changing. As
new research and experience broaden our knowledge, changes in practice,
treatment and drug therapy may become necessary or appropriate. Readers
are advised to check the most current information provided (i) on procedures
featured or (ii) by the manufacturer of each product to be administered,
to verify the recommended dose or formula, the method and duration of
administration, and contraindications. It is the responsibility of the
practitioner, relying on their own experience and knowledge of the patient,
to make diagnoses, to determine dosages and the best treatment for each
individual patient, and to take all appropriate safety precautions.
To the fullest extent of the law, neither the publisher nor the editors
assumes any liability for any injury and/or damage.

Every effort has been made by the Publisher to obtain permission to reproduce
material written by Harold M. Frost taken from the first edition of the book.
The Publisher

ELSEVIER your source for books,
journals and multimedia
in the health sciences
www.elsevierhealth.com

Working together to grow
libraries in developing countries

www.elsevier.com | www.bookaid.org | www.sabre.org

ELSEVIER   BOOK AID International   Sabre Foundation

The
publisher's
policy is to use
**paper manufactured
from sustainable forests**

Printed in China

Contents

Contributors

Kim Bennell BAppSc(Physio), PhD
Associate Professor and Director, Centre for Sports Medicine Research and Education, School of Physiotherapy, University of Melbourne, Australia

Grant Bigg-Wither MBChB, FRANZCR
Department of Medical Imaging, St Vincent's Hospital, Darlinghurst, Australia

Nikolai Bogduk MD, PhD, DSc, Dip Anat, Dip Pain Med, FFPM (ANZCA)
Professor of Pain Medicine, University of Newcastle, Royal Newcastle Hospital, Newcastle, Australia

Robert Boland BAppSc, GradDipManipTher, PhD
Lecturer, School of Physiotherapy, Faculty of Health Sciences, University of Sydney, Australia

Janet Carr EdD FACP
Honorary Associate Professor, School of Physiotherapy, Faculty of Health Sciences, University of Sydney, Australia

Philip G. Conaghan MBBS, FRACP
Senior Lecturer and Honorary Consultant Rheumatologist, University of Leeds and Leeds General Infirmary, Leeds, UK

Richard O. Day AM, MD, FRACP
Professor of Clinical Pharmacology, Department of Clinical Pharmacology, St Vincent's Hospital, Darlinghurst, Australia

Mark Elkins B Phty, B Arts, M Hlth Sci
Research Physiotherapist, Royal Prince Alfred Hospital, Camperdown, Australia

Harold M. Frost MD
Orthopaedic Surgeon, Southern Colorado Clinic, Pueblo, USA

Elizabeth M. Gass DipPhty, BAppSc, MAppSc (Cumb), PhD, MPAA
Associate Professor, School of Physiotherapy and Exercise Science, Faculty of Health Sciences, Griffith University, Queensland, Australia

Michalene Goodsell MAppSc, GradDipManipTher
Unanderra Physiotherapy Centre, Unanderra, Australia

David Gronow MBBS, FFARACS, FANZCA, FFPMANZCA, FChPMRACP
Director, Sydney Pain Management Centre, Parramatta, Australia

Robert Herbert BAppSc, MAppSc, PhD
Senior Lecturer, School of Physiotherapy, Faculty of Health Sciences, University of Sydney, Australia

Paul Kelly MSc (Hon.CausaSyd) DipPhty GradDip ManipTher (Cumb) MAppSc (Cumb)
St Vincent's Clinic, Darlinghurst, Australia

Karim Khan MD, PhD, FACSP
Assistant Professor, Department of Family Practice and School of Human Kinetics, University of British Columbia, Vancouver, Canada

Jane Latimer BAppSc, GradDipAppSc, PhD
Senior Lecturer, School of Physiotherapy, Faculty of Health Sciences, University of Sydney, Australia

Michael Lee BE, BAppSc, MBiomedE
School of Exercise and Sport Science, Faculty of
Health Sciences, University of Sydney, Australia

Christopher G. Maher PhD, BAppSc, GradDipAppSc
Associate Professor, School of Physiotherapy,
Faculty of Health Sciences, University of Sydney,
Australia

Susan Mercer BPhty (Hons), PhD, FNZCP
Senior Lecturer, Department of Anatomy and
Structural Biology, University of Otago, Dunedin,
New Zealand

Anne Moseley BAppSc (Physio), GradDipAppSc
(ExSpSc), PhD
Lecturer, Rehabilitation Studies Unit, Faculty of
Medicine, University of Sydney, Australia

Michael K. Nicholas BSc, MSc (Hons), MPsychol, PhD
Associate Professor, Pain Management and
Research Centre, University of Sydney at Royal
North Shore Hospital, St Leonards, Australia

Kathryn M. Refshauge DipPhty, GradDipManipTher
(Cumb), MBiomedE (NSW), PhD, MAPA, MPAA
Professor, School of Physiotherapy, Faculty of
Health Sciences, University of Sydney,
Australia

Roberta Shepherd EdD, FACP
Honorary Professor, School of Physiotherapy,
Faculty of Health Sciences, University of Sydney,
Australia

Catherine Sherrington BAppSc, MPH, PhD
Research Fellow, Prince of Wales Medical
Research Institute, Randwick, Australia

Lois Tonkin Dip Psy
Pain Management and Research Centre, Royal
North Shore Hospital, St Leonards, Australia

Foreword

It is always a salutary experience to read the second edition of a popular textbook, not only for a more contemporary account of the topics covered, but especially to see how (or if) the thinking of the authors and editors has changed during the interim. This is especially important when the text concerned focuses on clinical management and current practice in any of the health disciplines. If all that we readers get is essentially more of the same accompanied by an increase in volume and updated references (although the latter are useful), then the reader can be forgiven for wondering why another forest has been sacrificed to such little effect. I am pleased to say that this is not the case for the second edition of Kathryn Refshauge and Elizabeth Gass's book *Musculoskeletal Physiotherapy*.

The text certainly provides updated and current reference lists and continues the excellent approach toward evidence-based physical treatment of musculoskeletal disorders which was such a distinctive feature of the first edition. However, it does so in a way which allows for and indeed demands the reinterpretation of information, experience and data in clinical physiotherapy. This is not just more of the same.

In my foreword to the first edition I highlighted the approach to practice to which my contemporaries and I were exposed by our physiotherapy education/training of 40 years ago, in the words: 'The classical approach to the physical treatment of musculoskeletal disorders always relied on the referring doctor's diagnosis and a rather perfunctory examination, followed by treatment according "to the book". The reliance on the clinical judgements of authoritive forebears and their detailed prescriptions for patient management provided warm security for the physiotherapist, but cold comfort to the captive patient.'

A major goal of Refshauge and Gass, as evident in the first edition, was to ensure that an intimate relationship was shown to exist between science and practice. This has been further augmented in the second edition. *Musculoskeletal Physiotherapy* remains an 'active book', one which shies away from prescription, demands an intellectual response from the reader and insists on a rational, logical but always caring approach to physical treatment. Underneath the science, the editors and authors of this text really care what happens to patients and insist that physiotherapists retain this as the core of their patient treatment philosophy and approach.

As with the first edition, the chapters of this multiauthored book focus on the rationale behind examination, history-taking, diagnosis and finally physical treatment and pain management. This book is eminently readable and the authors and editors are to be commended for ensuring a consistency in style and approach evident throughout the work. There is a real but important difference between strong support for a concept or approach (in this case a rational, science-based orientation) and adopting an authoritarian, preaching style. It is interesting to note how far physiotherapy has travelled from the personality/guru-dominated approaches so characteristic of mid twentieth-century methodologies. It is to be hoped that those so passionate in this attack do not themselves fall into the same trap.

Musculoskeletal Physiotherapy (second edition) continues as a superb textbook for students and thinking practitioners of physiotherapy. It provides for the appropriate interpretation of contemporary knowledge and allows practitioners the scope for the logical application of physical treatment. I trust that other readers will enjoy and be challenged by it as much as I have been.

Lance Twomey AM
President and Vice-Chancellor
Curtin University of Technology
Perth, Australia

Preface

Writing the second edition has been challenging in surprising ways – ways that we had not expected when we embarked on the journey to update the original text. We knew a second edition was due, but finding time seemed impossible in our busy lives. We also didn't expect that there would be so much to update. But the evidence-based practice revolution in physiotherapy has really blossomed in the 10 years or more since the first edition, and so many more changes were required than originally anticipated. Much of the underlying sciences in Chapter 2 and the imaging in Chapter 3 required updating, but not major revision, although we included a new and exciting section by Kim Bennell and Karim Khan on the application to physiotherapy practice of research into bone density. Chapter 4, Principles of examination and measurement, required a new section, The accuracy of diagnostic tests, because there is a wealth of information now available including, for example, likelihood ratios of various tests. This information has then been applied in Chapters 5 and 6, where information about diagnosing serious pathology has included presentation of data in the form of likelihood ratios. Chapter 5 is quite different from the first edition, and now presents those questionnaires that are commonly used to measure pain and disability, accuracy of diagnosis of pathology, identification of yellow flags (i.e. indicators of poor prognosis) and cognitive factors. Chapter 6 has also changed dramatically, with inclusion of information about the measurement of various procedures and outcomes as an appendix to the chapter. Information about reliability and validity of each test has also been included here. Chapter 7 now includes a contribution from the Centre for Evidence-Based Practice. We are particularly fortunate that the Centre is based in our School of Physiotherapy at the University of Sydney. This is an excellent contribution helping the reader to understand how to read and interpret clinical trials. The chapter that consisted of case studies has been replaced by a new chapter on persisting (or chronic) pain, with an excellent overview of cognitive-behavioural therapy.

The task of completing the second edition was therefore far harder than anticipated, and a much bigger job than we had planned. However, it was also far more rewarding as we again grappled with new issues and the best way to present them for our students and for practising clinicians.

Kathryn Refshauge and Elizabeth Gass

Chapter 1

The context of musculoskeletal physiotherapy practice

K.M. Refshauge and E.M. Gass

THE NEED FOR THIS BOOK

To speak of need is to imply a goal, a means of achieving the goal and a means of measuring deficiency from the goal (Wilkin et al., 1992). A critical goal in musculoskeletal physiotherapy is to possess a sound theoretical basis for a clinical practice which demonstrably achieves relevant and effective outcomes. Achievement of this goal means overcoming deficiencies in both the musculoskeletal physiotherapy theory base and in demonstration of clinical effectiveness. In musculoskeletal physiotherapy the gap between the goal and the measured deficiencies is constantly narrowing.

Many former textbooks on musculoskeletal physiotherapy, while serving the important function of describing practical procedures, were frequently anecdotal, often including incorrect and unsubstantiated information, and describing practical procedures in isolation. In this revised edition current scientific knowledge underlying physiotherapy practice is interpreted and analysed for clinical use, although it is acknowledged that not all clinical practice can currently be fully substantiated.

Information that is well described and easily accessible elsewhere, such as how to perform passive motion procedures for assessment or treatment, will rarely be covered in detail (for examples, see Kaltenborn, 1980; Grieve, 1984; Maitland, 1986; Magee, 1987). Rather, this text focuses on an evaluation of examination procedures, the interpretation of tests and evaluation of management strategies. Occasionally procedures are described to enable evaluation and to avoid constant cross-referencing. Knowledge is drawn from related areas to develop a considered interpretation that is both current and clinically applicable. The use of information is illustrated with clinical examples, this contextual relevance giving the information a realistic perspective.

Examination and treatment of spinal musculoskeletal conditions are discussed, using examples relating to upper and lower quadrants, i.e. the cervical spine and shoulder, the lumbar spine and hip, and the sacroiliac joint and lumbar spine. Although much information is relevant to the peripheral regions, and some illustrations use the periphery for clarification, the periphery will not be dealt with separately.

THE MUSCULOSKELETAL PHYSIOTHERAPY PARADIGM

The goal of possessing a sound theoretical base for musculoskeletal physiotherapy clinical practice implies a close relationship between science and practice. The extent to which one considers that physiotherapy practice is based on science depends to some degree on one's view of what constitutes 'science'. This book does not explore the relationship between physiotherapy and science, but some relevant issues are raised. James Gordon (1987), in a fascinating exposition, explored the way in which science provides a guiding theoretical model, and the tenet that practical needs determine the validity of the theoretical model, using neurological physiotherapy as the example.

A discussion of the development of 'scientific' thought is relevant here to place in context the development of musculoskeletal physiotherapy. Many philosophers have proffered theories about the development of scientific thought (Kuhn, 1974; Popper, 1974; Chalmers, 1983). One of these is Kuhn and his theory of scientific revolutions. The development of musculoskeletal physiotherapy could be likened to these 'scientific revolutions'.

Kuhn (1974) and others propose that we operate using a theoretical framework and set of assumptions. Kuhn termed this 'scientific' framework a paradigm. He further suggests that in reality scientists

direct their work to solving questions determined by, or relevant to, the paradigm. When problems considered important within a discipline can no longer be solved using the current paradigm, a new theoretical framework and set of assumptions is adopted. Kuhn termed this a 'paradigm shift'. There are many examples of paradigm shifts in the historical development of scientific disciplines. A famous example is within the field of astronomy. In medieval times it was assumed that the earth was the centre of the universe, and that all the planets including the sun orbited the earth. In the seventeenth century it became important to solve the problem of the current calendar being inconsistent with the lunar year. Galileo was employed to solve this vexatious problem (Burke, 1985). The results of his work are well-known: the original assumption about the earth being the centre of the universe was no longer tenable. This led to a scientific (and personal for Galileo) crisis or revolution, and ultimately to a paradigm shift. Other examples can be found in the development of Charles Darwin's theories on evolution or Einstein's work on relativity.

A paradigm shift generally results in adopting more appropriate assumptions, although these are not necessarily 'correct' or even 'more correct'. Consequently a paradigm shift also results in a change in the questions that scientists and members of a discipline consider important.

The reason for discussing Kuhn's theories about paradigms and how they shift is that this philosophy provides a particularly apt perspective for interpreting growth of knowledge in physiotherapy. When considering past and future changes in physiotherapy knowledge and practice, it is attractive to believe that we currently operate within a paradigm. This paradigm will most probably shift in the future; however, this book is concerned with our current understanding of science and physiotherapy practice.

The various authors in this book have explored the paradigm of contemporary physiotherapy practice. Current scientific knowledge is interpreted and analysed for use in clinical practice. This, of necessity, involves evaluating prevailing approaches to examination and treatment. This in turn involves attempting to identify assumptions underlying physiotherapy practice. Some assumptions are explicit (such as that a reduction in spinal pain leads to return of normal function), but many are implicit, and therefore very difficult to identify. When identified, these assumptions are evaluated. We make it clear that such a process is not intended to be negative, but is an attempt at identification and analysis of the philosophy underlying physiotherapy practice.

PHYSIOTHERAPY PRACTICE

At any instant, the practice of physiotherapy may appear to be clearly defined and static. This is probably particularly true from the perspective of undergraduate students. The following brief summary of the development of physiotherapy highlights the enormous changes that have actually taken place in physiotherapy practice.

The first descriptions of practice allied to physiotherapy refer to the use of 'therapeutic gymnastics' and 'gymnastic medicine' as preventive and curative treatments in the time of Herodicus (approximately 480 BC), Hippocrates (460–370 BC) and later Galen (AD 129–210). Even in these early times there was controversy about the delineation of roles of physicians and gymnasts in the delivery of these treatments (Berryman, 1987).

The practice of manual therapies did not change substantially until the twentieth century. In 1920 the Chartered Society of Massage and Medical Gymnastics emerged in the UK, amalgamating several small groups that had apparently originated from an initial group formed in 1894, consisting at that time of eight women. The aim of the Chartered Society of Massage and Medical Gymnastics was to bind together those who practised physical treatment in an honourable way (Mennell, 1934). A similar association was formed in the USA, the American Women's Physical Therapeutic Association (now the American Physical Therapy Association) that, in 1921, aimed to establish and maintain a professional and scientific standard and disseminate information through medical and professional articles (American Women's Physical Therapeutic Association, 1921).

The First and Second World Wars increased the demand for treatments to deal with stiff joints, weak muscles and associated functional deficits following fractures and gunshot and shrapnel wounds

(May, 1954). The poliomyelitis epidemic in the 1950s further increased this demand (May, 1954). Those carrying out physical treatments at this time worked closely under the guidance of medical practitioners. The 6-month training course was entirely technical, and predominantly equipped physiotherapists to perform massage and exercise, such as the Swedish Remedial Exercise System (Palmer, 1918; Mennell, 1934). The types of massage and remedial exercises prescribed in the 1920s make interesting reading; however, one wonders whether current practice is actually any more firmly based on theory.

The writings of many physiotherapists, in particular those of Geoffrey Maitland, profoundly influenced the further development of musculoskeletal physiotherapy practice (Maitland, 1964; Kaltenborn, 1980). Although the emphasis in these first editions was on manipulative treatment, Maitland proposed an extensive system of examination of patients and advocated basing treatment decisions on the patient's signs and symptoms rather than on the diagnosis. The preface to Maitland's first edition emphasized that all physiotherapy treatments described in the book would require medical referral (Maitland, 1964). In a foreword to a subsequent edition (Brewerton, 1977) the question was posed whether it is sufficient for physiotherapists to apply heat, ice or active exercise when patients have stiff or painful joints, or whether something more specific to restoration of joint movement should be used. The author prophesied that controlled trials would be needed to resolve such a question and noted that, since it might be many years before adequate answers were produced, it was essential to achieve an assessment based on clinical judgement and experience (Brewerton, 1977).

Throughout many editions of the books written by Maitland (1964, 1968, 1973, 1981, 1986) the emphasis was not only on describing a system of manoeuvres and techniques for assessment and treatment of joints, but also on evaluating results of treatment and prescribing adequate treatment doses. Maitland suggested constant monitoring of changes in the patient's signs and symptoms and introduced the concept of 'irritability' to assist in dose prescription. New concepts of 'comparable joint sign' and 'accessory joint movement' were also described, and suggested as tools to enable more specific examination and treatment of spinal musculoskeletal disorders. Maitland and his peers thus applied a challenge to accepted musculoskeletal physiotherapy practice.

More recently the trend to evidence-based practice has heavily influenced all health professionals including physiotherapists. Approximately 5 years ago the early evidence-based practice movement, originating predominantly in medicine, stressed the importance of basing clinical decisions upon research evidence, particularly randomized controlled clinical trials (Sackett, 1997a, b). This move to evidence-based practice has had a strong impact in physiotherapy, both as a stimulus for research that is more focused and relevant to physiotherapists, and as a guiding principle underlying examination and treatment of patients. The evidence to date gives strong support to many of our examination procedures and treatments for musculoskeletal conditions.

An evidence-based approach has raised some concern about implementation, with some authors suggesting that it signals a move away from decisions being made largely on the basis of clinical findings and pathology (Crombie, 1997) towards decisions being made on the basis of available research evidence (Crombie, 1997; Sackett et al., 1997a, b). The approach to evidence-based practice has encouraged debate, particularly in the area of what constitutes evidence (Jones and Higgs, 2000). It has been suggested that we should define evidence as 'knowledge that has been derived from a variety of sources that has been subject to testing and found to be credible' (Jones and Higgs, 2000). Thus clinical experience can be a legitimate source of knowledge, and in fact the best evidence is likely to be that derived from scientific enquiry but informed by knowledge based on clinical experience.

Interestingly, in medicine there has also been vigorous debate about the possible conflicts between the clinical evidence base and the public health evidence base (Cassell, 1997; Churchill, 1997; Frankel and Smith, 1997; Kernick, 1997; Maynard, 1997; Sackett, 1997a, b; Wolfe, 1997). This debate focuses on the cost-utility of clinical decisions and the possible dilemma of having evidence to support a certain individual clinical management approach, and having public health evidence about population outcomes and costs which might work against

implementation of the evidence-based individual treatment approach. These issues may become important in physiotherapy in the near future as health costs continue to rise.

Education of physiotherapy students closely parallels these advances in theoretical frameworks and practical skills. These advances form the foundation for our current practice as independent professionals.

CONTEXT OF CURRENT PRACTICE: ASSUMPTIONS AND THEORETICAL MODELS

The context of physiotherapy practice is heavily influenced by the overall health and social context. These broader contexts will vary and be influenced by a myriad of factors, including:

- political environment
- community health needs
- availability of resources
- demographic trends
- incidence/prevalence of certain diseases and conditions
- need for accountability
- trend for evidence-based practice.

One of the biggest changes in the delivery of health care in recent times is the shift towards community-based practice, with more emphasis on education and advice and less emphasis on 'one on one' therapeutic interactions. This trend is likely to continue. Physiotherapists must therefore assume a larger role in developing and implementing public health strategies, for example by encouraging good bone health throughout the lifespan, prescribing and monitoring exercise for many chronic conditions such as chronic low back pain, arthritis, diabetes and sarcopenia in older people, and implement strategies to prevent falls. By knowing how treatments achieve their outcomes, we can then improve key aspects of patient management such as who will benefit most from a particular treatment and how further to target and improve the treatment, its dose and evaluation of the outcome. By adhering to principles of inquiry and reflective practice we can avoid using treatments in a routine way, often described as 'mythical' or 'ritualistic'. It is the role of educational institutions and professional associations to take account of predicted changes in health care needs and to ensure that physiotherapists are able to meet these needs effectively.

The current paradigm within which musculoskeletal physiotherapy is situated includes consideration of:

- knowledge of tissue/organ response to injury, disuse and overuse
- knowledge of prognostic factors, particularly those in the psychosocial domain
- effective, reliable, valid, sensitive and specific assessment procedures and outcome measures that are also responsive
- evidence base for the use of certain procedures and dosages
- patients' goals
- how best to maximize function and prevent or minimize dysfunction
- epidemiological and public health data and strategies.

Clinical decisions made by physiotherapists must be predicated upon the available knowledge base, and rely on the ability to make a diagnosis, prescribe effective management and prevention strategies and predict prognosis and a time frame for achievement of objectives. The assumptions underlying such clinical decisions in musculoskeletal physiotherapy are often difficult to identify, but probably include assumptions adopted from fields such as physiology, biomechanics and other disciplines within the health and medical sciences. It may be valuable, however, to attempt to identify some assumptions, to gain a clearer insight into the basis of current musculoskeletal physiotherapy practice.

Some readily identifiable assumptions include:

1. Non-specific mechanical pain is musculoskeletal in origin.
2. Pain and pain behaviour exhibited by the patient are signals that the musculoskeletal system is disordered.
3. Musculoskeletal tissues and organs behave in a predictable way when damaged and, provided

that the environment is adequate, will follow a prescribed healing and repair process.
4. Both the patient and the physiotherapist have key roles in achieving goals of treatment. Except in extreme circumstances, a partnership approach is generally assumed to help achieve stated treatment goals.
5. Treatments aimed at affecting the musculoskeletal system will primarily affect the musculoskeletal tissues.
6. Prevention of certain musculoskeletal disorders is possible. This remains an assumption because there is a lack of knowledge of cause and effect of various factors. Some examples of prevention include interventions aimed at altering segmental alignment (or posture) to prevent future pain, or altering the amount of foot pronation to prevent future lower limb or spinal pain. Since there is little evidence about cause and effect of these characteristics, such interventions remain based on assumption.

These assumptions may seem trite or even ridiculous. Paradigms shift, however, when fundamental 'truths' such as these no longer hold. It is extremely difficult to recognize implicit assumptions because they are often considered to be known facts; however, identification of common assumptions can provide a basis for challenge and growth. It is useful to recognize that physiotherapists operate in today's paradigm, and that the basis of musculoskeletal physiotherapy may change radically even within a decade if, and as, the paradigm shifts. It is difficult to predict the next major change in a discipline when one is so firmly entrenched in current practice.

The writers and editors of this book have faced the challenge of explicit identification of the scientific basis for musculoskeletal physiotherapy practice. The process of facing this challenge has been stimulating, thought-provoking and, at times, uncomfortable and sobering. Physiotherapists are encouraged to read, reflect on and question the material presented in this book, because this material is thought to represent the current foundation of musculoskeletal physiotherapy practice.

REFERENCES

American Women's Physical Therapeutic Association (1921). Constitution. *Phys. Ther.*, **1**, 5.

Berryman, J.W. (1987). The tradition of the 'six things non-natural': exercise and medicine from Hippocrates through ante-bellum America. *Exerc. Sport Sci. Rev.*, **17**, 515–559.

Brewerton, D.A. (1977). Foreword. In: *Peripheral Manipulation*, 2nd edn, ed. G.D. Maitland, pp. 1–9. London: Butterworths.

Burke, J. (1985). *The Day the Universe Changed*. London: British Broadcasting Corporation.

Cassell, J. (1997). Evidence-based medicine and treatment choices. *Lancet*, **349**, 570–571.

Chalmers, A.F. (1983). *What is This Thing Called Science: An Assessment of the Nature and Status of Science and its Methods*, 2nd edn. St Lucia, Queensland: University of Queensland Press.

Churchill, D. (1997). Evidence-based medicine and treatment choices. *Lancet*, **349**, 571–572.

Crombie, I.K. (1997). The limits of evidence-based medicine. *Pain Forum*, **7**, 63–65.

Frankel, S. and Smith, G.D. (1997). Evidence-based medicine and treatment choices. *Lancet*, **349**, 571.

Gordon, J. (1987). Assumptions underlying physical therapy intervention: theoretical and historical perspectives. In: *Movement Science. Foundations for Physical Therapy in Rehabilitation*, ed. J.H. Carr, R.B. Shepherd, J. Gordon et al., pp. 1–31. London: Heinemann Physiotherapy.

Grieve, G.P. (1984). *Mobilisation of the Spine*, 4th edn. London: Churchill Livingstone.

Jones, M. and Higgs, J. (2000). Will evidence-based practice take the reasoning out of practice? In: *Clinical Reasoning for the Health Professions*, 2nd edn, ed. J. Higgs & M. Jones, pp. 307–315. Oxford: Butterworth-Heinemann.

Kaltenborn, F.M. (1980). *Mobilization of the Extremity Joints*, 3rd edn. Oslo: Olaf Norlis Bokhandel.

Kernick, D.P. (1997). Evidence-based medicine and treatment choices. *Lancet*, **349**, 570.

Kuhn, T.S. (1974). *The Structure of Scientific Revolutions*, 2nd edn. Chicago: University of Chicago Press.

Magee, D.J. (1987). *Orthopaedic Physical Assessment*. London: W.B. Saunders.

Maitland, G.D. (1964). *Vertebral Manipulation*. London: Butterworths.

Maitland, G.D. (1968). *Vertebral Manipulation*, 2nd edn. London: Butterworths.

Maitland, G.D. (1973). *Vertebral Manipulation*, 3rd edn. London: Butterworths.

Maitland, G.D. (1981). *Vertebral Manipulation*, 4th edn. London: Butterworths.

Maitland, G.D. (1986). *Vertebral Manipulation*, 5th edn. London: Butterworths.

May, F. (1954). The changing face of physical medicine. *Austr. J. Physiother.*, **1**, 6–10.

Maynard, A. (1997). Evidence-based medicine and treatment choices. *Lancet*, **349**, 572–573.

Mennell, J. (1934). *Physical Treatment by Movement, Manipulation and Massage*. London: Churchill.

Palmer, M.D. (1918). *Lessons on Massage including Swedish Remedial Gymnastics and Bandaging*. London: Baillière, Tindall and Cox.

Popper, K.R. (1974). *Conjectures and Refutations: The Growth of Scientific Knowledge*, 5th edn. London: Routledge and Kegan Paul.

Sackett, D.L. (1997a). Evidence-based medicine and treatment choices. *Lancet*, **349**, 570.

Sackett, D.L. (1997b). Foreword. In: *The Evidence-based Medicine Workbook, Critical Appraisal for Evaluating Clinical Problem Solving*, ed. R.A. Dixon, J.F. Monroe & P.B. Silcocks, pp. vii–viii. Oxford: Butterworth-Heinemann.

Wilkin, D., Hallam, L. and Doggett, M.A. (1992). *Measures of Need and Outcome for Primary Health Care*. Oxford: Oxford University Press.

Wolfe, J. (1997). Evidence-based medicine and treatment choices. *Lancet*, **349**, 572.

Chapter 2

Theoretical basis underlying clinical decisions

E.M. Gass and K.M. Refshauge

When the role of physiotherapists became one of autonomous professional practice instead of simply the application of technical skills there also came the requirement to make independent clinical judgements. The ability to make effective clinical judgements requires a high level of background knowledge. This chapter therefore contains background information considered fundamental to the practice of musculoskeletal physiotherapy. The areas of information included are: acute and chronic pain, physiology and clinical pharmacology, biomechanics, adaptation of various tissues, including bone, muscle and other connective tissue, skill learning following musculoskeletal lesions and the theories concerning clinical reasoning. The extensive and rapid growth of knowledge in each of these areas means that a full review of each is impossible here. We hope that interest will be kindled so that the reader will pursue the reading recommended in each section for a more comprehensive understanding of each area of knowledge. The integration of theory to clinical practice is explicit in some instances within this chapter or is implicit in material presented in other chapters within this book.

Clinical reasoning in physiotherapy

K.M. Refshauge

Clinical reasoning has, no doubt, been occurring for as long as health professionals have treated patients, but was only identified as a separate and essential skill in good clinical practice at the end of the twentieth century (Elstein et al., 1978). Clinical reasoning, sometimes known as decision-making, making clinical judgements or problem-solving (Grant et al., 1988), describes the process of collecting and interpreting information from the patient and formulating predictions about outcomes. The process is heavily influenced by the individual therapist's knowledge base, beliefs or values, and skills associated with clinical practice. Reflecting on new experiences or knowledge allows integration of new information with the existing knowledge base in the context of the person's beliefs.

The clinical reasoning literature is replete with unresolved issues. Many theories have been proposed to describe the way in which clinicians reason, but the process used remains obscure, although it has been argued that different processes may be used in different contexts (Higgs and Jones, 1995). Perhaps reference to research in psychology, especially that on cognition and thinking, could be applied to reasoning with clinical problems. However, the few studies to investigate the issue have shown that introducing explicit study of clinical reasoning into education programmes has not led to clearly positive outcomes (Bowden, 1988). Several reasons have been proposed to account for the lack of positive outcomes, including a disparity between espoused theory and the actual teaching and assessment methods used (Bowden, 1988). Since then, there have been many advances in clinical reasoning education, but any improvement in outcomes has yet to be studied. Nevertheless, clinical reasoning is now an integral part of most education programmes. The aspects of clinical reasoning most relevant to this book are probably the theories describing clinical reasoning and the influence of knowledge and belief systems on the reasoning process.

CLINICAL REASONING THEORY

Reasoning processes, and specifically the clinical reasoning process, have been studied extensively, investigations being predominantly based on either normative theories of decision-making or actual decision behaviour. Normative theories emphasize what clinicians should do. These theories assume that there is an optimal solution to a problem and often use mathematical techniques, such as probability theories, to reach this optimal solution. It is further assumed that, with the addition of new information, clinicians will revise their understanding of the probability of their hypotheses about the patient. A hypothesis, in this context, refers to a supposition made about a diagnosis or treatment that will be modified according to the data subsequently collected. However, it is generally agreed that humans do not reason optimally (Browning et al., 1988; Grant, 1991).

Other investigations have been directed towards describing actual decision behaviour. These investigations do not assume that there is an optimal decision, nor prescribe an optimal method for reaching a solution to a problem. Rather, this line of inquiry seeks to describe how clinicians reason or use knowledge.

From investigations based on both normative theories and actual decision behaviour, three major models have emerged to explain reasoning in the clinical context:

1. hypotheticodeductive reasoning (Elstein et al., 1978; Jones, 1992)
2. pattern recognition (Scadding, 1967; Barrows and Feltovich, 1987)
3. problem-solving (Bashook, 1976; Paton, 1985).

Other models have been proposed such as the phenomenological model (Mattingly, 1991), backward and forward reasoning models (Ridderikhoff, 1989; Patel and Groen, 1991) and models emphasizing intuition (Benner and Tanner, 1987; Rew and Barrow, 1987). It is most likely that no single model accounts for reasoning in all situations, and that either a more complex model is required or a combination of these proposed models is more representative than a single model.

Hypotheticodeductive reasoning has been investigated in relation to many cognitive tasks, including aspects of clinical reasoning, such as diagnosis. The original hypotheticodeductive reasoning models describe the clinical reasoning process as largely sequential; that clinicians collect information, then form hypotheses about specific aspects of the problem, then confirm or reject these hypotheses. The view that reasoning occurs sequentially (e.g. data acquisition followed by problem identification) underestimates the complexity of the process. Galė and Marsden (1982) provide convincing evidence that clinicians actively evaluate and interpret information during data collection rather than after data collection is complete. In the clinical context, medical practitioners have been most frequently studied, with a consequent high regard for diagnosis (or 'correct' outcome). Although physiotherapists may appear to adopt similar clinical reasoning processes, they probably place greater emphasis on treatment and subsequent evaluation, and ultimate solution to the patient's problem, than do these medical models, and therefore the notion of a single 'correct' outcome is inappropriate. Studies designed to describe the use of hypotheticodeductive reasoning in solving abstract tasks also found that people tend to use verification strategies almost exclusively (Gilhooly, 1988). In other words, clinicians tend to engage in a line of questioning or physical testing that would confirm favoured hypotheses about diagnosis and treatment rather than pursue a line of investigation leading to rejection of alternative hypotheses.

The pattern-recognition model suggests that information collected from the patient is compared with existing knowledge and experience until the problem is recognized as a familiar one, with a consequently determined management strategy. This infers that prior to recognizing the pattern, the clinician passively receives information. However, research in psychology demonstrates that humans do not passively receive information; rather they actively structure it and continually interpret it (Gale and Marsden, 1982).

Finally, clinical reasoning skills are often referred to as problem-solving skills. The implication that problem-solving skills are generalizable was taken further by introducing problem-based curricula. Although there are advantages in such curricula, the advantages do not appear to relate to better problem-solving skills (Norman and Schmidt, 1992). Browning et al. (1988) tested the correlation between general problem-solving test scores and clinical performance measures, finding no correlation between the two. This preliminary finding for health professionals confirms the findings of studies in other fields (Glass and Holyoak, 1986). Problem-solving is context-specific, requiring rules and knowledge related to the task and context (Glass and Holyoak, 1986).

All the above theories attempt to describe how clinicians currently reason. Another approach might be to find the best way to reason, so that optimal reasoning may be achieved. Investigations into optimal reasoning are found in the literature of mathematics-based sciences and artificial intelligence. Optimal reasoning is therefore usually described in relation to either solving problems with a known best solution (best possible outcome), or in relation to the 'genius' (best possible reasoning process). The former is usually based on mathematical problem-solving techniques, with a known best outcome, which is unlike clinical practice. The latter, exploration of the best possible process, suggests that the 'genius' has a vast knowledge base, often in disparate knowledge areas, makes extensive links between these knowledge areas, and does not accept information at face value (Gilhooly, 1988). These characteristics are probably highly relevant to clinical reasoning and clinical practice.

It is still unclear whether all clinicians reason in the same way. The nature of clinical reasoning does not lend itself to rigorous investigation since, of necessity, studies are based on either the outcome (e.g. correct diagnosis) or reflection (recalling later what the clinician was thinking at the time the information was given). Therefore perhaps the best we can hope for is a theory or model that seems reasonable and consistent. It is most likely that clinicians use all the models described and possibly other unidentified processes, since no single model would be appropriate in all circumstances. For example, sometimes a key piece of information is immediately recognized as representing a particular condition (pattern recognition), whereas in less familiar cases, a modified hypotheticodeductive reasoning process may be used. Once the general rules for particular classes of clinical problems have been learnt, perhaps problem-solving using learned rules is part of the process.

THE ROLE OF KNOWLEDGE IN CLINICAL REASONING

Although overlapping substantially, there may be significant differences between scientific, professional and personal knowledge. Knowledge is generally considered to be a person's range of information, which includes knowledge from the scientific discipline and profession to which the person belongs, as well as from experiences of one's own and others. An individual's knowledge base is therefore unique.

To be most useful knowledge needs to be not only broad-based, but also constantly evolving, adequately comprehensive, relevant, accurate, accessible (able to be retrieved for use) and well organized. It appears that a well-organized knowledge base enables the recall of all interrelated information, thus providing a more comprehensive view of a problem. There is increasing evidence that the relevance and depth of knowledge content, the structure of individuals' knowledge bases, and learners' ability to organize knowledge in a meaningful way are of major importance to clinical reasoning ability (Bordage and Lemieux, 1986; Grant and Marsden, 1987; Grant et al., 1988; Norman, 1988; Patel and Groen, 1991; Jones, 1992).

There is currently no doubt about the major role of knowledge in effective clinical reasoning and clinical practice. A compelling question that arises from this understanding is, when striving to improve one's own or another's reasoning process, is it enough to address the knowledge base? The answer to this question may rest in the broader definition of knowledge, i.e. what is considered 'factual' information and what is considered a reasoned deduction about information. Improvement in clinical reasoning probably requires increasing the volume of 'factual' knowledge, as well as making better links between knowledge areas. The process of logical deduction seems to be implicit in making links between items of information. In addition, the impact of each individual's beliefs and values on the interpretation of information should not be overlooked.

A discussion about either the value or the process of increasing the size of an individual's knowledge base is probably unnecessary here. Suffice it to say that being acquainted with disseminated information is important to retain professional currency. However, we now demand our students and practising clinicians to be logical in their thinking and in their use of information. But, what do we mean by logic? Logic is generally defined as the science of reasoning or the chain of reasoning. People do not ordinarily reason using putative (or mathematical/statistical) logic. Rather they tend to rely on their belief systems, and simpler ways of solving problems, providing solutions even in the absence of adequate information (Gilhooly, 1988). In addition, it could be argued that each profession has a 'professional logic', i.e. information is interpreted in a way that is unique to that profession, usually based on empirical evidence, experience and clinical wisdom (for example, pushing on a painful vertebra will reduce pain). The links and interpretations made are not necessarily 'logical' – usually, they could not be deduced from the data alone, as could a problem in geometry from knowledge of deriving theorems from first principles. This is not logic in the pure sense, and must be learnt as the novice joins the profession. To this extent, 'professional logic', or making links, could in fact be considered to be part of 'professional knowledge', and therefore must be learnt from others rather than deduced. When making new links, or evaluating information in a new way, some deduction and logic may be involved. This is often how progress is made in professional practice but probably occurs infrequently.

The other important feature of individuals' reasoning is the system of beliefs and values to which they subscribe, and against which they compare information. If new knowledge or ideas are incongruent with their belief system, individuals may reject the new information. This is consistent with the common tendency to exhibit a confirmatory bias (Elstein et al., 1978; Gilhooly, 1988). Several studies have demonstrated that, in all fields including the health sciences, confirmatory bias is common, that people tend to accept information that supports their beliefs, and reject or ignore information that conflicts with their beliefs. For example, if a physiotherapist strongly believes that segmental alignment is important in the aetiology of back pain, the intervention offered may often include postural correction. There will be a tendency to ignore evidence demonstrating lack of effectiveness of such intervention. In this instance, the physiotherapist may look for other reasons if the intervention fails, e.g. non-compliance with the exercise programme or inadequate dosage of exercise.

CONCLUSION

The identification of clinical reasoning as a separate skill has been a major influence in causing changes in physiotherapy education. Probably the single most important feature in determining the quality of one's clinical reasoning is the knowledge base, in terms of both type and extent of knowledge. Obviously, if one has no knowledge, one has nothing with which to reason. The other important feature is the individual's belief system. An inappropriate belief system can impede integration of new and evaluation of old knowledge.

Acute and chronic pain

D. Gronow

The anatomy and physiology of pain perception are areas from which many of us tend to shy away. Our initial teaching in this area was often laborious and not relevant to our subsequent professional practice. Indeed, many early theories of pain perception failed to explain the clinical experience of pain perception.

The *nociceptive* system is a protective or defensive system which enables the body to recognize and defend itself from harmful or potentially harmful stimuli. Pain is commonly defined as an unpleasant sensory and emotional experience associated with actual or potential tissue damage, or described in terms of such damage. Such a definition highlights the two components of pain. The first is the biological function of the body's recognition of a noxious (painful) stimulus. The second is the experience and expression of this stimulus which involves the emotional, cognitive, developmental, behavioural and cultural aspects of pain behaviour. Pain behaviour allows us to show the suffering being experienced which may not be related directly to the level of nociceptive stimulus. The sensation of nociception is always unpleasant, and invokes an emotional experience. The response to this experience is shaped by an individual's ability to communicate this experience and his or her adaptability to the current environment. In practice, for example, no two patients with a similar injury, such as a Colles fracture, present with the same pain complaints or behaviour. It is tempting to attribute these differences in pain behaviour to differences in pain tolerance rather than looking for the cause of the suffering. The fundamentals of nociception help us to understand how the signals of noxious stimuli reach the central nervous system to produce a pain response. Nociception can therefore be described as the biological recognition of such a stimulus.

Our understanding of the nociceptive process is progressing rapidly, but is still incomplete. Melzack and Wall (1965), describing the gate theory of pain, rekindled the interest of the scientific world in the theory of pain and nociception. The gate theory introduced the idea of modulation of the nociceptive stimulus in the dorsal horn of the spinal cord by the effect of non-noxious stimuli (e.g. touch, proprioception) or descending inhibition reducing the central perception of nociception.

The rapidity of the increase in knowledge in this area and its important clinical application can be illustrated by our growth in understanding of the mechanisms and site of action of morphine. It was not until 1973 that the opiate receptor in the brain was identified (Pert and Sydner, 1973). In 1976 binding sites in the dorsal horn of the spinal cord were described. More recently opiate receptors were found to be formed on peripheral nerves in inflamed tissue, suggesting that morphine and other opiates may have a peripheral mechanism of action in some inflammatory pain states. The use of intra-articular morphine in arthroscopy has been shown to reduce joint pain with no systemic effects. This, of course, is contrary to our classical teaching. Each of these basic science discoveries has advanced the understanding of nociception and altered the clinical course of management of various pain states. Considerable research is being undertaken to develop specific pharmacological substances to take advantage of this knowledge. A new group of peripherally acting opioids that do not cross the blood–brain barrier would give a new dimension in the management of certain inflammatory musculoskeletal pain states. Thus the importance of our knowledge and understanding of nociception and pain perception will continue to help in our clinical decision-making.

Nociception can be divided into the peripheral recognition of the stimulus, the modulation of that stimulus in the spinal cord, in particular the dorsal horn, and the central interaction allowing localization of the stimulus and the behavioural and learnt responses. Over the last two decades much of the work has been directed at understanding the dorsal horn responses to nociception, initially in acute pain and in understanding the changes in some chronic pain states, particularly following peripheral nerve injury. More recently studied are the peripheral receptor responses and the changes that may occur in acute and chronic pain. A brief outline of the nociceptive experience will hopefully entice the reader to gain further knowledge in this area.

Peripheral nerves are divided into those carrying non-noxious and noxious information. The non-noxious nerves, typically those that respond to sensation such as touch, vibration, heat and proprioception, are classified as responding to mechanical and thermal stimulation. Noxious nerves respond to strong stimulation by heat (thermal), mechanical (such as pinprick) and chemical stimuli, e.g. inflammation. These nerves normally have a high threshold to stimulation with pathways to the dorsal horn via the small-diameter unmyelinated C fibres and the small-diameter myelinated A-delta fibres. The distribution of the termination of these nerves in deep tissue is still under debate. In the joint, free nerve endings of the small-diameter fibres have been demonstrated in the fibrous capsule, adipose tissue, ligaments, menisci and periosteum but their presence is disputed in the synovial and cartilage tissue.

In the pathological state following tissue damage or nerve injury hyperalgesia (an increased response to noxious stimuli), allodynia (where a non-noxious stimulus is felt to be painful) or persistent pain (prolongation of the response to brief stimulation) may develop. During the early stages of tissue damage when acute inflammation is still present, peripheral neural mechanisms contribute to the development of ongoing pain. After healing has occurred, however, spinal mechanisms are increasingly involved in the persistence of pain.

Sensitization of both non-noxious and noxious afferents occurs in the inflamed joint. This sensitization lowers the threshold to noxious stimuli, also causing non-noxious afferents to respond as if to a noxious response. Thus the normal range of movement or loading of an inflamed joint will be perceived as being painful. In addition there will be an increased barrage into the dorsal horn causing further changes.

Further, it has been postulated that there are a group of mechano-insensitive afferents or 'silent nociceptors' which become functional in the inflamed joint.

Protracted afferent input, particularly with stimulation through the C-fibre receptors and afferents, will cause sensitization of other peripheral afferents which will enhance the peripheral response to any stimuli. In turn this ongoing input will alter the dorsal horn responsiveness to produce a state of secondary hyperalgesia (i.e. increased responsiveness to the same level of noxious input) and hyperaesthesia. This area of responsiveness can be in a much wider area than the original stimulus or injury and is often non-dermatomal. Such a state partly accounts for prolongation of the postinjury response to pain and may explain the maintenance of some pain states.

The prostaglandins (PGE_1, PGE_2 and PGI_2), bradykinin, serotonin, leukotrienes, substance P and histamine are known to sensitize the peripheral afferents, altering their threshold to stimulation and their intracellular processing and, as mentioned above, can cause the production of new receptors that are responsive to application of opiate (and therefore possibly of others).

Prolonged or repetitive noxious stimulation of C fibres leads to sensitization of neurons in the dorsal horn, leading to the phenomenon of 'wind-up'. Wind-up is characterized by these dorsal horn cells developing reduced thresholds, prolonged afterdischarges and increased spontaneous activity with expansion of peripheral fields. At least two receptors in the dorsal horn are implicated in this process. These are neurokinin-1 (NK1) activated by substance P and N-methyl-D-aspartate (NMDA) which is activated by the amino acid neurotransmitters glutamate and aspartate. Substance P and glutamate can coexist in primary peripheral afferents, being released on noxious stimulation. Activation of the NMDA receptor allows Ca^{2+} ions to enter the neuron, increasing intracellular Ca^{2+} and precipitating a series of events. Through mechanisms such as the formation of nitric oxide (NO) and changes in gene expression, the responsiveness of the neuron will be further altered. These changes in Ca^{2+} and NO alter synaptic transmission and may account for the development of chronic pain states of hyperalgesia, allodynia and wind-up. If therapeutic approaches could be developed that would interfere with this process, then such pain states may be reversed.

The implication is that, even by reducing peripheral nociceptive input which occurs naturally with tissue healing, the magnitude of the painful response may not reduce. This can have important clinical considerations in the management of acute pain states. Importantly, reduction of this spinal effect improves the recovery time. Providing adequate analgesia at the time of the acute injury response has been shown to reduce the wind-up effect in the dorsal horn and lead to quicker return of normal function. Providing adequate analgesia at the time of physiotherapy is an important consideration in clinical practice.

Many mechanisms operate to reduce the excitatory responsiveness of the dorsal horn and spinal systems. These inhibitory systems have a complex interaction. One inhibitory system acts via the opiate receptors and explains the ability for both endogenous and exogenous opioids to reduce dorsal horn activity and the perception of pain. In addition, descending pathways from the brain may reduce or inhibit spinal cord activity via action of noradrenaline (norepinephrine), serotonin and enkephalin, thus improving the spinal effect of analgesia. The central control mechanisms synapsing on to the dorsal horn are influenced via these inhibitory systems by such states as relaxation and agitation, providing possible application in clinical practice.

The ascending pathways to the higher levels within the central nervous system are even more complex. Classically, these pathways ascend in the spinothalamic tract. However, other reported pathways have been noted to contain or have the ability to contain nociceptive input. Although their clinical relevance is not yet known, we are aware that after cordotomy or tractotomy of the spinothalamic tract one can still develop pain states that are very resistant to treatment. The thalamus is an important major relay site for nociceptive information, but not necessarily all nociceptive information is relayed through the thalamus. Fibres will then project to some extent to the cortex and to the limbic system where the emotional, memory and learning component of pain perception is caused. The role of the cortex in the perception of pain is unclear. Although pain must be perceived as a result of activity in the corticoneurons, focal stimulation of the cortex rarely results in pain, and lesions of the cortex of the brain rarely affect pain perception. The frontal cortex may have a role in the affective motivational aspects of pain, although this is not the only area where this occurs. Interestingly, frontal lobotomy was first used to treat phantom limb pain in amputees after the First World War. Further work will enhance understanding of the role of the cortex. Positron emission tomography is now being used to localize the region of cortex activity during noxious stimulation.

It is hoped that this section has produced an awareness in the reader of the importance of the basic sciences of pain, nociception and pain perception in the understanding and treatment of the patient in pain. References to other texts are recommended to further the understanding of this area of science and to provide a basis for thoughtful informed physiotherapy practice and research.

Physiology and clinical pharmacology: inflammation, pain and anti-inflammatory drugs and analgesics

P.G. Conaghan and R.O. Day

INFLAMMATION

In clinical practice the signs of inflammation are heat, redness, swelling, pain and loss of function. Inflammation represents the response of living tissues to injury. Acute inflammation involves:

1. Increased blood supply in the region of injury. Inflammatory mediators or the traumatizing agent itself act on smooth muscle in the vessel walls to cause vasodilation. Sometimes there are stimuli for new vessel formation.

2. An increase in local capillary permeability. This process involves active contraction of the capillary lining cells or endothelium leading to gaps between cells, again in response to chemical mediators.

3. Exudation of vascular fluid. This inflammatory exudate follows the increased capillary permeability. It contains many plasma proteins and antibodies.

4. Migration of inflammatory cells out of the blood vessels into the surrounding tissue. This involves adhesion of cells in the blood stream (leukocytes such as neutrophil granulocytes, lymphocytes and monocytes) to the vascular endothelium and the subsequent 'squeezing' of the leukocytes through the intercellular junctions of the endothelium. Adhesion requires specific molecules on the surfaces of involved cells. Some of these adhesion molecules are constitutively expressed and others are only expressed in response to inflammatory mediators; certain cell types can then be selectively recruited. Migration also involves chemotaxis,

which is the directional movement of cells in response to inflammatory mediators.

5. Molecular mediators of inflammation. Many chemicals are released by cells and many plasma proteins are activated in inflammation. Examples of these mediators are histamine, which is released by mast cells, prostaglandins, which are formed from phospholipids in cell membranes, and bradykinin, formed by activation of a precursor molecule in plasma.

Acute inflammation may be followed by tissue death or necrosis, scarring or fibrosis, or chronic inflammation. The best example of chronic inflammation in musculoskeletal medicine is rheumatoid arthritis and because all classes of anti-inflammatory drugs are used to treat this condition, it is appropriate to discuss its underlying features.

RHEUMATOID ARTHRITIS

Rheumatoid arthritis is a chronic inflammatory arthritis that presents usually as a symmetrical destructive polyarthritis. It affects about 1% of the adult population, with females being more frequently affected than males. The aetiology of this condition is still unknown, although genetic and environmental factors play a role.

The normal joint has a thin lining layer or synovium overlying a thick fibrous joint capsule and cartilaginous articular bony surfaces. This synovium consists of cells termed synoviocytes overlying a matrix of extracellular proteins. The initial changes on light microscopy of the synovium in rheumatoid arthritis include thickening of the lining layer due to accumulation of cells and fluid. This thickened lining can be seen macroscopically and is called the pannus. Early in the disease white cells migrate into the joint lining from the blood vessels. The predominant leukocytes invading the synovium are lymphocytes, whereas the predominant leukocytes in the synovial fluid are neutrophil granulocytes. As well as infiltration of cells, there is proliferation of synoviocytes and local replication of lymphocytes and phagocytic cells or macrophages.

All the cells involved, especially the lymphocytes and macrophages, produce a group of soluble molecules called cytokines, which act as intercellular messengers over short distances. The most important of the cytokines involved are interleukin 1 (IL-1), tumour necrosis factor-α (TNF-α), interferon-γ, platelet-derived growth factor and IL-6. These molecules act as chemoattractants for more inflammatory cells and stimulate other cells such as fibroblasts to produce collagen and glycosaminoglycans, i.e. the proteins that make up the substance or matrix of the synovium. This increase in extracellular protein together with the cytokine effects leads to increased fluid retention within the inflamed synovium.

The initial inflammatory mediators activate an enzyme, phospholipase A_2, in cell membranes which consequently releases arachidonic acid. Arachidonic acid is then converted into prostaglandins by an enzyme called cyclooxygenase and then into leukotrienes via the lipoxygenase pathway. Prostaglandins and leukotrienes play an important role in amplifying the inflammatory response.

The thickened synovium or pannus grows slowly across the articular surface. As well as producing proteins that lay down material, fibroblasts and other cells produce a range of molecules which are important in local tissue destruction. Cytokines such as IL-1 are important in stimulating cells to produce these enzymes, which include collagenase and stromelysin which are important in breaking down collagen. Reactive oxygen molecules (called reactive oxygen species) are produced and play an important proinflammatory role. As disease progresses, the invading pannus causes destruction of cartilage and adjacent bone. These bony changes may be seen on radiographs and are called erosions. Soft tissues surrounding the inflamed synovium such as ligaments may also be involved in the inflammatory process and destroyed. Many ligament and tendon ruptures are associated with ongoing inflammation, resulting in many of the common deformities seen in rheumatoid arthritis.

The above is a necessarily brief description of the complex interaction between cells, cytokines and structural proteins.

CLINICAL PHARMACOLOGY

Before discussing any therapeutic agent, it is appropriate to consider not only how it works, its effects and side-effects (termed the pharmacodynamics) but also how it reaches its site of action and is metabolized by the body (the pharmacokinetics of the drug). Pharmacokinetics looks at drug absorption, distribution throughout different body compartments, metabolism and eventual excretion. Only a few key concepts of pharmacokinetics will be discussed.

The half-life ($t_{1/2}$) of a drug refers to the time required for the amount in the body to fall to 50%, and it is important when calculating dosage schedules. It is dependent on two other important parameters, drug clearance (C) and the volume of distribution (V). The terms are related by the following formula:

$$t_{1/2} = 0.7V/C$$

The volume of distribution gives an index of drug binding to tissues and plasma proteins and gives an indication of the initial or loading dose. It is important to remember that it is the free or unbound concentration of a drug that is active or available to bind to appropriate receptors. Drug clearance determines daily dosage and largely relates to hepatic metabolism and renal excretion of drugs. Some drugs undergo extensive metabolism on their first passage through the liver: this is referred to as a first-pass effect.

ANTI–INFLAMMATORY DRUGS

The anti-inflammatory drugs are usually classified into categories of steroidal and non-steroidal medications. The drugs will be discussed below under the categories:

1. glucocorticosteroids
2. non-steroidal anti-inflammatory drugs (NSAIDs)
3. disease-modifying antirheumatic drugs (DMARDs).

Rheumatoid arthritis patients will often use an NSAID and a DMARD, often with additional glucocorticosteroid.

Glucocorticosteroids

Glucocorticosteroids are produced naturally in the body by the cortex of the adrenal gland. The adrenal gland responds to hormones released by the pituitary gland which in its turn is responsive to hormonal commands from the hypothalamus in the brain. The hypothalamus secretes corticotrophin-releasing hormone which acts on the anterior pituitary gland to cause production of adrenocorticotrophic hormone (ACTH). ACTH, which is released with a diurnal rhythm, then acts on the adrenal cortex resulting in glucocorticoid production. Cortisol (or hydrocortisone) is the main glucocorticoid produced in humans.

A number of glucocorticosteroids are available for use, including cortisone, prednisolone, methyl-prednisolone, triamcinolone, betamethasone and dexamethasone. Some are only available for intramuscular or intravenous use. These glucocorticoids have different degrees of effect, for example on a milligram-for-milligram basis prednisolone is four times more potent than hydrocortisone.

Glucocorticosteroids are powerful immune-suppressant and anti-inflammatory drugs and have a large role in the treatment of inflammation-based conditions. Their modulation of immune and inflammatory conditions is an extension of the natural action of cortisol which is physiologically released at times of stress and illness. Many mechanisms of glucocorticoid action have been described and it is known that these corticosteroids bind to receptors in the cell cytoplasm and that the receptor–steroid complex enters the cell nucleus, modifying DNA transcription. In inflammatory states, exogenous glucocorticoids can inhibit the function and even decrease the circulating numbers of various leukocytes, especially lymphocytes and macrophages. They can reduce prostaglandin and leukotriene production and antagonize the effect of some proinflammatory cytokines.

Steroid therapy is usually given orally or intra-articularly. Intra-articular therapy is commonly used in inflammatory arthritis where a small number of joints are inflamed and not being controlled by systemic therapy. These injections may need to be repeated depending on the duration of response of an individual joint. Intra-articular steroids can also be used in other musculoskeletal problems, for example in inflammation secondary to rotator cuff tendon damage in the shoulder, or in lateral epicondylitis or tennis elbow. Glucocorticosteroids may damage cartilage and therefore the number of injections into a given joint is usually limited to three or four per year. Intravenous corticosteroids may be used when a very rapid effect is required in severe or life-threatening inflammatory conditions. Intramuscular steroids are occasionally used in intermittent doses as an alternative to continuous daily oral therapy.

Glucocorticoids have many adverse effects and these are listed in Table 2.1. The most important long-term adverse effects include weight gain, osteoporosis with concomitant increased risk of fracture and increased susceptibility to infection. It is obvious from this list of complications that a decision must be made when starting a patient on long-term oral steroids that there is a significant inflammatory component to the disease. Every effort is made to try to reduce the oral steroid dose to the minimum that has the required anti-inflammatory effect. The dose required of anti-inflammatory steroid varies with conditions. A common maintenance anti-inflammatory dose in rheumatoid arthritis would be in the range of 5–10 mg/day.

Long-term oral glucocorticoid therapy leads to suppression of the body's own hypothalamic–pituitary–adrenal axis. Consequently any attempt to reduce the dose of prednisolone is carried out slowly, often in a stepwise manner, or else the risk of hypocortisolaemia occurs.

Non-steroidal anti-inflammatory drugs

NSAIDs are drugs that work quickly to help reduce the symptoms and signs of inflammation such as

Table 2.1 Adverse effects of glucocorticosteroid therapy

Musculoskeletal	Osteoporosis
	Myopathy
	Avascular necrosis
	of femoral head
Immunological	Increased susceptibility
	to infection
Endocrine	Truncal obesity, moon-like face
	Hyperglycaemia or frank diabetes
	Acne
	Hirsutism
	Salt and water retention
Dermatological	Thinning of skin
	Increased fragility of skin
Cardiovascular	Hypertension
	Exacerbation of congestive
	cardiac failure
Gastrointestinal	Peptic ulceration
	Reduced rate of ulcer healing
	Pancreatitis
Neurological	Cataracts
	Psychosis
	Change in mood (especially
	with high doses)

Table 2.2 Common non-steroidal anti-inflammatory drugs

Class	Drug	Usual daily dose (mg/day)
2-Arylacetic acids	Indometacin[a]	50–150
	Diclofenac[a]	75–150
	Sulindac	200–400
2-Arylpropionic acids	Ibuprofen[a]	1200–3200
	Ketoprofen[a]	100–400
	Naproxen	375–1500
	Tiaprofenic acid[a]	200–600
Oxicams	Piroxicam	10–20
	Tenoxicam	10–20
	Meloxicam	10–20
Salicylates	Acetylsalicylic acid[a]	1200–5200
	Diflunisal	500–1000
COX-2 inhibitors	Celecoxib	200–400
	Rofecoxib	12.5–25

[a]These NSAIDs have short half-lives (<6 h). The others have half-lives >10 h.

pain, stiffness and swelling. Although anti-inflammatory, they do not modify the long-term course of a disease process, hence the differentiation with disease-modifying drugs. It should be noted, however, that there is some overlap between these categories. Common NSAIDs are classified according to their chemical derivation (Table 2.2). As well as being used as anti-inflammatory drugs, they can be used as analgesics, antipyretic agents and antithrombotic agents. They can be given orally, rectally and topically.

NSAIDs seem to work by preventing the formation of prostanoid derivatives by inhibiting cyclooxygenase. There are two cyclooxygenase enzymes, COX-1 and COX-2. COX-1 is important in producing prostaglandins with physiological functions such as protection of the gastrointestinal mucosa and vascular homeostasis; its levels are reasonably constant. However the COX-2 enzyme is upregulated at sites of inflammation and it is responsible for the production of inflammatory mediators. Many other mechanisms have, however, been

suggested for their mode of action because their anti-inflammatory actions are seen at drug concentrations greater than those required to inhibit cyclooxygenase. NSAIDs also interfere with the lipoxygenase pathway and the consequent formation of leukotrienes. There is evidence that they affect neutrophil leukocyte function, interfering with both the chemotactic response of the cell and the generation of reactive oxygen species by the cell membrane.

NSAIDs are generally mildly acidic and concentrate at sites of lowered pH, such as the sites of inflammation, and also in gastric and renal tissue. The latter findings are of note because of the side-effects of these drugs (Table 2.3). In terms of pharmacokinetics the drugs are all very well absorbed in the gastrointestinal tract and are highly plasma protein-bound with only a very small amount of the drug being available for equilibration in tissues. NSAIDs undergo only little first-pass effect.

All NSAIDs appear to be of equivalent efficacy but have different pharmacokinetic properties. They can be divided into those having short and long half-lives (Table 2.2). In general, the more potent anti-inflammatory NSAIDs are seen to have higher side-effect profiles, but this may only reflect

Table 2.3   Adverse effects of non–steroidal anti–inflammatory drugs (NSAIDs)

Gastrointestinal	Dyspepsia
	Peptic ulceration
	Gastritis
	Hepatitis
Renal	Reversible renal impairment
	Interstitial nephritis
Neurological	Confusion, especially in the elderly
	Headaches
Endocrine	Fluid retention
Cardiovascular	Exacerbation of congestive cardiac failure
Haematological	Interference with platelet function

their increased relative dosage. NSAIDs are required in smaller doses than aspirin to have equivalent anti-inflammatory potency.

The differential COX-1 and COX-2 functions led to the potential for developing new COX-2-selective agents. All existing NSAIDs inhibit both enzymes with varying selectivity. A new class of drugs, the coxibs, have high COX-2 selectivity and there is evidence that they reduce endoscope-visualized peptic ulcers. There is also some recent evidence that they reduce clinically serious gastrointestinal side-effects such as ulcers, perforations and bleeds.

Adverse effects of NSAIDs

The common adverse effects of NSAIDs are listed in Table 2.3. Of these side-effects the gastrointestinal ones are the most commonly encountered. Although the risk of peptic ulceration or complication of ulcers is small for an individual, the frequency of encountering problems increases with age, such that people over 65 years old have a much higher risk of gastrointestinal problems. The causes of toxicity are again thought to be due to inhibition of prostaglandin formation. In the kidney, where prostaglandins play an important role in regulating intrarenal blood flow and glomerular filtration, lack of prostaglandins secondary to NSAIDs can precipitate acute renal failure and hyperkalaemia, amongst other problems. Patients with pre-existing renal impairment are especially at risk of adverse effects.

There are also important clinical pharmacodynamic interactions with NSAIDs. NSAIDs can antagonize antihypertensive medications, including drugs that work via vasodilation and diuretic mechanisms. Hyperkalaemia may occur in conjunction with certain diuretics and antihypertensives. The concomitant use of warfarin, and perhaps alcohol, increases the risk of NSAID-induced gastrointestinal bleeding.

Topical NSAIDs

The topical use of NSAIDs has the potential to deliver drug locally without systemic side-effects. However concentrations achieved in the skin and muscle are variable and may depend on individual skin properties as well as frequency of topical administration. The evidence for the efficacy of topical NSAIDs in musculoskeletal problems is limited, often by poor clinical trial design. There is some evidence for short-term efficacy (2–4 weeks) of topical agents in knee and hand osteoarthritis. There are certainly reduced systemic side-effects, with rash and pruritus at the site of application being the commonest problems.

Disease–modifying antirheumatic drugs

As the name implies, these drugs are used in the treatment of rheumatoid arthritis and are seen to modify the course of the disease. A particular DMARD (or combination) is started early in the disease in an attempt to prevent permanent joint damage. These drugs are also known as the slow-acting antirheumatic drugs (SAARDs), referring to their slow onset of action, often 4–6 weeks. For most of these agents the exact mechanism by which they have their effect is unknown. The DMARDs are also used in inflammatory arthritides such as psoriatic arthritis and ankylosing spondylitis, although not all agents are effective in these other conditions.

Methotrexate

Methotrexate is a folate antagonist which was initially used in treating malignant disease. As with the other DMARDs, its mode of action is unclear. It acts as a folate antagonist by inhibiting the enzyme dihydrofolate reductase which reduces the amount of intracellular folate. This folate is required for synthesis of purine, important in cell replication. However, as well as being an antiproliferative agent, methotrexate is immunosuppressive and it is not clear which of these actions accounts for its activity as a disease suppressant. Although there are few data to compare directly the efficacy of the DMARDs, methotrexate is the quickest acting with onset of efficacy at about 3–5 weeks. Methotrexate is moderately well absorbed orally and can be given intramuscularly. It has an elimination half-life of 5–6 h. About 50% is excreted renally and therefore the drug can be toxically retained in the presence of chronic renal impairment.

Methotrexate is usually given in doses of 5–15 mg as a single weekly oral or intramuscular dose. Because it works against rapidly dividing cells, the side-effects involve the gastrointestinal tract and the bone marrow. Nausea and mouth ulcers occur in about 10% of people. Abnormal liver function tests may occur and this warrants regular blood testing. One of the serious complications of methotrexate therapy is hepatic fibrosis which may rarely lead to cirrhosis: this is related in some patients to previous liver damage or ongoing alcohol use. Effects on the bone marrow can reduce cell counts and frequent full blood counts are also part of monitoring. Pneumonitis may rarely occur with severe hypoxia.

Gold

Gold can be used for rheumatoid arthritis in an oral or intramuscular form. The intramuscular form is more commonly used and has a very good response rate but higher side-effect profile.

Intramuscular gold is normally given as a 10 mg test dose and then quickly increased up to a maintenance dose of 20–50 mg per week. This is continued up to a total dose of 1 g or until clinical improvement is seen, at which stage the dosage interval may be increased.

Side-effects of gold include skin rashes, which may or may not necessitate discontinuation of therapy, mouth ulcers, and sometimes bone marrow depression with low white cell and platelet counts. Gold can also affect the kidneys, causing proteinuria and even glomerulonephritis, so as well as regular blood screening, routine urine analysis is performed before each injection.

Oral gold or auranofin is given as a dose of 3 mg twice a day but does not seem to be as effective as the intramuscular form. It has a milder side-effect profile, with diarrhoea being the most frequent problem and renal side-effects much less common.

Sulfasalazine

Sulfasalazine is a combination of sulfapyridine, which is an antibacterial agent, and 5-aminosalicylic acid, which has anti-inflammatory properties. This drug is most commonly used for treatment of inflammatory bowel disease and it was subsequently found to be an effective disease-modifying agent. It is normally given in doses up to 1 g twice a day, and again, like other DMARDs, may require weeks before onset of action. The common side-effects of sulfasalazine include nausea and dyspepsia, along with rash. Very occasionally low white blood cell counts are seen and therefore regular blood monitoring is again required. Headache is another occasional side-effect.

Leflunomide

Leflunomide is a new DMARD that appears to act by selectively inhibiting new pyrimidine synthesis. This action prevents the multiplication of pro-inflammatory lymphocytes involved in rheumatoid arthritis. This oral medication has a very long half-life (15–18 days) and the usual maintenance dose is 10–20 mg once daily. The common side-effects include diarrhoea, nausea, rashes, hair loss, hypertension and liver function test abnormalities.

BIOLOGICAL THERAPIES

The importance of cytokines, or intercellular messengers, in promoting inflammation has been mentioned above. Novel antibody therapies are becoming available that inhibit some of the key cytokines, such as TNF-α or IL-1. These therapies are very expensive and given as regular intravenous infusions or subcutaneous injections. At present their use is limited to rheumatoid arthritis sufferers who have failed to respond to multiple DMARDs. Their side-effects include increased risk of infections, infusion reactions and injection site rashes. Among the rare, serious side-effects are serious infections such as tuberculosis and demyelinating diseases.

Hydroxychloroquine

Hydroxychloroquine is related to chloroquine which was first used as an antimalarial drug. It is probably the mildest acting of the DMARDs, but similarly it has a very good side-effect profile. It is normally given in a dose of 200–400 mg/day orally. The major but rare potential side-effect of hydroxychloroquine is damage to the retina; 6-monthly thorough eye examinations are required since patient symptoms are a poor guide to ongoing damage.

OTHER SECOND–LINE ANTIRHEUMATIC AGENTS

The agents listed above are the commonest agents used for the treatment of rheumatoid arthritis and other inflammatory arthritides. Other agents that are used uncommonly include penicillamine, cyclosporin A, azathioprine (which may be used as an adjunct to allow reduced dose of steroid) and cyclophosphamide.

Analgesics

It is useful to think of pharmacological therapy for pain according to the type of pain involved. There are many analgesic agents available. In nociceptive-type pain, paracetamol, aspirin, NSAIDs and opioids are all used. For neurogenic pain opioids are also used but other drugs such as dothiepin and other antidepressants or carbamazepine, an anticonvulsant, can be used. Members of the benzodiazepine family, e.g. diazepam, can be used as muscle relaxants, although they are of limited efficacy.

Aspirin and the NSAIDs are excellent analgesics as well as anti-inflammatory agents and their pharmacology has already been discussed. Paracetamol and the opioids will be discussed below.

Paracetamol

Paracetamol, also known as acetaminophen, is a very weak anti-inflammatory agent but is probably equal to aspirin in analgesic properties. Although it is also thought to work by inhibiting prostaglandin synthesis, its site of action seems to be more in the central nervous system than at peripheral sites of inflammation. It is well absorbed orally and reaches maximum blood concentrations between 15 min and 2 h after dosing. It is extensively metabolized by the liver and therefore it can accumulate in chronic liver disease. Paracetamol does not have the same degree of adverse effects as the more potent anti-inflammatory agents, and its most serious side-effect is acute hepatic necrosis in overdose situations. The presence of alcohol enhances this overdose-induced hepatic toxicity. Paracetamol is usually recommended in doses of less than 4 g/day because of possible hepatic toxicity in long-term studies.

Opioids

As the name suggests, these drugs are derived from the opium poppy. These agents are not frequently used in acute musculoskeletal pain and only a few are discussed but other short- and long-acting oral agents are available. They all work by acting on endogenous opioid receptors, though not all are active at each subtype of receptor.

Morphine

Morphine is derived from opium and is a very potent analgesic and euphoria-producing agent. Although oral preparations are available and are used extensively in palliative care, the drug undergoes sustantial first-pass effect after oral dosing and so the parenteral route of administration is commonly used. It has a half-life of 2.5–3 h and for an otherwise fit 70-kg adult would be given intramuscularly in a dose of 5–15 mg at 3–4-hourly intervals.

Morphine has substantial side-effects and the drug should be individualized with these in mind. It acts centrally to produce nausea and vomiting and depresses respiratory drive. It reduces gastrointestinal motility leading to constipation and acts as a vasodilator to reduce blood pressure. Physical dependence can occur with regular use.

Pethidine

Unlike morphine, pethidine is a synthetic narcotic but it works in a similar way. Again it is well absorbed orally with a short half-life but undergoes extensive first-pass metabolism and so is used parenterally. A dose of 50–150 mg intramuscularly every 3–4 h is used in a 70-kg adult. The side-effects are very similar to those of morphine. However, norpethidine, which is a breakdown product of pethidine metabolism, can cause convulsions and other central nervous system adverse effects. This metabolite accumulates in renal impairment so care must be exercised in patients with this problem and in the elderly. Pethidine is not recommended for use in chronic situations.

Codeine

Codeine is another opium derivative, although less potent than morphine. It is available in tablets on its own or in combination with paracetamol or aspirin. It is not as extensively metabolized on first pass through the liver as morphine or pethidine and so it is often given in oral preparations. It is metabolized in part to morphine and this probably explains its analgesic efficacy. The daily dose will depend on whether it is used alone or in combination. The major side-effect at common dosage is constipation.

Biomechanics of joint movements

M. Lee

Studying joint movements can tell us a great deal about the way the musculoskeletal system is working. If a child has a disordered movement control system, then joint movements may be jerky, or may be abnormally fast or slow. A person with a group of muscles showing abnormal mechanical behaviour may have one of more joints that show a smaller or larger amount of movement than normal. Pathological changes to the structural elements of an intervertebral joint may produce alterations in the pattern of joint movement.

DETERMINANTS OF JOINT MOVEMENT

The rotation at a joint is the relative rotation between the segments on either side of the joint. Each segment will rotate according to the net torque applied to the segment and the inertia of the segment (Winter, 1990). Considering torques about an axis at the centre of mass of the segment, the torques applied to the segment can be classified according to whether they originate from active or passive sources. The total passive torque includes contributions from ligaments, joint capsule, fascia and skin, as well as torque produced by the passive muscles. The magnitude of the passive torque exerted by a particular structure may depend on the angle of the joints involved. The active source of torque is the contraction of muscles and in most instances has the potential to produce larger torques. The magnitude of the torque is chiefly dependent on the level of activation, as determined by the motor control system, but the upper limits of muscle torque do depend on joint angles. Hence, the rotation at a joint during normal activities is largely controlled by the motor control system. However, in individuals with conditions involving abnormally high passive torques, the passive torque could be the dominant factor. For example, a man who has had a fracture of the tibia and fibula involving the talocrural joint may experience abnormal passive stiffness at this joint after the fracture has healed. This abnormal passive stiffness may prevent the man from actively dorsiflexing his foot during walking to the angle that would have been present prior to the fracture.

In addition to rotation, there can be translations between the segments that comprise the joint. Translations will partly occur in association with rotation, but may also occur independently of rotations. Such translations will, however, be different for each pair of points on the two segments (Meriam and Kraige, 1993). The relative movement at the contact point of the joint surfaces is perhaps of most interest to physiotherapists. The magnitude of the relative displacement at this point is determined by the bone-on-bone contact force, especially the components tangential to the contact surface, and the stiffness of the joint in each direction of possible translation. In active movements, the bone-on-bone force is strongly related to the muscle force, but could also have a significant contribution from segment weights (Winter, 1990). When the therapist moves a joint with the patient remaining passive, the therapist's force, the segment weight and the joint stiffness are the major determinants of joint movement at the contact point.

In the following sections we shall examine some aspects of joint movements: how motion between any two segments can be described, intersegmental kinematics; the motion between the two surfaces of a joint, joint surface kinematics; the resistance of a joint to passive movement, passive joint dynamics; and a special condition of abnormal movement, instability. Although there will not be any further discussion of the determinants of joint movements, the reader should remember that a disorder of active movement could reflect a dysfunction of the person's motor control system and/or an abnormality of the passive properties of the joint.

INTERSEGMENTAL KINEMATICS

How do we describe the movement between two adjacent body segments? There are a number of aspects that need to be included if we are to identify those elements of joint movement that are likely to be signs of a disorder of the musculoskeletal system. The major elements involved are the amount and pattern of movement.

During movement of a limb, it appears as though the limb segments rotate around the joints. The most complete method for describing joint movements begins with this basic observation. The first parameter to be defined when describing a joint movement is the axis, the line in space around which the joint rotation occurs. In the case of human joints that behave as 'hinge' joints, such as the elbow, we can define the pattern of joint movement by simply defining the three-dimensional location of the joint axis. The amount of movement can be measured as

the angle of rotation about the axis. This axis of movement is sometimes known as the helical axis of motion (Woltring et al., 1985; Panjabi and White, 2001). In practice very few joints, if any, have an axis that remains completely fixed in space throughout the entire range of movement. As rotation occurs the axis may change its location, moving to a new location with the new axis parallel to the initial location. Another possibility is that the axis may change to a slightly different orientation in relation to the bones. Therefore to characterize fully the pattern of movement at a joint we need to locate the axis of motion at each instant during the movement through the range of motion.

So far we have considered a joint motion involving rotation around an axis, where the axis can be fixed or where it changes its position or orientation during the range of motion. Another possible movement also exists. Sometimes a joint moves in such a way that, as well as the main rotation about the axis, there are also very small amounts of movement along the axis. For example, during knee flexion with the thigh in a fixed position, the axis of motion lies in an approximately medial–lateral orientation. During flexion there may be slight medial or lateral translations of the tibia in relation to the fixed femur. Although the amount of this type of movement would be expected to be small, a complete description of joint movement requires that we incorporate this translation as one of the parameters describing the joint movement. In fact, although this movement may be small, it is conceivable that when damage to the joint capsule and ligaments occurs, the amount of translation along the axis of motion may be a sensitive indicator of abnormal joint motion.

We can now see that there are three parameters required for complete description of the movement at a joint:

1. location of the axis of motion in three dimensions, including information about how this location changes during the movement
2. amount of rotation – the angle through which the joint rotation occurs around the axis of motion during the movement
3. amount of translation – the displacement (if any) that occurs along the axis of motion during the movement.

Knowledge of the normal pattern and amount of movement allows us to detect abnormalities of movement. If we knew that the axis was normally fixed in a particular direction throughout the movement, then any movement involving a differently oriented axis, or in which the axis moved during the range of movement, could be regarded as showing an abnormal pattern.

Inevitably we are not able to obtain complete information about movement of a joint and an approximate description of joint motion is given. The first aspect of approximation occurs in the way we describe the changes in axis position throughout a movement. Usually we do not know the location of the axis at every part of the range of motion. In fact, we do not know the axis location at any given instant. In practice, each axis location is derived by knowing the location of the body segments on either side of the joint on two occasions (A and B) in time, where these two occasions are separated by a finite angle. A procedure is then applied to calculate the location of an axis of motion, around which rotation seems to have occurred between the two positions (Spoor and Veldpaus, 1980). This axis is known as the finite helical axis of motion between positions A and B (Woltring et al., 1985). The degree to which this finite axis approximates the locations of the instantaneous axes as the joint moves between A and B depends on how close A and B are together. In some cases A may correspond to the position of full flexion and B may correspond to the position of full extension. In such a situation, the finite axis between A and B tells us nothing about the variation of axis location during the movement and may tell us little about the pattern of movement at all.

The second aspect of approximation in describing joint motion occurs in the way we describe the axis. Imagine that we located a knee flexion axis and found it to lie in a horizontal, medial–lateral direction. If we view this axis from the front, the axis will be a horizontal line. If we view from the side, looking at motion in a sagittal plane, where the axis passes through a mid sagittal plane it will appear as a point in that plane. Any such point on the axis of rotation is known as a centre of rotation for the movement. Provided the axis is perpendicular to the plane, the location of the centre of rotation in a plane can accurately represent the axis. However, if the axis passes obliquely through the plane, then it cannot be fully represented by one point in the mid sagittal plane. To be an accurate representation of the axis of motion, we need to know the orientation of the axis as it passes through the centre of rotation. If we are fully to define the pattern of movement, we must also note whether there is any translation along the axis during rotation. In addition, as with the axis of rotation, we need to know this information on as many occasions as possible during the range of motion.

The axis-of-rotation method, whether used in its complete form or simplified to centre of rotation, is most useful for describing movements that occur in a single fixed plane. If a movement is complex, the axis may move into orientations that are oblique to those corresponding to previous parts of the movement. Although the axis-of-rotation method remains a valid way of describing such movements, it is less convenient to use because of the need to employ a three-dimensional method to show the positions and orientations of the axes.

To deal more conveniently with complex three-dimensional movements, a simpler method of joint movement description is often used. In particular, much of the detail of the pattern of movement is usually omitted. The method used involves considering the joint motion as comprising components of rotation in each of the three cardinal planes (sagittal, frontal and horizontal) and three components of translation (anteroposterior, medial–lateral, cephalocaudal). For physiological movements, where rotation is the desired motion, one of the rotations is designated as the main movement. All other movements, including rotation in other planes and translations in any direction, are called coupled movements (Panjabi and White, 2001). For example, if we attempt to produce right lateral bending at a normal C4–C5 intervertebral joint, right axial rotation will occur as well as the desired right lateral bending (Harrison et al., 1988). In this case the main movement is right lateral bending, and the right axial rotation is a coupled movement. Note that this approach to describing joint movement gives a simplified, but quantitative method of describing the pattern and amount of motion. For example, Goel et al. (1985) measured the main and coupled motions to assess the effect of discectomy on the kinematics of the whole lumbar spine. They applied torques in each of the cardinal planes in turn, and measured the resulting main and coupled rotations and the three coupled translations. For a 3 Nm right lateral bending load applied to an intact specimen, the main rotation was 12° with a coupled lateral translation to the side of movement of 8 mm. The other coupled rotations and translations were found to be an order of magnitude smaller: less than 1 mm or degree. These data give us useful information about the normal pattern and extent of lumbar lateral flexion.

JOINT SURFACE KINEMATICS

Intersegmental movements make up part of the picture of joint movements. Another aspect of joint motion is the movement of one joint surface in relation to another. An anatomist, MacConaill, has developed a complicated system of classification and description of joint types and movements that emphasizes the anatomical aspects of joints (MacConaill, 1964). In considering the kinematics of joint surfaces, we will just consider one small aspect of MacConaill's ideas.

MacConaill focused very much on the shape of joint surfaces. He declared that there were only two different joint surface shapes: ovoid (egg-shaped; convex in all directions or concave in all directions) and sellar (saddle-shaped; convex in one direction and concave in another direction). Most joints comprise two ovoid surfaces, one concave and one convex. MacConaill divided the movements between the joint surfaces into three categories: spin, roll and slide. When spin occurs there is essentially minimal movement through space of the body segments. Rotation occurs around an axis that coincides with the line of the segment, while the axis of motion remains in a fixed position. On the other hand, both roll and slide are associated with translation of the body segment through space. When roll occurs there is rotation of the segment about an axis that is located at the point of contact between the joint surfaces. Slide involves translation of the body segment without rotation.

In a typical joint, roll and slide occur together. If roll occurs alone then the point of contact between the surfaces moves (such as when a ball rolls on a table). The combination of roll and slide allows the point of contact to remain approximately stationary.

The roll alone may tend to move the point of contact in one direction, but if this is combined with a slide in the opposite direction the point of contact can remain in one place. This combination of movements is desirable if the amount of cartilage-covered area of one joint surface is small, such as in the case of the glenoid fossa that forms one surface of the glenohumeral joint. Passive movements produced by a physiotherapist probably involve slide movements between the joint surfaces without the degree of concomitant roll that would occur in a physiological movement, for example anteroposterior glides at the glenohumeral joint (Maitland, 1991). Therefore joint movements produced in this manner may not normally occur during physiological motion. A focus on joint surface movements is a feature of the approach taken by Kaltenborn (1980) to manual therapy of joints.

PASSIVE JOINT DYNAMICS

Passive joint movements are often divided into two categories (Maitland, 1986). Passive physiological movements involve the same sorts of movement patterns as active movements, but are performed by the therapist while the patient is passive. Passive accessory movements occur when the therapist moves the joint in a way that is not normally done by the patient's muscles. The physiotherapist attempts to translate a body segment during accessory movements, rather than rotate it. Here we will briefly discuss the resistance to these passive movements, considering separately the cases of passive physiological and passive accessory movement.

For physiological movements, the torque versus angle curve is usually similar to that shown in Figure 2.1 (Berme et al., 1985). Depending on the joint and the direction of movement, the low-stiffness region AB may be of variable length. Generally there will be a substantial low-stiffness region because joints are designed to allow physiological movements to occur freely within a certain range. At the highly mobile glenohumeral joint the low-stiffness zone AB is relatively large for most movements (Engin, 1979) while at the ankle joint this zone is much smaller (Chesworth and Vandervoort, 1989).

For accessory movements, because translation is being produced, we can describe the passive

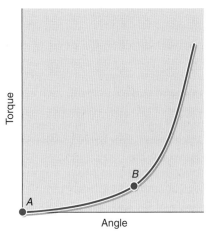

Figure 2.1 Resistance of typical physiological movement.

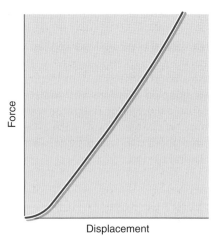

Figure 2.2 Force versus displacement curve expected for typical accessory movement.

resistance to movement using a force versus displacement graph. For these movements it appears that there is only a minimal low-stiffness phase, which is probably caused by compression of compliant soft tissue overlying the bone. Although very few data are available, it seems likely that in accessory movements there is resistance to the entire movement, with the resisting force probably increasing approximately linearly with the amount of translation, as shown in Figure 2.2 (Farahmand et al., 1998; McQuade et al., 1999).

In both cases, the stiffness of the movement is the gradient of the curve: the torque versus angle curve for physiological movements, and the force versus displacement curve for accessory movements. For both physiological and accessory movements little information is available about which anatomical structures are responsible for the stiffness measured (or perceived) at the skin surface. It is often assumed that muscles provide most of the resistance to physiological movements, and accessory movements are resisted mostly by ligaments and joint capsule. There is some evidence, largely based on animal studies, to support a major role for muscles in resisting passive physiological movements (Johns and Wright, 1962; Barnett and Cobbold, 1969; Akeson et al., 1974; Riener and Edrich, 1999). However, there is little evidence to implicate any specific tissues in the resistance to passive accessory movements. In the case of the accessory movements in the spine, the therapist is not necessarily able to

produce pure translation of the vertebra to which she or he applies a force, nor is she or he able to stabilize adjacent vertebrae so that movement only occurs at one or two intervertebral joints. Indeed, research indicates that when a force is applied to, for example, an L3 vertebra, then appreciable intervertebral movements occur as far away as T8 (Lee and Svensson, 1993). In this situation there will be contributions to the movement resistance from a large number of structures. Therefore the clinical meaning of the behaviour of resistance will be difficult to determine.

INSTABILITY

There is one particular case of abnormal joint movement that is worthy of special consideration here – instability. A major issue to consider in relation to instability is one of definition. The term 'instability' related to joint movements is used in many different ways in the clinical literature and these different uses involve quite different meanings. As a result there is considerable confusion about the concept of instability. The confusion can be partly resolved by identifying the distinctly different ways in which the term 'instability' is used and using different terms for each separate variant, with corresponding different operational definitions. Two such terms could be *mechanical (true) instability* and *clinical instability*.

The key to understanding mechanical instability lies in consideration of the changes in potential energy of a joint system. Therefore, before we consider instability further we need to understand how the potential energy of a joint system can be changed. In relation to a joint there is one major form of potential energy, elastic potential energy. The amount of elastic potential energy possessed by a body depends on the amount of elastic deformation. In the case of a joint, the elastic deformation is the stretch of the spring-like soft tissues around the joint. For a linearly elastic tissue, the potential energy stored when it is deformed is equal to $\frac{1}{2}kx^2$, where k is the stiffness and x is the amount of elastic deformation. Where a bone is restrained (at a joint) by a number of soft tissues, such as ligaments and muscles, the total potential energy is the potential energy stored in all of those restraining structures. According to a principle first elaborated by Euler in 1748 (Beeson, 1992), a system such as a joint will tend to come to rest in a position in which the total stored potential energy is least.

Mechanical instability can now be defined as the situation where small joint movements result in a decrease in total system potential energy. Where there is mechanical instability, small initial movements will result in further movement away from the initial position. The movement continues until finally a position of stability is reached and the potential energy is at a minimum. Conversely, in the case where mechanical stability exists, small initial movements result in an increase in potential energy and the joint tends to move to lower its potential energy and return to its original position. Consider the example shown in Figure 2.3. A post is restrained by four elastic cables A, B, C and D. If the post is displaced in the direction of the arrow, then restraints A and B will become stretched and will increase their store of potential energy. Therefore, according to our definition, the post is stable. If the post is released, it will tend to return to the original vertical position.

In a joint, some of the structures that restrain movement may be deficient as the result of trauma, disease or other factors and there is a decreased tendency for the joint to return to its original position after a small perturbation. Consider the case shown in Figure 2.4, which is a better representation of a peripheral joint.

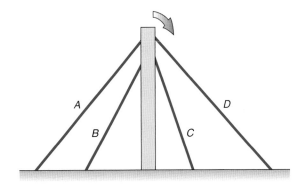

Figure 2.3   Example of a stable system.

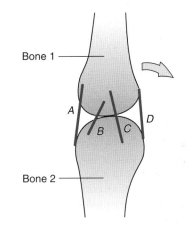

Figure 2.4   Simple representation of a peripheral joint.

There are two bones, held together by tissues that can act as restraints to joint movement. Imagine that bone 1 can move and bone 2 is fixed. There are a number of restraining tissues (A, B, C and D, representing ligaments, joint capsule, etc.) that are tending to hold the joint in position. However, if one of the key restraints is weak or missing (such as A), then we may find that we can move bone 1 to the right through a small distance and it will not return to its original position. Movement to the right will cause restraint B to experience an increase in tension, increasing its potential energy. However the shape of the joint surfaces means that as bone 1 moves to the right, it can also move downwards, as indicated by the arrow. Hence restraints C and D may shorten substantially, decreasing their potential energy, and giving a net decline in the potential energy of the joint system. This is then an unstable situation, and bone 1 will continue to move away from the initial position. Eventually, restraints C and

D will become completely slack and further movement will result in no decrease in their potential energy (since it is already zero), while the increase in tension in restraint *B* will continue. Hence, the total potential energy would start to rise again and a new stable equilibrium position has been reached.

It is well known that some peripheral joints show an instability not unlike that which has just been described. For example, in some individuals the glenohumeral joint can be unstable, with dislocation resulting if the humerus is moved too far in a particular way (Levine and Flatow, 2000). In the example above (shown in Fig. 2.4) a passive accessory movement was shown to produce instability. Instability can also occur in active physiological movements. In an active movement muscles provide much of the resistance that tends to restore the joint to the initial position. An activated muscle behaves much like a spring, whose stiffness increases with the degree of activation (Ettema and Huijing, 1994; Gardner-Morse and Stokes, 2001). It is possible that a sudden change in activation of a muscle when an external load is being applied may allow a joint to move quickly away from the neutral position with minimal resistance. This phenomenon could, rightly, also be called instability.

Clinical instability is a much simpler concept, but does not really involve instability at all! A more correct term would be pathological hypermobility.

This term is most often applied to the spine. In this context the term instability usually means excessive movement at an intervertebral joint, which is likely to compromise the spinal cord. A person who has damage to the structures that restrain intervertebral movement (caused by disease or trauma) can show an amount of intervertebral movement that could endanger the spinal cord so that surgical stabilization is required. The judgement as to whether instability exists is often made on the basis of the amount of coupled intervertebral anteroposterior translation that is exhibited during movement through the full flexion–extension range. Cases of clinical instability show hypermobility but may not show the decreasing potential energy that is the characteristic of true mechanical instability.

The term instability is also used quite differently, meaning neither mechanical instability nor clinical instability (for example, Kirkaldy-Willis and Farfan, 1982; Tropp et al., 1984; Richie, 2001). In addition, there are many instances of use of the term instability where it is not clear how the term is operationally defined (Hodges and Richardson, 1996). In a number of these cases, the authors possibly just mean 'abnormal control of joint movement', reflected in the magnitude or timing of muscle activation, without necessarily observing the actual joint movements that result from this apparent abnormality.

Bone: recent concepts in bone damage, modelling and remodelling

H.M. Frost

INTRODUCTION

This section summarizes recent developments in bone research that finally seem ready for physical therapists, coaches, trainers and other health professionals to apply to clinical practice. Definition of key terms is provided in Table 2.4. Values for some important parameters are also provided. The following facts should be noted:

1. Our daily mechanical usage (MU) provides the loads that cause strains and stress in bones (Martin and Burr, 1989; Burr and Martin, 1992). Strains are deformations (Table 2.4); stress is the internal force in bone that resists them. Increased vigour of MU means larger forces on bones, not more frequent ones.

2. The largest bone loads and strains come from muscles, not body weight. On a soccer player's femur those loads can briefly exceed five times body weight (Frost, 1986; Martin and Burr, 1989; Burr and Martin, 1992).

3. Bone fractures at about 25 000 microstrain (Martin and Burr, 1989; Burr and Martin, 1992).

4. Two biological mechanisms, modelling and remodelling, help to control a bone's architecture, mass and strength, and to fit it to its MU, minimize its fatigue damage and keep strains below its fracture strain (Fig. 2.5).

5. Each mechanism responds to stimuli in its own way but both use osteoclasts and osteoblasts to do it (Frost, 1986; Jee, 1989; Martin and Burr, 1989; Burr and Martin, 1992).

6. Modelling can add to and strengthen bone and remodelling can remove it when a mechanical need for it ceases, but neither can do the other's work.

MICRODAMAGE

Repeated load–deload cycles (as in running) cause microscopic damage or microdamage in bone (Frost, 1986; Martin and Burr, 1989; Parfitt, 1990; Schnitzler, 1993). This damage increases with the size and number of the loads and can weaken bone enough to let normal MU cause stress fractures and spontaneous fractures. Excessive microdamage always causes such fractures (Frost, 1986; Burr and Martin, 1992).

Bone has a microdamage threshold well below its fracture strain and can repair lesser but not larger amounts. At 2000 microstrain it can take over 40 years of normal activities to fracture a bone in fatigue, but less than 2 months at 4000 microstrain. Doubling the size of the strains in that 2000–4000 microstrain region increases microdamage hundreds of times (Pattin and Carter, 1991; Frost, 1993). The remodelling mechanism (see below) normally repairs microdamage by removing and replacing damaged bone with new bone (Frost, 1986; Burr, 1993).

Creating too much microdamage, depressing its repair or both can cause stress fractures and spontaneous fractures. Small amounts of microdamage seldom cause pain but enough microdamage to threaten a fracture usually causes bone pain during MU. This can happen in particular conditions, such as osteoporosis, at particular sites, such as around artificial joints and teeth, and can affect particularly active groups such as aggressive athletes and military trainees (Frost, 1986).

Table 2.4 Definitions of key terms used for bone involvement in musculoskeletal physiotherapy

Fracture strain	The strain at which normal lamellar bone usually fractures (its ultimate strength). Equal to about 25 000 microstrain (a little more in children and less in adults), it corresponds to a compression or tension stress of about 16 000 lbf/in^2 or 130 MPa
MESm[a]	The minimum effective strain range that controls modelling. Where typical peak strains exceed a modelling threshold range (MESm), modelling increases bone strength and mass. Where strains stay below that range, mechanically controlled modelling stays off (in humans, centred near 1000 microstrain)[b]
MESr[a]	The minimum effective strain range that controls remodelling. A strain threshold range at and above which remodelling begins to conserve bone, but below which it removes bone (in humans, centred near 50–100 microstrain)[b]
Microdamage threshold	The strain range at and above which more new microdamage arises than its repair mechanism can handle, so it begins to accumulate (for bone, centred near 3000 microstrain)
Microstrain	A measure of deformation, which can be in tension, compression, shear, bending and/or torque; 25 000 microstrain in compression equals a 2.5% shortening of a bone, e.g. from 100% to 97.5% of its original length; 1500 microstrain in compression (or tension) equals 0.15% shortening (or stretching) of a bone, e.g. from 100% to 99.85% or (100.15%) of its original length. Whereas strain can be measured directly in tissues, stress must be inferred from other measurements
MU	Mechanical usage of the skeleton, with far more emphasis on the size of the resulting bone loads or forces than on their number and frequency

[a]These MES ranges correspond to the natural criteria that determine if too little or too much bone exists for its usual mechanical usage. If they differ in different people, that could make some people unusually resistant to injury and others unusually susceptible to it.
[b]Studies of *in vivo* bone strains revealed these thresholds and suggested their approximate values with respect to the fracture strain of bone. As their systematic study began relatively recently, the above values may need revision in the future.

MODELLING: STRENGTHENING AND ADDING BONE

Strains in or above an MESm range (Table 2.4) can make modelling drifts (henceforth called 'modelling') begin to strengthen bone by adding more to it and/or changing its shape and size (Frost, 1990a; Jee et al., 1991). These changes usually reduce further strains towards the bottom of this MESm range, an arrangement that makes bones very strong. Since the MESm normally lies below the microdamage threshold of bone (Table 2.4), modelling keeps strains below that threshold also (Jee et al., 1991; Frost, 1992).

In summary, global modelling can add to and strengthen bone but does not normally remove and weaken it. During normal MU, the MESm indicates whether and where a bone needs strengthening.

REMODELLING AND CONSERVING OR REMOVING BONE

Over approximately 4 months a typical remodelling basic multicellular unit (BMU) replaces a small packet of older bone with new bone (Frost, 1986; Martin and Burr, 1989; Heaney, 1993), for example, the secondary osteon. By changing how much bone completed BMUs resorb and make, remodelling can conserve or remove bone but does not normally add to it (Frost, 1990b). Here 'remodelling' means by BMUs. Remodelling normally repairs microdamage, an important if belatedly accepted function (Frost, 1986; Burr, 1993; Heaney, 1993; Parfitt, 1993). Remodelling usually removes bone where strains stay below an MESr strain range, as in disuse (Table 2.4), but conserves it where strains exceed that range (Frost, 1990b; Burr and Martin, 1992).

In summary, global remodelling can remove or conserve but does not normally add to and strengthen bone. It also repairs microdamage. The MESr distinguishes mechanically needed from unneeded bone during normal MU.

There are a number of questions which should be asked by physiotherapists working in the musculoskeletal area:

1. Which mechanisms determine bone mass and strength? In children longitudinal bone growth adds new trabecular bone and length to cortical bone. Then modelling can thicken and strengthen both, while remodelling can conserve or remove them. Adults lack longitudinal growth and effective cortical bone modelling, so remodelling mostly controls conservation of the bone mass and strength they accumulated during growth (Frost, 1986, 1993; Jee, 1989). Hence this is a reason to encourage children to accumulate good bone banks (see next).

2. What controls those mechanisms? MU exerts the most important control over them.

    (a) For bone mass and strength. In children increased MU tends to increase the above additions and to reduce losses from remodelling, so bone mass and strength increase. Disuse reduces such gains and increases the losses, so bone mass and strength decrease. In adults who lack longitudinal growth and efficient modelling of cortical bone, the remodelling responses to MU control most conservation and losses of bone (Frost, 1986, 1992; Burr and Martin, 1992).

    Throughout life the largest loads and strains have far more influence on bone mass and strength than small ones. This gives weight lifters stronger bones than marathon runners (Frost, 1986).

    MU effects dominate non-mechanical ones long thought to be more important, but which can help or hinder the MU ones (Frost, 1986; Jee and Frost, 1992). Examples of non-mechanical influences include: vitamin D, calcium and protein in the diet; the adrenal cortical, growth, parathyroid and sex hormones; homeostatic needs; genetics, some drugs.

    (b) For microdamage. Some hormones, drugs and diseases can depress microdamage repair in bone, and in fibrous tissues (Frost, 1986; Schnitzler, 1993), causing stress fractures, tendon and ligament ruptures and aseptic necroses of the hip, knee and humeral head (Frost, 1986). Although agents that improve microdamage repair should exist, future research must find and prove them.

3. What are the explanations for some of the problems encountered in sports medicine? True bone pain in athletes, special forces trainees or patients with other problems usually reflects increased microdamage, which may cause local inflammation also. Greatly reducing the vigour of the MU that caused this pain usually lets microdamage repair catch up to the need, but that can take many months (Frost, 1992).

4. How long does it take for adaptation to occur? Throughout life a BMU needs at least 4 months to repair a bit of microdamage. In children, modelling needs similar time to react effectively to increased vigour of MU (Frost, 1986, 1990a, b). Many factors (ageing, disease, genetic influences, drugs) can prolong those times but so far nothing has been found to shorten them, including drugs, hormones and, sorry to say, all treatment methods in use in physical therapy and rehabilitation medicine, and by athletic coaches and trainers. Although agents that could shorten them should exist, future research must find and prove them also.

5. How can adaptation be maximized? First, the vigour of the MU that caused the microdamage should be greatly decreased. This should be done for the months bone needs to adapt to the need. The vigour of new strenuous activity should be increased slowly towards maximum, over 6–12 months (Frost, 1986). Physiotherapists should also know that aggressive training can sometimes increase muscle strength faster than bone, tendon and ligament can adapt to it. This regimen has obvious applications to the post-operative management of bone and ligament repair and reconstruction.

6. How can one distinguish microdamage in fibrous tissues? Distinguishing true bone pain from the pain caused by excessive microdamage

in ligament, tendon and fascia (Charley horse, fasciitis, shin splints, tendinitis) requires diagnostic acumen and experience and, even with this, is not always possible. Excessive fibrous tissue microdamage usually results from any regimen based upon the time frame for adaptation of bone outlined in the answer to question 4.

7. How does research guide us with healing problems? Small strains, in the MESm region, of a healing fracture or spinal fusion probably improve their healing (Frost, 1989). Achieving this outcome can pose problems, however, because very small loads cause such small strains in healing tissues, and apply trivial loads to them, but they may accrue more from this phenomenon than from the gross joint and limb motion itself.

8. Are there other roles for bone remodelling? In the past many assumed that the major function of remodelling lay in controlling the blood calcium and acid–base status (homeostasis). However, this is not so (Jee and Frost, 1992), although some clinicians do not yet understand this. The role of remodelling in microdamage repair and control of bone conservation and loss for mechanical requirements usually dominates its homeostatic function (Martin and Burr, 1989; Jee et al., 1991; Jee and Frost, 1992; Burr, 1993; Parfitt, 1993).

Bone: application of research to physiotherapy practice

K. Bennell and K. Khan

Bone is a unique tissue with the principal responsibility of supporting loads that are imposed on it. Osteoporotic fractures occur in bone that is weakened due to low bone mass and microarchitectural deterioration. This is an increasing public health problem with one in two women and one in three men over the age of 65 years at risk of osteoporotic fracture. Musculoskeletal physiotherapists are often involved in the prevention, diagnosis and rehabilitation of such fractures. Furthermore, many therapists will be managing patients for other conditions who are at risk of osteoporotic fracture. This chapter will provide a brief overview of factors determining bone strength, how bone strength is measured clinically and how bone responds to mechanical loading.

WHAT FACTORS DETERMINE BONE STRENGTH?

The key mechanical function of bone is to resist fracture. Bone strength is determined by both its intrinsic material properties (mass, density, stiffness and strength) and its gross geometric characteristics (size, shape, cortical thickness, cross-sectional area and trabecular architecture; Carter et al., 1976; Currey, 2001; Forwood, 2001).

Material properties of bone

The organic and inorganic components of bone determine its material properties. The organic component, primarily type I collagen, provides tensile strength. Abnormal collagen matrix leaves bone brittle, irrespective of the amount of bone mineral present. The inorganic component, mineral, resists compressive forces. Functional tests under controlled conditions using a defined volume of bone can be used to measure the material behaviour of bone as a tissue. When a load, or stress, is applied, the bone is deformed. This deformation is referred to as strain.

Stress and strain

Stress, the force applied per unit area, can be classified as tensile, compressive, torsional or shear. Strain describes the deformation of a material without regard to its structural geometry and refers to the percentage change in bone length. Strain is greatest at the point of highest loading and dissipates along the length of the long bone. For example, during walking or running, the highest measurable strain would occur at the calcaneus and distal tibia. In addition, during locomotion the greatest strain is generated at the cortex under compression. Strains measured directly during physical activity in humans using strain gauges reveal complex patterns (Burr et al., 1996; Milgrom et al., 2000).

The intrinsic material properties of bone include the concepts of stiffness and strength. The amount of force required to deform a structure is termed its *stiffness* and is represented by the slope of the stress–strain curve. The strength of the structure can be defined as the load at the yield or failure points, or as the ultimate load, depending on the circumstances. Strength is an intrinsic property of bone and is independent of its size.

Bone mineral mass

Bone mass is a determinant of bone material properties; the distribution of bone mass and bone geometry are connected to bone strength and stiffness. Further, the strength and stiffness of bone is a function of density. Although bone mass is only one component of overall bone strength (Mosekilde, 1993), it does explain more than 80% of that variable (Johnston and Slemenda, 1993). Because bone mass is highly correlated with

dual-energy X-ray absorptiometry (DXA) results, this technique is used to measure bone mass and give an estimate of fracture risk in humans. DXA technology and its clinical implications are discussed further below.

Structural properties of bone

Geometric characteristics of bone include size, shape, cortical thickness, cross-sectional area and trabecular architecture. For tension and compression loads, the strength of a bone is proportional to the bone cross-sectional area. Hence, a larger bone is more resistant to fracture as it distributes the internal forces over a larger surface area, resulting in lower stresses (Hayes and Gerhart, 1985). With respect to bending loads, both the cross-sectional area and the distribution of bone tissue around a neutral axis are important geometrical features. The area moment of inertia is the index that takes into account these two factors in bending. A larger area moment of inertia means that the bone tissue is distributed further away from the neutral axis (the axis where the stresses and strains are zero) and is more efficient in resisting bending.

The length of a bone also influences its strength in bending. The longer the bone, the greater the magnitude of the bending moment caused by the application of a force. For this reason, the long bones of the lower extremity are subjected to high bending moments and hence high tensile and compressive stresses (Nordin and Frankel, 1989).

HOW IS BONE STRENGTH MEASURED CLINICALLY?

Bone mineral density (BMD) is used as a surrogate measure to diagnose and grade osteoporosis and to predict an individual's short-term fracture risk. DXA is currently the bone densitometry technique of choice. DXA measures the transmission through bone and soft tissue of a dual-photon beam from an X-ray source (see Ch. 3). It can evaluate BMD at axial and peripheral sites with excellent measurement precision, greater image resolution, lower radiation dose and reduced scanning time compared with its predecessors.

All absorptiometry techniques convert a three-dimensional body into a two-dimensional image providing an integrated measure of both cortical and trabecular bone. The measurement of BMD is calculated by dividing the total bone mineral content (BMC) in grams by the projected area of the specified region. It is therefore not a true volumetric density but an area density expressed in g/cm^2.

Physiotherapists need to be able to interpret DXA scans as the results can guide patient management. The most useful BMD scores are the Z- and T-scores. The Z-score compares the person's BMD with that of an age-matched group (calculated as the deviation from the mean result for the age- and sex-matched group divided by the standard deviation of the group). This score indicates whether one is losing bone more rapidly than one's peers. The T-score is similarly defined but uses the deviation from the mean peak bone density of a young, healthy sex-matched group. The World Health Organization has defined bone mass clinically based on T-scores (WHO Study Group, 1994) and has categorized it into normal, osteopenia, osteoporosis and established osteoporosis (Table 2.5). DXA-derived BMD scores have been shown clinically to predict fracture risk relatively well.

Table 2.5 Diagnostic criteria for osteoporosis (WHO Study Group, 1994)

Classification	DXA result
Normal	BMD greater than 1 standard deviation (SD) below the mean of young adults (T-score above −1)
Osteopenia	BMD between 1 and 2.5 SD below the mean of young adults (T-score −1 to −2.5)
Osteoporosis	BMD more than 2.5 SD below the mean of young adults (T-score below −2.5)
Severe or established osteoporosis	BMD more than 2.5 SD below the mean of young adults plus one or more fragility fractures

DXA, dual-energy X-ray absorptiometry; BMD, bone mass density.

WHAT ARE THE RISK FACTORS FOR OSTEOPOROTIC FRACTURES?

Bone density and falls are two major determinants of the risk of fracture (Petersen et al., 1996; Lespessailles et al., 1998). An individual's peak bone mass is reached around the late teens and early 20s with up to 60% acquired during the pubertal years (Young et al., 1995; Bailey, 1997). A slow rate of bone loss starts after this time in both sexes and superimposed on this is an accelerated loss of bone in women at the menopause when oestrogen production ceases. Here rates of loss may be as great as 5–6% per year and are highest in the years immediately postmenopause (Riggs and Melton, 1986; Fig. 2.5). It is now thought that one's peak bone mass is a better predictor of the risk of osteoporosis in later life than the amount of bone lost with age. Therefore, in addition to steps for minimizing bone loss, prevention strategies for osteoporosis are focusing on maximizing peak bone mass.

Approximately 60–80% of our peak bone mass is determined by our genes (Zmuda et al., 1999). Other determinants include hormones, mechanical loading, nutrition, body composition and lifestyle factors such as smoking and alcohol intake. Physiotherapists need to be aware of risk factors for osteoporosis as well as medical conditions and pharmacological agents that predispose to secondary osteoporosis (Box 2.1).

A greater propensity to fall will increase the risk of fracture (Parkkari et al., 1999). Falls occur

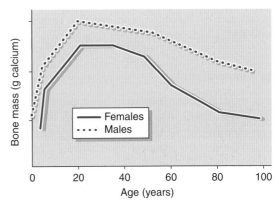

Figure 2.5 Changes in bone density with age in men and women.

Box 2.1   Risk factors for osteoporosis

- Family history of osteoporosis
- Early menopause without hormone replacement therapy
- Sedentary lifestyle
- Inadequate calcium and vitamin D intake
- Cigarette smoking
- Excessive alcohol
- High caffeine intake
- Amenorrhoea – loss of menstrual periods
- Anorexia
- Thin body type
- Rheumatological conditions, e.g. rheumatoid arthritis, ankylosing spondylitis
- Endocrine disorders, e.g. Cushing's syndrome, primary hyperparathyroidism, thyrotoxicosis
- Malignancy
- Gastrointestinal disorders (malabsorption, liver disease, partial gastrectomy)
- Certain drugs (corticosteroids, heparin)

---

frequently in individuals over the age of 65 years (Hill et al., 1999) and in residents in institutionalized care (Tinetti et al., 1988; Campbell et al., 1989). Many risk factors for fall initiation have been identified. These can be classified into intrinsic factors, for example, poor eyesight, reduced balance and reduced lower limb strength and extrinsic factors such as home hazards, multiple drug use and inappropriate footwear (Lord et al., 1991, 1994).

WHAT IS THE RESPONSE OF BONE TO MECHANICAL LOADING?

The skeleton is subjected to forces produced by gravity (weight-bearing), by muscles, and by other external factors. Bone tissue is an anisotropic material, which means that its behaviour varies depending on the direction of the applied load. The skeleton's response to a load depends on the strain magnitude, rate, distribution and cycles in the target bone as well as the rest period between loading cycles (Burr et al., 2002). Much of what we know about the influence of functional loads on bone comes from research with animal models where the applied load can be precisely controlled. The mechanical variables that influence bone are:

- *Strain magnitude*: early work using the turkey ulna clearly showed that bone formation

increased with larger strain magnitudes (Rubin and Lanyon, 1985). Activities that elicit high peak forces (or high strain magnitude) may have a greater effect on bone mass than activities associated with a large number of loading cycles (Whalen et al., 1988).

- *Strain rate*: the rate at which strain develops and releases determines bone's adaptive response. Higher strain rates are most effective for a maximal adaptive bone response (Turner et al., 1995; Mosley and Lanyon, 1998). Umemura and colleagues (1995) compared jump training with running training in rats and found that jumping was associated with a higher strain rate and magnitude and was more effective than running for eliciting a positive bone response.

- *Strain distribution*: it has been hypothesized that unusual strains of uneven distribution are more likely to stimulate osteogenesis than repetitive strains that result from everyday activity (Lanyon, 1984).

- *Strain cycles*: although a minimum number of loading cycles is required for a positive bone response, the number of strain cycles appears to be less important for bone adaptation than strain magnitude or strain rate (Rubin and Lanyon, 1984; Lanyon, 1987; Umemura et al., 1997).

- *Rest periods*: recent work has shown that bone cells desensitize soon after a loading session is initiated. Bone cells then require a recovery period before they can respond again to their mechanical environment. The anabolic effect of loading appears to be greater when the stimulus is broken down into smaller bouts separated by recovery periods than when the loading stimulus is delivered in a single uninterrupted bout. In previously stimulated bone cells, mechanosensitivity was restored after approximately 4–8 h of load-free recovery (Robling et al., 2000, 2001, 2002). Furthermore, a 30 s rest between loading cycles appears to be more effective than 3 s of rest within the one loading session (Umemura et al., 2002).

Mechanostat

It is not fully understood how bone responds to mechanical loads. It has been suggested that this response is controlled by a 'mechanostat' that endeavours to keep bone strain at an optimal level by adjusting bone structure (Frost, 1983; Turner, 1999). It is thought that bone strains resulting from mechanical loading are transduced into a cellular signal. Osteocytes have been proposed as the bone cells responsible for sensing strain and transmitting signals (Aarden et al., 1994). The cellular signals are then compared with the optimal strain for that region. If the signal falls within the optimal strain range, no adaptive response will occur and a state of remodelling or modelling equilibrium ensues. However, if the strains are above or below the optimal range, a state of overuse or disuse is perceived. This results in an appropriate response with net bone gain or loss in order to readjust bone strains.

Modelling and remodelling

Bone modelling and remodelling are the processes that lead to changes in bone geometry and mass. Bone modelling is an organized bone cell activity that allows bone growth and adjusts bone strength through the strategically placed, non-adjacent activity of osteoblasts and osteoclasts (Frost, 1990). Modelling improves bone strength not only by adding mass, but also by expanding the outer (periosteal) and inner (endocortical) diameters of bone.

Remodelling is a continuous, sequential process of breakdown and repair of microscopic cavities in bone. Remodelling occurs on both periosteal and endosteal surfaces within cortical bone and on the surface of trabeculae. Both osteoclasts (bone-resorbing cells) and osteoblasts (bone-forming cells) are involved in remodelling, organized into discrete packets called basic multicellular units (Frost, 1991).

Remodelling occurs in five stages: (1) quiescence; (2) activation; (3) resorption; (4) reversal; and (5) formation. A small area of bone surface is converted from rest to activity by an initiating stimulus, which may be hormonal, chemical or physical. Osteoclast precursors are then recruited to the bone surface where they fuse to form multinucleated osteoclasts. These cells form a cavity by resorbing bone. A 1–2-week interval between termination of the resorptive processes and commencent of formation is known as the reversal phase. During this time, the bone site is weakened. Therefore continued mechanical loading during the reversal phase could result in microdamage accumulation and the beginning of a stress fracture.

Repair of the resorption cavity is performed by osteoblasts and occurs in two stages, matrix synthesis and mineralization. First, a layer of type 1 collagen bone matrix, known as an osteoid seam, is deposited. After 5–10 days of maturation, the new matrix begins to mineralize with crystals of hydroxyapatite deposited within and between the collagen fibrils.

A key feature of remodelling is that it replaces damaged tissue with an equal amount of new bone tissue in the healthy skeleton. In the ageing and osteoporotic skeleton, however, the balance between the amount of bone resorbed and formed is shifted in favour of resorption, so that insufficient bone is formed to refill the resorption cavity. A net loss of bone results, and eventually bone strength and integrity are compromised.

EXERCISE PRESCRIPTION FOR BONE LOADING

While it is clear that mechanical loading influences bone material and structural properties, it is not known whether exercise reduces fracture rates – the ultimate goal. The fact that there are no randomized controlled trials to answer this question reflects inherent methodological difficulties. However, large-scale epidemiological studies suggest that physical activity is associated with a lower risk of fracture in both men and women (Turner et al., 1995; Joakimsen et al., 1999; Kujala et al., 2000).

The skeletal effects of exercise at different ages

It is presently thought that exercise in childhood and adolescence produces much higher gains in bone mass than does exercise in adulthood (Conroy et al., 1993; Morris et al., 1997; Bass et al., 1998; Bradney et al., 1998; Heinonen et al., 2000; McKay et al., 2000). The optimal time to maximize the skeletal effects with exercise appears to be during the early pubertal years rather than pre- or post-puberty (Heinonen et al., 2000; MacKelvie et al., 2001). In addition, it appears that childhood exercise stimulates the bone modelling process, expanding the bone size to produce a larger, possibly stronger bone (Haapasalo et al., 1996; Bradney et al., 1998; Petit et al., 2002). This phenomenon is generally not possible once growth has ceased.

It is not known whether the skeletal benefits achieved during the growing years can be maintained into later life when fractures occur. Short-term detraining studies (Kontulainen et al., 2001; Fuchs and Snow, 2002) and cross-sectional studies in retired athletes (Khan et al., 1996; Bass et al., 1998) suggest that this might be possible, although this issue needs to be further clarified (Karlsson et al., 2000).

Exercise in adulthood is important to conserve bone and to minimize bone loss with age (Wolff et al., 1999; Kelley et al., 2000). In adulthood, exercise must be continued in order to maintain exercise-induced BMD levels (Dalsky et al., 1988). Attrition rates from exercise are high even in supervised clinical trials (Bassey and Ramsdale, 1994; Kerschan et al., 1998). This reinforces the importance of developing strategies to improve compliance and encourage lifelong participation in physical activity.

Types of exercise for bone loading

In humans, high-impact exercises which generate ground reaction forces greater than twice body weight are more osteogenic than low-impact exercises (Bassey and Ramsdale, 1994; Heinonen et al., 1998, 2000). These are appropriate for younger individuals for whom jumping-type activities can be safely performed.

Since lean mass (Flicker et al., 1995; Young et al., 1995) and muscle strength (Madsen et al., 1993) are positively correlated with bone density, weight training has been advocated for skeletal health (Gleeson et al., 1990; Snow-Harter et al., 1992; Lohmann et al., 1995; Hartard et al., 1996). Loss of muscle mass and strength with age is well documented (Harries and Bassey, 1990; Rutherford and

Jones, 1992). Progressive weight training even in the frail elderly can lead to large strength gains (Fiatarone et al., 1990). One recent study also showed that stronger back extensor muscles were associated with a lower rate of subsequent vertebral fracture in postmenopausal women (Sinaki et al., 2002). In an elegant unilateral exercise study, Kerr et al. (1996) compared two strength-training regimes that differed in the number of repetitions and the weight lifted. The strength programme (high loads, low repetitions) significantly increased bone density at the hip and forearm sites whereas the endurance programme (low loads, high repetitions) had no effect.

Walking is frequently recommended in clinical practice to maintain skeletal integrity but generally the results of walking trials have not demonstrated significant effects on densitometry-derived bone density (Hatori et al., 1993; Martin and Notelovitz, 1993; Ebrahim et al., 1997; Humphries et al., 2000). This may relate to the fact that walking imparts relatively low-magnitude, repetitive and customary strain to the skeleton. While walking has numerous health benefits, some of which may influence fracture risk, it should not be prescribed as the exercise of choice for *skeletal loading* in healthy ambulant individuals. Whether walking is effective in those with restricted mobility is yet to be researched.

Non-weight-bearing activities such as cycling and swimming do not stimulate bone adaptation despite increases in muscle strength (Orwoll et al., 1989; Rico et al., 1993; Taaffe et al., 1995). This suggests that these activities do not generate sufficient strain to reach the threshold for bone adaptation.

Exercise dosage

The exact exercise dose required for maximal skeletal effects is not yet known. For an elderly or previously sedentary population, exercise should be gradually introduced to minimize fatigue and prevent soreness (Forwood and Larsen, 2000). Exercise should be performed two to three times per week. Animal studies suggest that this is as effective for bone as daily loading (Raab-Cullen et al., 1994).

For aerobic exercise, sessions should last between 15 and 60 min. The average conditioning intensity recommended for adults without fragility fractures is between 70 and 80% of their functional capacity. Individuals with a low functional capacity may initiate a programme at 40–60% (Forwood and Larsen, 2000).

Adults commencing a weight-training programme may perform a few weeks of familiarization (Kerr et al., 1996), followed by a single set of 8–10 repetitions at an intensity of 40–60% of 1 RM. This can be progressed to 80%, even in the very elderly (Fiatarone et al., 1994; ACSM, 1998). Programmes should include 8–10 exercises involving the major muscle groups. Supervision, particularly in the beginning, and attention to safe lifting technique are paramount.

Periodic progression of exercise dosage is needed, otherwise bone adaptation will cease. Increasing the intensity or weight-bearing is more effective than increasing the duration of the exercise. A periodic increase in a step-like fashion may be better than progression in a linear fashion (Forwood and Larsen, 2000). Nevertheless, there comes a point where gains in bone mass will slow and eventually plateau.

TREATMENT OF INDIVIDUALS WITH LOW BONE DENSITY

In osteoporotic and older patients the exercise focus shifts from specifically loading bone to preventing falls and improving flexibility, muscle strength, posture and function. Factors that will influence the choice of treatment programme include the patient's age, previous fractures, comorbid musculoskeletal or medical conditions, lifestyle, interests and current fitness level. Exercises to avoid in osteoporotic patients include high-impact loading, abrupt or explosive movements, trunk flexion, twisting movements and dynamic abdominal exercises. Only a small number of studies have evaluated the effect of exercise specifically in individuals with diagnosed osteopenia or osteoporosis (Sinaki and Mikkelsen, 1984; Ayalon et al., 1987; Bravo et al., 1996; Hartard et al., 1996; Preisinger et al., 1996; Kronhed and Moller, 1998; Malmros et al., 1998; Carter et al., 2001). Overall, the results support a role for exercise in improving falls risk factors, function and quality of life and in reducing pain. Of those studies that included bone density as an outcome measure, most reported skeletal benefits with exercise. However, the type of exercise also needs to be considered. One older study showed that, over 1–2 years, back flexion exercises were associated with a greater prevalence of wedging or compression of spinal vertebrae compared with back extension exercises (Sinaki and Mikkelsen, 1984).

SUMMARY

Musculoskeletal physiotherapists commonly encounter patients in whom bone strength may be compromised. It is important that reductions in skeletal integrity are given due consideration in clinical decision-making. Physiotherapists need to understand which factors place an individual at risk of fracture, how osteoporosis is diagnosed and how bone responds to mechanical loading.

Adaptations of muscle and connective tissue

R. Herbert

Muscles and connective tissues perform fundamentally important roles. First, and most obviously, muscles actively generate forces which move body segments. Muscle forces interact with gravitational forces and forces associated with the acceleration of body segments to produce controlled movement. When muscles become unable to generate tension appropriately, normal motor performance may be impaired.

Muscles and connective tissues also perform an equally important passive role. They function to constrain the movement of joints within normal ranges. Muscles need not always actively contract to perform this role, as it is possible that some muscles generate functionally significant amounts of passive tension with the amounts of stretch they experience during task performance. Of course muscles and connective tissue must not overly constrain joint motion – joints cannot function effectively if they are rigid. Clearly muscles and connective tissues must prevent excessive movement at joints, but they must also permit sufficient movement for effective task performance.

DISORDERS OF MECHANICAL PROPERTIES OF MUSCLES AND CONNECTIVE TISSUES

Many diseases act directly on nerves, muscles or connective tissues. Also, trauma can damage the nervous system or tear muscles or connective tissues. The effects of disease and trauma on mechanical properties of muscles and connective tissues are covered extensively in neurology, orthopaedic and rheumatology texts (see, for example, Walton, 1974, 1985; Guttman, 1976; Hughes, 1977; Mastaglia and Walton, 1982; Dyck et al., 1984; Millikan et al., 1987; Woo and Buckwalter, 1988; Vinken et al., 1990; Sunderland, 1991). Diagnosis and treatment of these problems is primarily the role of neurologists, orthopaedic surgeons and rheumatologists.

This section focuses on a *secondary* cause of disorders of mechanical properties of muscles and connective tissues: tissue adaptation. The mechanical properties of muscles and connective tissues adapt to the stresses imposed on the tissues. For example, when muscles are repeatedly required to generate large forces they hypertrophy, and they become more able to generate force. Likewise, it is thought that muscles that are frequently exposed to a high degree of stretch adapt by becoming longer and more extensible. In healthy people, this adaptability ensures that muscle strength is matched to demands for force production and that the extensibility of soft tissues is sufficient to permit the joint motion required for normal function. Unfortunately adaptability is a two-edged sword. When, as a result of disease or trauma, muscles and connective tissues are exposed to abnormally altered patterns of use (typically *disuse*), they adapt accordingly. Muscles and connective tissues may respond to disuse by becoming short and inextensible, and muscles may become less able to produce or sustain force. Such adaptations are frequently deleterious to function. In fact, the secondary adaptations are often far more disabling than the initial disease or trauma.

By way of example, a person with a recent rotator cuff tear may be capable of full arm elevation, but may choose not to elevate the arm because movement of the shoulder causes pain. A similar circumstance might arise in a person with rheumatoid arthritis affecting shoulder joints. In these examples, shoulder joints are effectively immobilized by pain. A likely consequence is that muscles will adapt by becoming weak and muscles and connective tissues that span shoulder joints will become inextensible, restricting shoulder motion. In these examples the secondary adaptations may impair function. Such impairments may persist even when the muscle tear has healed or when there is remission from the arthritis.

Presented with one of these scenarios, a physiotherapist might try to prevent or treat weakness and stiffness of shoulder muscles by prescribing exercise designed to normalize the mechanical environment of muscles and connective tissues. The aim of exercise (and other physiotherapy interventions designed to treat weakness or increased joint stiffness) is to induce the tissues to adapt in a way that restores function. It is important to recognize that the role of the physiotherapist is not usually in the treatment of the primary disease or trauma. Physiotherapists cannot directly repair rotator cuff tears or modulate the inflammatory response in rheumatoid arthritis. Instead, physiotherapy intervention is aimed at preventing or reversing deleterious secondary adaptations of the mechanical properties of muscles and connective tissues.

Rational prescription of exercise or other interventions requires an understanding of the sorts of deleterious adaptations that are likely to occur and how the tissues adapt their mechanical properties to different mechanical environments. That is the focus of the remainder of this section.

DISUSE WEAKNESS AND TRAINING

When muscles are immobilized in casts, or by traction, bedrest or pain, they become deprived of the tension which they normally experience, that is, they experience disuse. In response, disused muscles lose the ability to generate tension, and the person becomes weak (for reviews, see St-Pierre and Gardiner, 1987; Herbert, 1993a). The time course of the development of this process is highly variable, especially in the heterogeneous population of patients with whom physiotherapists usually deal, but mean strength losses of 30–60% with 5 weeks of bedrest or cast immobilization are typical (Herbert, 1993a). Chronic low-level disuse, such as may occur in response to arthritic disease, may induce equally significant strength losses. This degree of weakness is likely to impair motor function in many people, particularly those whose strength prior to the period of immobilization only marginally exceeded their requirements for normal function.

Disuse is often accompanied by clinically observable wasting of tissues. The circumference of disused limbs decreases, in the most extreme cases to apparently little more than the circumference of the underlying bones. Measures of limb circumference do not, however, provide a good measure of muscle atrophy (or, more specifically, of the decrease in muscle cross-sectional area, which is the most important determinant of muscle force-generating capacity) because tissues other than muscle also atrophy, and because there may be large differences in the amount of atrophy in different muscle groups crossing one joint (Davies and Sargeant, 1975; Ingemann-Hansen and Halkjaer-Kristensen, 1980; Young et al., 1982). Consequently it is not possible to obtain good clinical measures of muscle atrophy. For experimental purposes, reasonably reliable measures of muscle or muscle fibre cross-sectional area can be obtained by muscle biopsy, ultrasonography, computed tomography (CT) scans or nuclear magnetic resonance (NMR) imaging. Even with these techniques, valid measures are difficult to obtain, not least because of the complex architecture of most major human muscle groups (Fukunaga et al., 1992). The best available data suggest that the magnitude of the atrophy varies from muscle to muscle, and it probably also depends on the degree of disuse that the muscle experiences, the muscle's biochemical characteristics, and the length at which the muscle was immobilized (for reviews, see St-Pierre and Gardiner, 1987; Herbert, 1993a).

It might be expected that immobilization-induced decreases in muscle cross-sectional area would occur in proportion with the degree of muscle weakness, because in normal (non-immobilized) muscles tetanic tension is approximately proportional to muscle cross-sectional area. However, when decreases in muscle cross-sectional area have been measured, they have usually been found to be much less than the decrease in strength (McDougall et al., 1980; LeBlanc et al., 1988; Wigerstad-Lossing et al., 1988; Rutherford et al., 1990). There are several explanations as to why strength may decline much more than measures of muscle or fibre cross-sectional area would predict. Perhaps the most compelling is that, with disuse, people become less able to activate motor unit pools at sufficiently high frequencies to obtain near-tetanic muscle contractions. Some electro-myographic studies provide support for this hypothesis (Duchateau and Hainaut, 1987, 1990), although electromyographic studies may be biased by changes in tissue impedance and muscle fibre dimensions that accompany immobilization. A few animal studies suggest that immobilization (particularly immobilization in a shortened position) may decrease the specific tension of muscle, so that the amount of tension produced per unit of muscle cross-sectional area becomes less (Edgerton et al., 1975; Witzmann et al., 1982a). There is a more mundane explanation too. It could be that the methods used to measure muscle cross-sectional area underestimate the atrophy which occurs because they are incapable of accounting for complex muscle architectures.

To some degree, the losses of strength that accompany immobilization can be prevented by exercise. For example, Bamman et al. (1998) found that five sets of high-resistance leg press exercise (80–85% of 1 RM) performed every second day prevented losses of dynamic strength that other-wise occurred when healthy young adults were subjected to 2 weeks of bedrest. Stillwell et al. (1967) investigated the effects of performing iso-metric exercise (10×10 s isometric contractions hourly) within a unilateral long leg cast and found that exercise substantially reduced losses of iso-metric and dynamic strength losses.

Disuse adaptations of muscle cross-sectional area and muscle strength appear to be largely reversible, at least in some circumstances. One study found that, even without structured exercise the weight and tension-generating ability of rat hindlimb muscles returned to near-normal values within 28 days of termination of a 6-week period of immobilization (Witzmann et al., 1982b). This sug-gests that demands put upon the neuromuscular system in the performance or attempted perform-ance of everyday motor tasks provide a powerful stimulus for favourable adaptations to occur. Nevertheless there are clinical reports which sug-gest that some people still have less than normal strength several years following knee injury and reconstruction (Rutherford et al., 1990). It is widely believed, although not yet clearly demonstrated, that structured exercise provided by therapists can hasten recovery following a period of disuse, and,

where complete recovery would not have occurred, exercise can produce a better recovery of strength.

The effect of exercise for able-bodied subjects is less ambiguous. There is no doubt that well-designed training programmes can cause large and rapid increases in strength in able-bodied sub-jects. Over the past few decades an enormous volume of research has been directed towards expli-cating the mechanisms by which these strength increases are mediated. Despite a major research effort, however, the mechanisms remain uncertain.

One mechanism which certainly does mediate training-induced increases in muscle strength is muscle hypertrophy. Measures of fibre and muscle cross-sectional areas made before and after training using muscle biopsies or ultrasound, CT or MRI imaging procedures demonstrate hypertrophy with training (Narici et al., 1989). Typically, measurable muscle hypertrophy does not manifest until several weeks after the start of training (see McDonagh and Davies, 1984, for review).

In addition, it has been suggested that training may bring about an increased ability to activate muscle, and that this could increase voluntary force production. Evidence for this comes from studies which have measured changes in electro-myogram, motor neuron excitability or muscle fibre membrane excitability. Also, the observations that training responses are largely specific to the type of contractions employed in training, mani-fest contralaterally, and may be induced by imag-ined contractions all support the view that increases in strength are neurally mediated (Enoka, 1988; Sale, 1988, 1992; Yue and Cole, 1992). In contrast, meas-ures of muscle activation suggest that, at least dur-ing isometric contraction of isolated muscle groups, most subjects can almost fully activate their mus-cles prior to training (Jones and Rutherford, 1987; Gandevia and McKenzie, 1988), and that training does not increase voluntary drive to muscles (Herbert et al., 1998).

At a more behavioural level, the literature pro-vides some useful guidelines for the prescription of exercise aimed at increasing muscle strength (for reviews, see Atha, 1981; McDonagh and Davies, 1984; Herbert, 1993a). Most importantly, studies on able-bodied subjects clearly indicate that, if train-ing is to be effective, it must employ high-intensity contractions (McDonagh and Davies, 1984). As a rule of thumb, the most rapid increases in strength can be obtained when subjects train with weights no lighter than the weight they can just lift 10 times without resting (Berger, 1962). Less information is available for the prescription of isometric exercise, but it appears that the optimal isometric training programmes should also employ high but submaximal intensity contractions (Szeto et al., 1989; Khouw and Herbert, 1998). There is some evidence that both isometric and dynamic training programmes will be most effective if training is structured so that it induces fatigue (Davies and Young, 1983; Rooney et al., 1994). This can be done by ensuring that subjects continue lifting a training weight without rests until they can perform no further lifts (Rooney et al., 1994), or, for isometric exercise, by sustaining contractions (Davies and Young, 1983).

The response to training is often said to be training-specific. That is, the increases in strength are most evident with the type of contractions which were employed in training (for reviews, see Sale, 1988, 1992; Herbert 1993a). The implications of this phenomenon for training are discussed by Carr and Shepherd in Chapter 6.

ADAPTIVE MUSCLE SHORTENING

Clinicians have known for a long time that, under some conditions, an increase in the resistance of resting muscles to stretch may limit the amount of movement at joints. This phenomenon, perhaps one of the most functionally significant adaptations of muscle, has been called many things, including 'contracture', 'muscle shortening' and 'muscle tightness'.

Only in the past few decades have significant insights been gained into the nature of adaptive muscle shortening. Most of these insights have come from studies in which animals have been immobilized in casts (for reviews, see Gossman et al., 1982; Herbert, 1988, 1993b; O'Dwyer et al., 1989). Other models of muscle shortening (including congenital spasticity, the injection of tetanus toxin and bone-shortening procedures) have demonstrated changes in muscle which are broadly similar to those induced with cast immobilization, but it is not yet clear how well these models represent the problems of adaptive muscle shortening seen by physiotherapists in clinical practice.

When an animal's limb is immobilized so that some muscles are held in their most shortened position, the length of the muscle–tendon units decreases and the muscles become stiffer (Herbert and Balnave, 1993). Some of these changes can be attributed to changes in muscle tissue. Specifically, fibres of adaptively shortened muscles are usually found to have fewer sarcomeres in series and a greater proportion of their volume is comprised of connective tissue (Tabary et al., 1972; Williams and Goldspink, 1984; Jozsa et al., 1990; but see Heslinga and Huijing, 1993). The loss of sarcomeres must be associated with a loss of titin, a sarcomeric protein that binds myosin filaments to the z-line, and it is probably the loss of titin that causes the decrease in muscle extensibility (Toursel et al., 2002). Changes in muscle morphology such as these may be responsible for decreasing the length and increasing the stiffness of muscle tissue, and they affect the contractile properties of the muscle too. The effect of sarcomere loss is to cause fibres to develop their greatest active tensions at shorter lengths and over a shorter range of lengths (Williams and Goldspink, 1978; Witzmann et al., 1982a). Sarcomere number increases in fibres of muscles immobilized in a lengthened position, and this means that the length at which these muscles are best able to develop tension becomes greater than normal (Williams and Goldspink, 1978).

Changes in the tendinous portion of muscle have been much less investigated than the changes in muscle fibres. One of the first studies to look at adaptations of tendon length found significant length and compliance changes in the part of the tendon which blends with the muscle belly (the tendinous aponeurosis or tendon plate; Heslinga and Huijing, 1993) of immobilized rat gastrocnemius. In the immobilized rabbit soleus muscle, nearly two-thirds of the decrease in length of the muscle–tendon unit occurs in the tendon (Herbert and Crosbie, 1997). Perhaps this is not surprising, because in normal rabbit soleus muscle, as with many important human muscles, the tendon constitutes the greater part of the muscle–tendon unit's length.

One of the most important findings to come from studies on length adaptations in muscles is that the length of the muscle and tendon adapts to the position at which the muscle is habitually held – if the muscle is immobilized in a shortened position it becomes short, but if it is immobilized in a lengthened position it does not. Muscle shortening is, therefore, a response to deprivation of stretch, rather than to deprivation of movement. By implication, treatment aimed at preventing or treating adaptive muscle shortening should involve ensuring muscles receive adequate stretch. Little is known about what constitutes an adequate stretch to maintain the length of muscles, but animal studies suggest that relatively short durations of stretch (30 min every day in mouse soleus muscle) is adequate to maintain the length of muscles immobilized in a shortened position (Williams, 1990).

There have been many descriptions of the effects of stretch on range of motion in human studies, but relatively few studies have employed randomized designs to protect against bias. Of the few randomized studies, most have been conducted in rehabilitation environments. One trial on non-ambulatory nursing-home residents with knee flexion contractures showed that low-load prolonged stretch was substantially more effective in increasing joint range of motion than briefer high-load stretches (Light et al., 1984; but see also Steffen and Mollinger, 1995). In contrast, a recent study on spinal cord-injured subjects showed that 4 weeks of stretches applied to the plantarflexor muscles for 30 min each day did not make any difference to range of motion at the ankle (Harvey et al., 2000). Two studies failed to find any effect of positioning programmes on institutionalized adults with knee flexion contractures or stroke patients at risk of shoulder contractures, although this may reflect the small sample sizes in those studies (Dean et al., 2000; Fox et al., 2000). Serial casting produces increases in range of motion in head-injured adults with chronic plantarflexor contractures (Moseley, 1997), but splinting the hand in the functional position does not affect the length of extrinsic finger flexor muscles after stroke (Lannin et al., 2002).

REDUCED CONNECTIVE TISSUE EXTENSIBILITY

Connective tissues have sometimes been thought of as relatively incapable of adapting their mechanical properties. However, the connective tissues which surround joints can undergo functionally significant changes within the sorts of periods of immobilization which are commonly seen clinically.

Studies on immobilized rabbit joints indicate that, when taken together, the connective tissues which surround the knee (that is, all the tissues which cross the knee except muscle–tendon units and skin) become stiff in the flexion–extension direction with prolonged immobilization (for review, see Akeson et al., 1980). But immobilization also causes some ligaments to become less stiff (Noyes, 1977; see Woo, 1986, for a brief review). Together these findings translate, in clinical terms, to a loss of range of motion at the joint and an increase in joint laxity. These changes have been found to be at least partly reversible in animal studies (Akeson et al., 1977), although animal studies may not provide good models of chronic immobilization following injury, which is often seen clinically. There are many clinical cases where people develop intractably stiff joints, or permanently lax (and sometimes, therefore, unstable) joints.

Following injury, musculoskeletal injuries undergo repair. These repair processes are imperfect, at least in that a generic connective tissue – scar – is used to replace specialized connective tissues. Scar tissue performs a 'quick-fix' role by rapidly providing structural integrity to injured tissues, but it is often mechanically inferior to the original tissues (for a review, see Hardy, 1989). In particular, in binding together damaged parts of one tissue, scar may adhere injured tissues to other tissues (for example, muscle may adhere to skin or bone, and tendons may adhere to tendon sheaths), preventing the motion between tissues which must occur with normal joint movement. A consequence can be the loss of a normal range of joint movement.

Even long after injury and immobilization, muscle, tendon and ligament remain mechanically inferior to uninjured tissues – they tear at lower forces, and they are capable of absorbing less energy before tearing (for review, see Jarvinen and Lehto, 1993). However, injured muscles, tendons and ligaments undergo smaller losses of strength when the period of immobilization is minimized. This indicates that at least part of the decrease in tensile strength can be attributed to the effects of immobilization which followed injury. While some degree of immobilization is usually necessary to prevent further damage to injured tissues in the period immediately following injury, these findings suggest that the duration of immobilization should be kept as short as possible without risking further injury.

Regaining skill in motor performance

J. Carr and R. Shepherd

A THEORETICAL FRAMEWORK FOR SKILL LEARNING IN REHABILITATION

An understanding of human movement is fundamental to physiotherapy practice, hence research findings from the broad field of movement science have the potential to impact on the nature of that practice. Movement science is concerned with the phenomenon of human movement and incorporates many fields of enquiry such as functional anatomy, biomechanics, kinesiology, neurophysiology, muscle biology and work physiology. In addition, cognitive and ecological psychology explore the links between action and cognition and between action and the environment, and the field of motor learning investigates how individuals learn a new action and become skilled at it. The impact of recent advances in the field of human movement science provides the impetus for developing and testing new methods of movement rehabilitation for individuals with impairments of the neuromusculoskeletal system.

Clinical reasoning in physiotherapy practice also requires an understanding of the underlying impairments and adaptive mechanisms, the symptoms with which the individual presents and the processes involved in recovery, which include the regaining of skill in motor performance. Since movement is the principal means by which we interact with the environment, any breakdown of normal motor control, whether through disease, injury or disuse of the musculoskeletal system, will affect the individual's ability to produce goal-directed movements and interact with the environment. Clinical problem-solving also involves, therefore, an understanding of the importance of context and task in the organization of skilled movement, as well as of the naturally occurring musculoskeletal and biomechanical constraints. The individual with movement dysfunction is faced not only with having to cope with the demands normally imposed by tasks and the environment but also with the changing demands imposed by the damaged and recovering musculoskeletal system.

In rehabilitation, the physiotherapist is concerned not only with the physical treatment of symptoms (such as pain, joint stiffness or muscle weakness) but also with the restoration of health, physical fitness and optimal functional motor performance. This section is concerned with the theoretical basis of that part of clinical reasoning that has to do with the planning and implementation of restorative motor training; that is, training to regain skilled performance in those actions relevant to the individual recovering from a musculoskeletal lesion.

Physiotherapy intervention is based on theoretical assumptions regarding how movement is controlled and organized, what happens when the neuromusculoskeletal system is damaged and how recovery takes place. The last two decades have seen a substantial increase in the number of investigations into human movement, the results of which require a change in many of our underlying assumptions and, in many cases, a change in practice. Recent scientific investigations have provided new information related to such aspects of movement as its neural control and dyscontrol; skill learning; the biomechanical characteristics of functional motor tasks and the changes to these occurring when motor control is impaired and adaptive changes to soft tissue have developed; the effects of environmental factors on movement control; muscle adaptability; and the specificity effects of exercise and training. Such research enables the development of a scientific theoretical framework for rehabilitation and the generation of hypotheses which can be tested in the clinic. The results of clinical research, providing information about which methods are effective and which are not, form the basis for evidence-based practice.

A BRIEF HISTORICAL PERSPECTIVE

Rehabilitation in large part is a learning process in which individuals attempt to regain the ability to perform effectively previously well-learned skills, for example, reaching for an object, standing up from a seated position, walking or serving in tennis. Some individuals must master new skills, such as walking with crutches or a prosthesis, or ambulating by means of a wheelchair. Physiotherapists intervene in the learning process to facilitate the regaining of mastery in the performance of such actions.

Learning is an abstract concept and difficult to define. Generally motor learning is viewed as a set of processes involving practice and exercise leading to a relatively stable change in motor behaviour (Schmidt, 1988). It involves the acquisition of the ability to perform an action effectively in a flexible manner in different environmental contexts.

In the early 1970s, Gentile (1972) published a seminal article that examined learning as a function of the interaction of the individual and the environment in the pursuit of goal attainment. The focus of Gentile's article was on the understanding of movement as it becomes organized and differentiated in varying environmental contexts. This was shortly followed by other influential papers by, for example, Schmidt (1975), Marteniuk (1976) and Stelmach (1978), who viewed movement as the product of a centrally represented and generalized motor programme, i.e., an abstract representation of action stored in memory and retrieved when the action must be produced. This period

marked the beginning of an intense focus within the field of motor learning on understanding movement itself and on investigating issues of motor control. (For reviews of theories of skill learning and related experimental studies, see Magill (2001) and Gentile (2000).)

The study of motor control has been influenced in particular by the ecological perspectives of Gibson (1966) in the study of perceptual processes, and by the perspective of the Russian physiologist, Bernstein (1967). Out of this work developed a dynamical systems approach in which the structure of movement is seen as emergent, dynamic and responsive to both internal and external mechanisms.

In the Gibsonian view, vision is not only considered as an exteroceptive sense but also as an exproprioceptive sense, providing subjects with information about their own movements and playing an essential role in the regulation of action (Gibson, 1986). In order to investigate this theory, Lee and colleagues (Lee and Aronson, 1974; Lee and Lishman, 1975) had subjects stand on a stable floor surrounded by a movable chamber made of three walls and a ceiling. The question of interest was how subjects would respond when the surrounding chamber was moved. The investigators found that able-bodied adults swayed in relation to the movement of the room, i.e., when the wall in front approached them, subjects swayed backward and when the wall receded, subjects swayed forward. In some instances, small children overcorrected and fell over when the wall approached them. It appeared that subjects in both experiments were responding to visual inputs indicating they were falling even when other inputs (e.g. proprioception) would have provided contradictory (and, in this case, accurate) information.

Bernstein (1967) was instrumental in pointing out the need to understand the biomechanical or dynamic characteristics of linked segments, what he called the problem of coordinating and controlling a complex system of biokinetic links. He noted the need for movement organization to be in some way simplified. Such simplifications may involve constructing functional linkages or synergies (Gelfand et al., 1971; Turvey et al., 1982), or forming a simplified 'virtual' limb, as suggested for reaching to grasp (Greene, 1982; Arbib et al., 1986).

Bernstein recognized that the study of movement could not simply focus on those muscle forces produced by the individual but must also include inertial and reactive forces (1967). It is important in rehabilitation to be aware that, during active movement, the dynamic coupling that exists between body segments can bring about movement at joints which are distant from the site of active movement. That is to say, joint torques may result from mechanical linkage effects as well as from muscle contraction.

Following on from Bernstein, either directly or indirectly, much recent human movement research has concentrated on increasing our understanding of intersegmental dynamics. Investigations of actions such as the vertical jump and sit-to-stand have contributed to an understanding of the dynamic effects of the sequencing of segmental rotation (Gregoire et al., 1984; Bobbert and van Ingen Schenau, 1988; Shepherd and Gentile, 1994). Hypotheses have been generated regarding the function of biarticular compared to monoarticular muscles (Jacobs and van Ingen Schenau, 1992).

As a consequence of this theoretical and research effort, it is generally accepted that movements take place as the result of cooperative activity between the forces generated by muscles and segmental movement. This activity is dynamic and flexible, enabling the individual to be effective in different environmental contexts, and to modify the action according to changing task and other demands.

Increasing numbers of biomechanical studies are enabling the collection of normative data about common everyday, work-related and sporting actions. These studies inform rehabilitation by clarifying the optimal pattern of kinematic, kinetic and muscle activation patterns which are to be practised and learned by the person attempting to regain skilled performance. Such studies include: walking (Winter, 1991), stair climbing (Andriacchi et al., 1980), sit-to-stand (Pai and Rogers, 1991; Carr and Gentile, 1994; Shepherd and Gentile, 1994), running (Mann and Hagy, 1980; Hinrichs, 1990), squat-lifting (Scholz, 1993), jumping (Bobbert and van Ingen Schenau, 1988; Depena and Chung, 1988) and kicking (Young and Marteniuk, 1995). Biomechanical studies analysing commonly utilized exercises such as step-up exercises (Agahari et al., 1996) are also being carried out enabling more informed exercise prescription.

One current area of motor learning research which is of particular interest to rehabilitation examines the changes in movement kinematics, kinetics and muscle activation patterns that accompany motor learning. Such studies seek to explain whether or not changes in performance can be attributed to changes in motor pattern production. For example, Young and Marteniuk (1995) examined whether the redundant degrees of freedom inherent in a kicking task, a complex multijoint action, were simplified by some form of constraint across lower limb joints achieved as the task was learned or became more skilled. Their findings suggest that simplification occurred by constraining the phase relationships of interjoint moments and powers, results which appear to link learning with more effective coordination of intersegmental dynamics.

Movement rehabilitation as a clinical science is taking up the opportunities offered by recent research into human movement and the acquisition of skill. We proposed some years ago that neurorehabilitation should be based on this research and have illustrated how research findings and theoretical perspectives can be utilized in clinical practice (Carr and Shepherd, 1987, 1998, 2000, 2003). This perspective is increasingly being seen as critical to the rehabilitation of individuals following brain damage (Winstein and Knecht, 1990; Mulder, 1991; Malouin et al., 1992, Dean et al., 2000). This perspective is also, however, a useful one for the physiotherapist working with individuals with lesions of the musculoskeletal system. Wherever the lesion, whether it directly or indirectly affects the musculoskeletal system, the individual must manage to control a multisegmental linkage in order to accomplish the goals of everyday life. A lesion of the motor effector apparatus, because of the complex musculoskeletal linkages and interactive forces produced during movement, must affect neural control and the performance of everyday actions. After injury, adaptive processes occur not only in the musculoskeletal system but also in the neural system.

ADAPTIVE MOTOR BEHAVIOUR

Recovery involves physiological changes that take place as the lesioned system repairs itself after, for example, a muscle tear, ligament injury or surgery. Recovery also involves the individual regaining the ability to function effectively in recreation, daily living tasks, sport or workplace activity.

During the acute period, the individual starts to function adaptively. This may be enforced by bedrest, splinting or pain. Such adaptive motor behaviour may persist after the symptoms have gone, particularly if the length of disability, physical inactivity or immobilization is long. After back injury or joint replacement surgery, for example, an individual is likely to persist with those motor patterns that had emerged a considerable time prior to the injury or surgery, during the period of pain and stiffness. This seems to occur even if such patterns are not optimally effective.

Immediately after a lesion of the musculoskeletal system, the individual's attempts at action reflect the emergence of adaptive motor behaviours. Such adaptation may include a change in the pattern of swing phase of walking when a splint constrains the knee. This constraint demands altered biomechanics at unconstrained joints (ankle and hip, and joints of other leg) if function is to be maintained. Detailed biomechanical analyses of adaptations to gait occurring as a result of functional limitations imposed by surgery and prosthetic devices have been reported (Winter, 1991).

Adaptive movement seems to emerge out of what can be used of the lesioned system. To put it another way, the individual moves in the most effective way possible given the effects of the lesion (e.g. pain, stiffness), the biomechanical possibilities inherent in the musculoskeletal linkage and the requirements of the task and environment. The performance adaptations reflect, therefore, the flexibility available in the multisegmental system. Motor performance and degree of skill are also affected by adaptive changes occurring in soft tissue as a consequence of imposed physical inactivity and immobility.

SKILL LEARNING IN REHABILITATION: OPTIMIZATION OF FUNCTIONAL MOTOR PERFORMANCE

The major aim of physiotherapy, beyond the stage where treatment of specific symptoms may be the principal issue, is the restoration of optimal motor performance. It cannot be assumed that improvement in the presenting symptoms (e.g. pain, stiffness) will necessarily generalize into improved performance of functional actions. A descriptive study of subjects on average 12.7 months after total hip replacement (THR) surgery (Drabsch et al., 1998) reported improved performance of walking and sit-to-stand associated with biomechanical changes after a 6-week task-specific training programme. Before training subjects had demonstrated deficits in muscle strength and function.

Another study of subjects following THR (Westwood, 1992) showed that, although all subjects had been discharged from rehabilitation, they continued to stand up from a seat using their arms to assist in propelling the body mass vertically. The subjects who were given specific training in sit-to-stand over a period of 6 weeks were able to stand up without using their arms, whereas an untrained control group were still using their arms when measured at the end of training. Jevsevar and colleagues (1993) have shown that 15 subjects considered fully rehabilitated following knee arthroplasty had performance deficits during walking, stair ascent and descent and sit-to-stand that included decreased peak knee moments of force and decreased knee angular velocities.

In planning an exercise and training programme, the physiotherapist utilizes the results of research into motor learning or how people acquire skill in action. Training is planned to optimize motor performance to enable the individual to return to everyday life, the athlete to return to sport, the worker to the workplace, without repeating the injury some time after discharge.

Annett (1971) has defined skill as any activity that has become better organized through practice. Skilled action is defined in terms of consistency in attaining a goal with some economy of effort through movement patterns shaped by dimensions of the performer and configured to fit the environment (Gentile, 2000). Several factors have been shown to be important in the acquisition of skill, such as training specificity, feedback, practice with maximum repetitions (to increase strength and control), and practice of the task in various contexts to train flexibility of performance.

EXERCISE AND TRAINING SPECIFICITY

One of the most interesting areas of research in recent times pertinent to rehabilitation has developed out of investigations of the task- and context-specific effects of training. To regain skilful performance requires not only the ability to generate muscle forces but also to time muscle activations in order to control complex multisegmental linkages. Biomechanical and muscle-strengthening studies consistently report muscle activations and movement patterns that are specific to the action being tested and also to the context in which the action is being carried out.

Many studies report that the major changes accompanying strength training are seen in the training exercise itself (Sale and MacDougall, 1981; Morrissey et al., 1995). Conventional leg-extension exercises to strengthen quadriceps have been shown to increase the weight lifted (by 200%) whereas the isometric strength of the muscle increased very little (by 11%; Rutherford and Jones, 1986). Typically the major changes in load lifted are seen to occur early in the training period (Rutherford and Jones, 1986), suggesting that, since isometric strength did not increase much during this period, the early changes in performance may have been due to the individual becoming more skilled at weight-lifting rather than increasing intrinsic muscle strength. In other words, the earliest changes may be due to learning, suggesting that neural factors may play a primary role in the early stages of training (Hakkinen and Komi, 1983).

In an early study, Rasch and Morehouse (1957) reported that subjects who performed resisted elbow flexion exercises in standing increased the strength of these muscles in standing but less so in supine. From work on the specificity of postural adjustments (Cordo and Nashner, 1982), it becomes apparent that in performing the strengthening exercise in standing, the subjects in Rasch and Morehouse's study were learning a pattern of muscle activations, throughout the body and including the lower limbs, which were specific to weight-resisted elbow flexion in standing.

Although particular muscles, such as lower limb extensors, need to be strong enough to generate the necessary power for such varied actions as stair climbing, sit-to-stand and cycling, the context in which the muscles must generate force varies from action to action. This means that the pattern of muscle activation differs according to task and context. As Rutherford (1988) pointed out, particular neural connections that become established as a result of weight-lifting exercises for quadriceps may not be the connections necessary for other actions. It appears that the neural adaptations which occur as a result of training are themselves specific (Sale, 1988). This implies that training should involve exercises not only to restore muscle bulk and efficiency but also training to improve performance in those actions required in everyday life.

The effects of exercise have been found to be *velocity-specific* (Wooden et al., 1992), perhaps because of velocity-specific adaptations within the muscle (by altering force–velocity characteristics of the muscle) and/or the neural system (by altering the motoneuron recruitment pattern; Rutherford, 1988). Ellenbecker et al. (1988) reported that, although significant strength improvements in shoulder rotator muscles occurred through both concentric and isokinetic (fixed-speed, variable-resistance) training, tennis serving speed increased only in the concentrically trained group of subjects.

Exercise effects have also been reported to be *length-specific* (Kitai and Sale, 1989), with isometric training being followed by an increase in strength at the joint angle at which the exercise was practised (Lindh, 1979; Sale and MacDougall, 1981). There is some evidence from electromyography that there might be a greater increase in motor unit activation at the joint angles trained (Thepaut-Mathieu et al., 1985).

Considerable research interest has centred around the differential effects of *concentric* versus *eccentric* training. Komi and Buskirk, for example, (1972) reported that eccentric exercise was followed by a greater increase in strength than concentric exercise. In addition, a characteristic of human muscle action in functional activities is its use in stretch-shortening cycles (Asmussen and Bonde-Petersen, 1974; Bosco et al., 1982; Komi, 1986). It has been shown, principally in studies of the vertical jump, that eccentric muscle contraction immediately prior to the major concentric force generation can augment the amount of force delivered by the prime mover muscles.

Closed kinetic chain weight-bearing exercises are considered to be a more functional (and hence specific) way of strengthening lower limb extensor muscles than single-joint (open-chain) exercises, given that many significant actions involve movement of the lower limb over a fixed base of support (the foot or feet). Such actions include stair climbing and descent, stance phase of walking, standing up and sitting down.

Being a functional exercise implies that there will be transferability from positive exercise effects to improvement on performance of functional actions with similar dynamics (Oxendine, 1984; Gottlieb et al., 1988). The step-up exercise, used extensively following knee surgery, is a good example of such an exercise. It involves a concentric and an eccentric phase, with simultaneous extension at hip, knee and ankle joints (step-up) followed by flexion (step-down). Functional stresses and muscle activation patterns are therefore similar to those found in the functional actions above (Palmitier et al., 1991; Irrgang, 1993). Good transferability can be inferred from the results of studies in which step-up exercises have been included in a home-exercise programme. One such study reported improvement in walking performance with fewer falls in elderly people (Sherrington and Lord, 1997).

Repetitive sit-to-stand exercises, starting from a raised seat height and increasing force-generating demands by progressively lowering the seat, is another closed kinetic chain strengthening exercise which improves performance on this common action but which has the potential to transfer to actions with similar dynamic characteristics.

Where muscles are very weak, it is likely that any exercise that improves the muscle's ability to contract (single-joint, isometric, machine-assisted exercises, electrical stimulation) will have a beneficial effect on functional performance; it probably does not matter that the exercise is, in a functional sense, non-specific. The available evidence suggests, however, that after a certain threshold of strength is reached, exercise needs to be specific to the action being trained (Buchner et al., 1996).

The implication for rehabilitation from these studies is that practice of an action is necessary for there to be improvement in the performance of that action. This hypothesis is supported by a few rehabilitation or quasi-rehabilitation studies reported within the last decade. In one study of able-bodied young men (Godges et al., 1993), passive hip flexor stretching and training of an isolated movement (a trunk flexion exercise) did not improve the 'economy' of walking or running as inferred from the measurement of open-circuit spirometry with subjects running on a treadmill. That is, although passive hip flexor stretching improved hip extension range of motion and trunk flexor exercises improved trunk flexor muscle performance, these isolated improvements did not affect functional activities. As the authors suggest, 'coaching' of subjects may be required so that they can integrate the localized improvements in strength and flexibility into a more efficient pattern of, in this case, walking. Baker and colleagues (1991) showed that walking training (using a treadmill) following THR was associated with a decrease in double support time and a normalization of stance/swing ratio for the affected leg. In another study of subjects following THR (Henderson et al., 1992), a 6-month programme of walking and weight-bearing activities was followed by a significant increase in walking speed.

ATTENTION AND LEARNING

Action comprises not only motor factors but also perceptual-cognitive factors. The obvious conceptual links between knowing and doing, i.e. cognition and action, are increasingly being recognized in the movement and neurosciences. However, as Mulder (1991) points out, the emphasis in rehabilitation remains largely on the motor system and perceptual-cognitive aspects of function tend to be ignored. This is despite an increasing body of theoretical clinical literature in which the need to recognize and incorporate the action–cognition link in rehabilitation is advocated, i.e. cognition needs action and action itself is part of cognition (Mulder, 1991; Carr and Shepherd, 1998).

In everyday life, virtually every movement we make is linked to an intention. As we move we are selecting, from all the available information (both internally derived sensations and those coming from the environment) the most essential to the task at hand; we select what it is we must pay attention to (Wise and Desimone, 1988). It is unlikely, therefore, that skill in action will be (re)gained unless that action is practised under the appropriate environmental conditions. We are learning not only the appropriate motor pattern but also learning to select the most appropriate information in order to match the intention or the goal to the action and the environment (Higgins, 1972). One of the important functions of the therapist (as coach) is setting up the conditions of practice to facilitate this process.

INFORMATION: INSTRUCTION, DEMONSTRATION AND FEEDBACK

Information about performance that is available to the learner, before, during or after the performance, is an important factor in optimizing skill acquisition (Newell, 1981) and therefore is of practical importance for both therapist and patient in rehabilitation.

Commonly used methods for conveying information about the goal and appropriate action sequences are verbal instructions and demonstrations (Newell, 1981; Johnson, 1984; Gentile, 2000). Information may focus on kinematic description, for example, angular displacements, paths of body parts and timing of action sequences, which requires an understanding by the therapist of linked segment dynamics and the biomechanical necessities of the action to be learned.

Instructions are given in such a way as to present a clear goal and to reduce uncertainty. They should enable the person to focus attention on the critical features of the task. There is evidence that individuals perform better when an action is presented as a concrete task as opposed to an abstract task. These two types of task differ in the degree to which the required action is directed toward controlling physical interaction with the environment as opposed to producing movement for its own sake.

Leont'ev and Zaporozhets (1960) had patients with restricted range of motion of the elbow or shoulder as a result of injury raise their forearm or whole arm (depending on the site of injury) in four actions that varied from abstract to concrete. The actions were to raise the arm: (1) as far as possible with eyes shut; (2) as far as possible with eyes open; (3) to a specific point on a ruled screen; and (4) to grasp an object. The results indicated that the amplitude of movement increased progressively from task 1 to task 4, i.e. as the task became more concrete. Similar results have been reported in children with cerebral palsy who obtained a greater range of forearm supination when the task involved supinating the forearm to beat a drum than when they were instructed to perform the more abstract task of supination for its own sake (van der Weel et al., 1991).

The goal of the action and the movements to be executed can be demonstrated either live or on videotape. Empirical work on the effectiveness of demonstration, however, has been sporadic and the results equivocal. One of the reasons for equivocal results is that the videotaped demonstration is sometimes distant from actual practice in both time and place. Gonnella and colleagues (1981), however, demonstrated that self-instruction using an audiovisual medium was effective in enabling able-bodied subjects to learn the new skill of crutch walking. The hypothesis that subjects could learn the cognitive aspects of the motor task in one viewing of the film was supported and transfer of learning to the physical performance of the task was found to occur.

Feedback refers to the use of sensory information for the control of action and is a factor in the process of skill acquisition. It can be positive or negative, subjective or objective, and it may motivate the learner as well as provide information. However, given that accurate feedback is essential to learning, the therapist should confine the use of positive reinforcement, for example, 'good', to successful or near-successful trials, not as a reward for a good try.

Feedback can provide clues to the learner about how to improve the next attempt or give information about whether or not the goal is being achieved. Knowledge of results (KR) is information related to achievement of the goal of the action and is known to be one of the most potent variables in learning (Annett and Kay, 1957; Newell, 1976). A second type of feedback, commonly referred to as knowledge of performance (KP), provides information about how the movement was performed.

Both KP and KR can be augmented by the therapist verbally, through demonstration and through the use of electronic devices such as videotape, electromyography, forceplate system, exercise machine (stepping machines, treadmill, bicycle ergometer, rowing machines) and computerized training systems in which motor performance is linked to events on a monitor. Although the early stages of learning may require more immediate and frequent feedback, the therapist should gradually withdraw augmented feedback, enabling the individual to use naturally occurring feedback mechanisms and increase problem-solving ability.

PRACTICE

Practice can be considered as a continuum of procedures from overt practice at one extreme to covert or mental practice at the other (Johnson, 1984). As a general rule, skill in performance increases as a direct result of the amount of practice. It has been shown, for example, that repetition of a task can improve performance, although thousands of repetitions may be necessary (Crossman, 1959; Beggs and Howarth, 1972; Kottke, 1980; Canning, 1987). Repetitive practice is known to be important for learning to occur, as the repetitions enable the system to coordinate the muscular synergies which move the segmental linkage to accomplish the goal of action. However, repetitive practice of an action (or an exercise) with increasing load is also necessary to increase the strength of the muscle contractions to that necessary to accomplish the goal.

One focus of research that has considerable importance for rehabilitation is the whole-versus-part method of practice. As a general rule, it seems that the action should be practised in its entirety, particularly when one part of the action is to a large extent dependent on the performance of a preceding part. For example, several studies of sit-to-stand (Schenkman et al., 1990; Pai and Rogers, 1991; Shepherd and Gentile, 1994) have pointed to the importance of rotation forward of the upper body (trunk segment) at the hips in setting up the conditions for ascent into standing. The implication from these studies is that vertical movement of the body mass (by lower limb extension) is facilitated by momentum generated by the initial flexion of the trunk through functional linkages between joints involved in the action.

Performing the whole action seems important for giving the individual the idea of the action to be achieved as well as enabling practice of coordinating a functional linkage. However, when the individual is having difficulty activating muscles and generating and timing force, it may be necessary to practise simple exercises to elicit activity in a particular group of muscles, or to practise a modified action in order to strengthen a muscle group critical to performance. Part practice should, however, be followed by an attempt at performing the entire action (Johnson, 1984). Furthermore, variable practice, i.e. practice on a range of similar tasks, has been found to lead to better performance than consistent practice of the one task (Newell, 1981; Johnson, 1984; Schmidt, 1988). Gaining skill involves not only the development of a stable pattern but also the ability to modify that pattern according to environmental and other demands.

In order to facilitate optimal practice conditions and improve motor performance, the practice environment can be modified by the therapist, by for example:

- The use of an external support such as taping (McConnell, 1993) in order to facilitate a muscle or group of muscles to contract and generate force at a particular length for a specific action.

- The practice of standing up from a higher than average chair to decrease lower limb extensor muscle force requirements while still ensuring that the individual is strengthening the extensor muscles in the appropriate context.

- Ensuring that crutch walking is practised not only in the protected environment of the physiotherapy area but also in a busy corridor where people and objects in the environment are moving.

- Having patients with an injury to one hand practise bimanual tasks in order to facilitate cooperative control between hands and object and particularly to enhance timing (Castiello et al., 1993).

Of major current interest in physiotherapy is increasing the time spent by patients in exercise and practice since this is necessary to enable the regaining of skill in motor performance. Such methods include group exercise and training programmes involving circuit training around workstations. The use of a treadmill is a method of increasing walking practice and may be particularly effective in helping restore an effective gait pattern.

SUMMARY

The primary purpose of this part of the book is to stress the significance in musculoskeletal clinical practice of organizing interventions to optimize skill in performance. Optimizing motor performance is critical in the rehabilitation of any individual with a neuromusculoskeletal lesion that interferes with essential or desirable actions. In some cases,

an individual may need to practise a sporting activity in order to regain skill; in others, the most pressing need may be to strengthen lower limb extensor muscles to optimize stair climbing and descent. A novel task such as walking with crutches may need to be learned, or the manner in which a task must be performed in the workplace may need to be modified to ensure that the individual's back injury is not repeated. What seems certain at the present time is that the process of rehabilitation should include opportunities for task-oriented motor learning (through the training of specific actions) as well as exercises to increase muscle strength, flexibility, control and endurance, and aerobic exercise to increase cardiorespiratory fitness.

REFERENCES AND FURTHER READING

CLINICAL REASONING IN PHYSIOTHERAPY

Barrows, H.S. and Feltovich, P.J. (1987). The clinical reasoning process. *Med. Educ.*, **21**, 86–91.

Bashook, P.G. (1976). A conceptual framework for measuring clinical problem-solving. *J. Med. Educ.*, **51**, 109–114.

Benner, P. and Tanner, C. (1987). Clinical judgement: how expert nurses use intuition. *Am. J. Nurs.*, **January**, 23–31.

Bordage, G. and Lemieux, M. (1986). Some cognitive characteristics of medical students with and without diagnostic reasoning difficulties. In: *Proceedings of the 25th Annual Conference of Research in Medical Education of the American Association of Medical Colleges*, pp. 185–190. New Orleans, Louisiana.

Bowden, J. (1988). Achieving change in teaching practices. In: *Improving Learning: New Perspectives*, ed. P. Ramsden, pp. 255–267. London: Kogan Page.

Browning, C., Thomas, S. and Oates, J. (1988). Clinical decision making and clinical performance. In: *Proceedings of the 2nd International Health Sciences Education Conference*, Sydney.

Elstein, A.S., Shulman, L.S. and Sprafka, S.A. (1978). *Medical Problem Solving: An Analysis of Clinical Reasoning*. Cambridge, MA: Harvard University Press.

Gale, J. and Marsden, P. (1982). Clinical problem solving: the beginning of the process. *Med. Educ.*, **16**, 22–26.

Gilhooly, K.J. (1988). *Thinking: Directed, Undirected and Creative*, 2nd edn. London: Academic Press.

Glass, A.L. and Holyoak, K.J. (1986). *Cognition*, 2nd edn. New York: Random House.

Grant, R. (1991). Obsolence or lifelong education: choices and challenges. In: *Proceedings of the World Confederation for Physical Therapy 11th International Congress*, London.

Grant, J. and Marsden, P. (1987). The structure of memorized knowledge in students and clinicians: an explanation for diagnostic expertise. *Med. Educ.*, **21**, 92–98.

Grant, R., Jones, M. and Maitland, G.D. (1988). Clinical decision making in upper quadrant dysfunction. In: *Clinics in Physical Therapy – Physical Therapy of the Cervical and Thoracic Spine*, ed. R. Grant, pp. 51–79. New York: Churchill Livingstone.

Higgs, J. and Jones, M.A. (1995). *Clinical Reasoning in the Health Professions*. London: Butterworth-Heinemann.

Jones, M.A. (1992). Clinical reasoning in manual therapy. *Phys. Ther.*, **72**, 875–884.

Mattingly, C. (1991). The narrative nature of clinical reasoning. *Am. J. Occup. Ther.*, **45**, 998–1005.

Norman, G.R. (1988). Problem-solving skills, solving problems and problem-based learning. *Med. Educ.*, **22**, 279–286.

Norman, G.R. and Schmidt, H.G. (1992). The psychological basis of problem-based learning: a review of the evidence. *Acad. Med.*, **67**, 557–565.

Patel, V.L. and Groen, G.J. (1991). The general and specific nature of medical expertise: a critical look. In: *Toward a General Theory of Expertise: Prospects and Limits*, ed. A. Ericsson and J. Smith. New York: Cambridge University Press.

Paton, O.D. (1985). Clinical reasoning process in physical therapy. *Phys. Ther.*, **65**, 924–928.

Rew, L. and Barrow, E. (1987). Intuition: a neglected hallmark of nursing knowledge. *Adv. Nurs. Sci.*, **10**, 49–62.

Ridderikhoff, J. (1989). *Methods in Medicine: A Descriptive Study of Physicians' Behaviour*. Dordrecht: Kluwer Academic.

Scadding, J.G. (1967). Diagnosis: the clinician and the computer. *Lancet*, **i**, 877–882.

ACUTE AND CHRONIC PAIN

Dubner, R. and Hargreaves, K.M. (1989). The neurobiology of pain and its modulation. *Clin. J. Pain*, **5** (suppl. 2), S1–S6.

Hargreaves, K.M. and Joris, J.L. (1993). The peripheral analgesic effects of opioids. *Am. Pain Soc. J.*, **2**, 51–59.

Meller, S.T. and Gebhart, G.F. (1993). Nitric oxide (NO) and nociceptive processing in the spinal cord. *Pain*, **52**, 127–136.

Melzack, R. and Wall, P.D. (1965). Pain mechanism: a new theory. *Science*, **150**, 971.

Pert, C.B. and Sydner, S.H. (1973). Opiate receptor: demonstrated in nervous tissue. *Science*, **179**, 1011.

Schaible, H.G. and Grubb, B.D. (1993). Afferent and spinal mechanisms of joint pain. *Pain*, **55**, 5–15.

PHYSIOLOGY AND CLINICAL PHARMACOLOGY: INFLAMMATION, PAIN AND ANTI-INFLAMMATORY DRUGS AND ANALGESICS

Inflammation and basic pathology

Cotran, R.S., Kumar, V. and Collins, T. (eds) (1999). *Robbins Pathologic Basis of Disease*, 6th edn. Philadelphia: W.B. Saunders.

Rheumatology

Klippel, J.H. and Dieppe, P.A. (eds) (2000). *Rheumatology*, 2nd edn. London: Mosby.

Immunology

Roitt, I.M. and Delves, P. (2001). *Roitt's Essential Immunology*, 10th edn. Oxford: Blackwell Scientific.

Pharmacology

Hardman, J., Limbird, L. and Goodman-Gilman, A. (eds) (2001). *Goodman and Gilman's The Pharmacological Basis of Therapeutics*, 10th edn. New York: McGraw-Hill.

Anti-inflammatory drugs

Williams, K.M., Day, R.O. and Breit, S.N. (1993). Biochemical actions and clinical pharmacology of anti-inflammatory drugs. *Adv. Drug Res.*, **24**, 121–198.

Analgesics

Victorian Medical Postgraduate Foundation (1992). *Analgesic Guidelines*, 2nd edn. Intersegmental Kinematics.

BIOMECHANICS OF JOINT MOVEMENTS

Determinants of joint movement

MacConaill, M.A. (1964). Joint movements. *Physiotherapy*, **50**, 359–367.

Meriam, J.L. and Kraige, L.G. (1993). *Engineering Mechanics*. New York: Wiley.

Winter, D.A. (1990). *Biomechanics and Motor Control of Human Movement*. Brisbane: John Wiley.

Intersegmental kinematics

Goel, V.K., Goyal, S., Clark, C., Nishiyama, K. and Nye, T. (1985). Kinematics of the whole lumbar spine: effect of discectomy. *Spine*, **10**, 543–554.

Harrison, D.E., Harrison, D.D. and Troyanovich, S.J. (1998). Three-dimensional spinal coupling mechanics: part I. A review of the literature. *J. Manip. Physiol. Ther.*, **21**, 101–113.

Panjabi, M.M. and White, A.A. (2001). *Biomechanics in the Musculoskeletal System*. New York: Churchill Livingstone.

Spoor, C.W. and Veldpaus, F.E. (1980). Rigid body motion calculated from spatial co-ordinates of markers. *J. Biomech.* **13**, 391–393.

Veldpaus, F.E., Woltring, H.J. and Dortmans, L.J. (1988). A least-squares algorithm for the equiform transformation from spatial marker co-ordinates. *J. Biomech.*, **21**, 45–54.

Woltring, H.J., Huiskes, R., de Lange, A. and Veldpaus, F.E. (1985). Finite centroid and helical axis estimation from noisy landmark measurements in the study of human joint kinematics. *J. Biomech.*, **18**, 378–389.

Joint surface kinematics

Kaltenborn, F.M. (1980). *Mobilization of the Extremity Joints*. Oslo: Olaf Norlis Bokhandel Universitetsgaten.

MacConaill, M.A. and Basmajian, J.V. (1969). *Muscles and Movements*. Baltimore: Williams and Wilkins.

Maitland, G.D. (1991). *Peripheral Manipulation*. London: Butterworth-Heinemann.

Williams, P.L., Warwick, R., Dyson, M. and Bannister, L.H. (1989). *Gray's Anatomy*, 37th edn. Edinburgh: Churchill Livingstone.

Passive joint dynamics

Akeson, W.H., Woo, S.L.Y., Amiel, D. and Matthews, J.V. (1974). Biomechanical and biochemical changes in the periarticular connective tissue during contracture development in the immobilised rabbit knee. *Connect. Tissue Res.*, **2**, 315–323.

Barnett, C.H., and Cobbold, A.F. (1969). Muscle tension and joint mobility. *Ann. Rheum. Dis.*, **28**, 652–654.

Berme, N., Engin, A.E. and de Silva, K.M.C. (1985). *Biomechanics of Normal and Pathological Human Articulating Joints*. Dordrecht: Martinus Nijhoff.

Chesworth, B.M. and Vandervoort, A.A. (1989). Age and passive ankle stiffness in healthy women. *Phys. Ther.*, **69**, 217–224.

Engin, A.L. (1979). On the biomechanics of the shoulder complex. *J. Biomech.*, **13**, 579–590.

Farahmand, F., Tahmasbi, M.N. and Amis, A.A. (1998). Lateral force-displacement behaviour of the human patella and its variation with knee flexion – a biomechanical study in vitro. *J. Biomech.*, **31**, 1147–1152.

Herbert, R. (1993). Preventing and treating stiff joints. In: *Key Issues in Musculoskeletal Physiotherapy*, ed. J. Crosbie and J. McConnell, pp. 114–141. Sydney: Butterworth-Heinemann.

Johns, R.J. and Wright, V. (1962). Relative importance of various tissues in joint stiffness. *J. Appl. Physiol.*, **17**, 824–828.

Lee, M. (2003). *Human Dynamics for Physiotherapists*. Sydney: Zygal.

Lee, M. and Svensson, N.L. (1993). Effect of frequency on response of the spine to lumbar posteroanterior forces. *J. Manip. Physiol. Ther.*, **16**, 439–446.

Maitland, G.D. (1986). *Vertebral Manipulation*. London: Butterworth-Heinemann.

McQuade, K.J., Shelley, I. and Cvitkovic, J. (1999). Patterns of stiffness during clinical examination of the glenohumeral joint. *Clin. Biomech.*, **14**, 620–627.

Riener, R. and Edrich, T. (1999). Identification of passive elastic joint moments in the lower extremities. *J. Biomech.*, **13**, 539–544.

Instability

Beeson, D. (1992). *Maupertuis: An Intellectual Biography.* Oxford: The Voltaire Foundation.

Crisco, J.J. and Panjabi, M.M. (1991). The intersegmental and multisegmental muscles of the lumbar spine. A biomechanical model comparing lateral stabilizing potential. *Spine*, **16**, 793–799.

Ettema, G.J. and Huijing, P.A. (1994). Skeletal muscle stiffness in static and dynamic contractions. *J. Biomech.*, **27**, 1361–1368.

Gardner-Morse, M.G. and Stokes, I.A. (2001). Trunk stiffness increases with steady-state effort. *J. Biomech.*, **34**, 457–463.

Hodges, P.W. and Richardson, C.A. (1996). Inefficient muscular stabilization of the lumbar spine associated with low back pain: a motor control evaluation of transversus abdominis. *Spine*, **21**, 2640–2650.

Kirkaldy-Willis, W.H. and Farfan, H.F. (1982). Instability of the lumbar spine. *Clin. Orthop. Rel. Res.*, **165**, 110–123.

Lee, M. (2004). *Introduction to the Analysis of Human Movement*, 4th edn. Sydney: Zygal.

Levine, W.N. and Flatow, E.L. (2000). The pathophysiology of shoulder instability. *Am. J. Sports Med.*, **28**, 910–917.

Pope, M.H. and Panjabi, M.M. (1985). Biomechanical definitions of spinal instability. *Spine*, **10**, 55–56.

Richie, D.H. (2001). Functional instability of the ankle and the role of neuromuscular control: a comprehensive review. *J. Foot Ankle Surg.*, **40**, 240–251.

Tropp, H., Ekstrand, J. and Gillquist, J. (1984). Stabilometry in functional instability of the ankle and its value in predicting injury. *Med. Sci. Sports Exerc.*, **16**, 64–66.

White, A.A. and Panjabi, M.M. (1990). *Clinical Biomechanics of the Spine*, 2nd edn. Sydney: J.B. Lippincott.

BONE: RECENT CONCEPTS IN BONE DAMAGE, MODELLING AND REMODELLING

Biewener, A.A. (1993). Safety factors in bone strength. *Calcif. Tissue Int.*, **53** (suppl.), 68–74.

Burr, D.B. (1993). Remodelling and the repair of fatigue damage. *Calcif. Tissue Int.*, **53** (suppl.), 75–81.

Burr, D.B. and Martin, R.B. (1992). Mechanisms of bone adaptation to the mechanical environment. *Triangle (Ciba-Geigy)*, **31**, 59–76.

Frost, H.M. (1986). *Intermediary Organisation of the Skeleton*, vols I and II. Boca Raton: CRC Press.

Frost, H.M. (1989). The biology of fracture healing. *Clin. Orthop. Relat. Res., Part I*, **248**, 283–293; Part II, **248**, 294–309.

Frost, H.M. (1990a). Structural adaptations to mechanical usage (SATMU): 1. Redefining Wolff's law: the bone modeling problem. *Anat. Rec.*, **226**, 403–413.

Frost, H.M. (1990b). Structural adaptations to mechanical usage (SATMU): 2. Redefining Wolff's law: the bone remodeling problem. *Anat. Rec.*, **226**, 414–422.

Frost, H.M. (1992). Perspectives: bone's mechanical usage windows. *Bone Miner.*, **19**, 257–271.

Frost, H.M. (1993). Suggested fundamental concepts in skeletal physiology. *Calcif. Tissue Int.*, **52**, 1–4.

Heaney, R.P. (1993). Is there a role for bone quality in fragility fractures? *Calcif. Tissue Int.*, **53** (suppl.), 3–6.

Jee, W.S.S. (1989). The skeletal tissues. In: *Cell and Tissue Biology. A Textbook of Histology*, ed. L. Weiss, pp. 211–259, Baltimore: Urban and Schwartzenberg.

Jee, W.S.S. and Frost, H.M. (1992). Skeletal adaptations during growth. *Triangle (Ciba-Geigy)*, **31**, 77–88.

Jee, W.S.S., Li, X.J. and Ke, H.Z. (1991). The skeletal adaptation to mechanical usage in the rat. *Cells Matter Suppl.*, **1**, 131–142.

Martin, R.B. and Burr, D.B. (1989). *Structure, Function and Adaptation of Compact Bone*. New York: Raven Press.

Parfitt, A.M. (1990). Bone-forming cells in clinical conditions. In: *Bone*, vol. I: *The Osteoblast and Osteocyte*, ed. B.K. Hall, pp. 351–429. West Caldwell, NJ: Telford Press.

Parfitt, A.M. (1993). Bone age mineral density, and fatigue damage. *Calcif. Tissue Int.*, **53** (suppl.), 82–86.

Pattin, C.A. and Carter, D.R. (1991). *Bone Mechanical Energy Dissipation during Cyclic Loading* (Transactions of the Orthopaedic Research Society, 37th Annual Meeting), p. 129.

Schnitzler, C.M. (1993). Bone quality: a determinant for certain risk factors for bone fragility. *Calcif. Tissue Int.*, **53** (suppl.), 27–31.

BONE: APPLICATION OF RESEARCH TO PHYSIOTHERAPY PRACTICE

Aarden, E.M., Burger, E.H. and Nijweide, P.J. (1994). Function of osteocytes in bone. *J. Cell Biochem.*, **55**, 287–299.

ACSM (1998). Position stand on exercise and physical activity for older adults. *Med. Sci. Sports Exerc.*, **30**, 992–1008.

Ayalon, J., Simkin, A., Leichter, et al. (1987). Dynamic bone loading exercises for postmenopausal women: effect on the density of the distal radius. *Arch. Phys. Med. Rehabil.*, **68**, 280–283.

Bailey, D.A. (1997). The Saskatchewan pediatric bone mineral accrual study – bone mineral acquisition during the growing years. *Int. J. Sports Med.*, **18**, S191–S194.

Bass, S., Pearce, G., Bradney, M. et al. (1998). Exercise before puberty may confer residual benefits in bone density in adulthood: studies in active prepubertal and retired female gymnasts. *J. Bone Miner. Res.*, **13**, 500–507.

Bassey, E.J. and Ramsdale, S.J. (1994). Increase in femoral bone density in young women following high impact exercise. *Osteoporosis Int.*, **4**, 72–75.

Bennell, K., Khan, K. and McKay, H. (2000). The role of physiotherapy in the prevention and management of osteoporosis. *Manual Ther.*, **5**, 198–213.

Bradney, M., Pearce, G., Naughton, G. et al. (1998). Moderate exercise during growth in prepubertal boys – changes in bone mass, size, volumetric density, and bone strength – a controlled prospective study. *J. Bone Miner. Res.*, **13**, 1814–1821.

Bravo, G., Gauthier, P., Roy, P.M. et al. (1996). Comparison of a group- versus a home-based exercise program in osteopenic women. *J. Aging Phys. Activity*, **4**, 151–164.

Burr, D.B., Milgrom, C., Fyhrie, D. et al. (1996). In vivo measurement of human tibial strains during vigorous activity. *Bone*, **18**, 405–410.

Burr, D.B., Robling, A.G. and Turner, C.H. (2002). Effects of biomechanical stress on bones in animals. *Bone*, **30**, 781–786.

Campbell, A.J., Borrie, M.J. and Spears, G.F. (1989). Risk factors for falls in a community-based prospective study of people 70 years and older. *J. Gerontol.*, **44**, M112–M117.

Carter, D.R., Hayes, W.C. and Schurman, D.J. (1976). Fatigue life of compact bone – 11. Effects of microstructure and density. *J. Biomech.*, **9**, 211–218.

Carter, N.D., Khan, K.M., Petit, M.A. et al. (2001). Results of a 10 week community based strength and balance training programme to reduce fall risk factors: a randomised controlled trial in 65–75 year old women with osteoporosis. *Br. J. Sports Med.*, **35**, 348–351.

Conroy, B.P., Kraemer, W.J., Maresh, C.M. et al. (1993). Bone mineral density in elite junior Olympic weight lifters. *Med. Sci. Sports Exerc.*, **25**, 1103–1109.

Currey, J.D. (2001). Bone strength: what are we trying to measure? *Calcif. Tissue Int.*, **68**, 205–210.

Dalsky, G.P., Stocke, K.S., Ehansi, A.A. et al. (1988). Weight-bearing exercise training and lumbar bone mineral content in postmenopausal women. *Ann. Intern. Med.*, **108**, 824–828.

Ebrahim, S., Thompson, P., Baskaran, V. et al. (1997). Randomized placebo-controlled trial of brisk walking in the prevention of postmenopausal osteoporosis. *Age Ageing*, **26**, 253–260.

Fiatarone, M., Marks, E., Ryan, N. et al. (1990). High-intensity training in nonagenarians. *J.A.M.A.*, **263**, 3029–3034.

Fiatarone, M.A., O'Neill, E.F., Ryan, N.D. et al. (1994). Exercise training and nutritional supplementation for physical frailty in very elderly people. *N. Engl. J. Med.*, **330**, 1769–1775.

Flicker, L., Hopper, J.L., Rodgers, L. et al. (1995). Bone density determinants in elderly women: a twin study. *J. Bone Miner. Res.*, **10**, 1607–1613.

Forwood, M.R. (2001). Mechanical effects on the skeleton: are there clinical implications? *Osteoporosis Int.*, **12**, 77–83.

Forwood, M. and Larsen, J. (2000). Exercise recommendations for osteoporosis: a position statement for the Australian and New Zealand Bone and Mineral Society. *Aust. Family Phys.*, **29**, 761–764.

Frost, H.M. (1983). A determinant of bone architecture. The minimum effective strain. *Clin. Orthop. Rel. Res.*, **175**, 286–292.

Frost, H.M. (1990). Structural adaptations to mechanical usage (SATMU): redefining Wolff's law. *Anat. Rec.*, **226**, 403–422.

Frost, H.M. (1991). Some ABC's of skeletal patho-physiology. 6. The growth/modeling/remodeling distinction. *Calcif. Tissue Int.*, **49**, 301–302.

Fuchs, R.K. and Snow, C.M. (2002). Gains in hip bone mass from high-impact training are maintained: a randomized controlled trial in children. *J. Pediatr.*, **141**, 357–362.

Gleeson, P., Protas, E., LeBlanc, A. et al. (1990). Effects of weight lifting on bone mineral density in premenopausal women. *J. Bone Miner. Res.*, **5**, 153–158.

Haapasalo, H., Sievanen, H., Kannus, P. et al. (1996). Dimensions and estimated mechanical characteristics of the humerus after long-term tennis loading. *J. Bone Miner. Res.*, **11**, 864–872.

Harries, U.J. and Bassey, E.J. (1990). Torque-velocity relationships for the knee extensors in women in their 3rd and 7th decades. *Eur. J. Appl. Physiol.*, **60**, 187–190.

Hartard, M., Haber, P., Ilieva, D. et al. (1996). Systematic strength training as a model of therapeutic intervention. *Am. J. Phys. Med. Rehabil.*, **75**, 21–28.

Hatori, M., Hasegawa, A., Adachi, H. et al. (1993). The effects of walking at the anaerobic threshold level on vertebral bone loss in postmenopausal women. *Calcif. Tissue Int.*, **52**, 411–414.

Hayes, W.C. and Gerhart, T.N. (1985). Biomechanics of bone: applications for assessment of bone strength. *Bone Miner. Res.*, **3**, 259–294.

Heinonen, A., Kannus, P., Sievanen, H. et al. (1996). Randomised, controlled trial of effect of high-impact exercise on selected risk factors for osteoporotic fractures. *Lancet*, **348**, 1343–1347.

Heinonen, A., Oja, P., Sievanen, H. et al. (1998). Effect of two training regimens on bone mineral density in healthy perimenopausal women: a randomised, controlled trial. *J. Bone Miner. Res.*, **13**, 483–490.

Heinonen, A., Sievanen, H., Kannus, P. et al. (2000). High-impact exercise and bones of growing girls: a 9-month controlled trial. *Osteoporosis Int.*, **11**, 1010–1017.

Hill, K., Schwarz, J., Flicker, L. et al. (1999). Falls among healthy, community-dwelling, older women: a prospective study of frequency, circumstances, consequences and prediction accuracy. *Aust. NZ J. Public Health*, **23**, 41–48.

Humphries, B., Newton, R.U., Bronks, R. et al. (2000). Effect of exercise intensity on bone density, strength, and calcium turnover in older women. *Med. Sci. Sports Exerc.*, **32**, 1043–1050.

Joakimsen, R.M., Fonnebo, V., Magnus, J.H. et al. (1999). The Truomso study – physical activity and the incidence of fractures in a middle-aged population. *J. Bone Miner. Res.*, **13**, 1149–1157.

Johnston, J. and Slemenda, C. (1993). Determinants of peak bone mass. *Osteoporosis Int.* (suppl. 1), S54–S55.

Karlsson, M.K., Linden, C., Karlsson, C. et al. (2000). Exercise during growth and bone mineral density and fractures in old age. *Lancet*, **355**, 469–470.

Kelley, G.A., Kelley, K.S. and Tran, Z.V. (2000). Exercise and bone mineral density in men: a meta-analysis. *J. Appl. Physiol.*, **88**, 1730–1736.

Kerr, D., Morton, A., Dick, I. et al. (1996). Exercise effects on bone mass in postmenopausal women are site-specific and load-dependent. *J. Bone Miner. Res.*, **11**(2), 218–225.

Kerschan, K., Alacamlioglu, Y., Kollmitzer, J. et al. (1998). Functional impact of unvarying exercise program in women after menopause. *Am. J. Phys. Med. Rehabil.*, **77**, 326–332.

Khan, K.M., Green, R.M., Saul, A. et al. (1996). Retired elite female ballet dancers and nonathletic controls have similar bone mineral density at weightbearing sites. *J. Bone Miner. Res.*, **11**, 1566–1574.

Kontulainen, S., Kannus, P., Haapasalo, H. et al. (2001). Good maintenance of exercise-induced bone gain with decreased training of female tennis and squash players: a prospective 5-year follow-up study of young and old starters and controls. *J. Bone Miner. Res.*, **16**, 195–201.

Kronhed, A. and Moller, M. (1998). Effects of physical exercise on bone mass, balance skill and aerobic capacity in women and men with low bone mineral density, after one year of training – a prospective study. *Scand. J. Med. Sci. Sports*, **8**, 290–298.

Kujala, U.M., Kaprio, J., Kannus, P. et al. (2000). Physical activity and osteoporotic hip fracture risk in men. *Arch. Intern. Med.*, **160**, 705–708.

Lanyon, L.E. (1984). Functional strain as a determinant for bone remodeling. *Calcif. Tissue Int.*, **36**, S56–S61.

Lanyon, L.E. (1987). Functional strain in bone tissue as an objective, and controlling stimulus for adaptive bone remodelling. *J. Biomech.*, **20**, 1083–1093.

Lespessailles, E., Jullien, A., Eynard, E. et al. (1998). Biomechanical properties of human os calcanei: relationships with bone density and fractal evaluation of bone microarchitecture. *J. Biomech.*, **31**, 817–824.

Lohmann, T., Going, S., Pamenter, R. et al. (1995). Effects of resistance training on regional and total bone mineral density in premenopausal women: a randomized prospective study. *J. Bone Miner. Res.*, **10**(7), 1015–1024.

Lord, S.R., Clark, R.D. and Webster, I.W. (1991). Physiological factors associated with falls in an elderly population. *J. Geriatr. Soc.*, **39**, 1194–1200.

Lord, S.R., Sambrook, P.N., Gilbert, C. et al. (1994). Postural stability, falls and fractures in the elderly: results from the Dubbo Osteoporosis Epidemiology Study. *Med. J. Aust.*, **160**, 684–691.

MacKelvie, K.J., McKay, H.A., Khan, K.M. et al. (2001). A school-based exercise intervention augments bone mineral accrual in early pubertal girls. *J. Pediatr.*, **139**, 501–508.

Madsen, O.R., Schaadt, O., Bliddal, H. et al. (1993). Relationship between quadriceps strength and bone mineral density of the proximal tibia and distal forearm in women. *J. Bone Miner. Res.*, **8**, 1439–1444.

Malmros, B., Mortenson, L., Jensen, M.B. et al. (1998). Postive effects of physiotherapy on chronic pain and performance in osteoporosis. *Osteoporosis Int.*, **8**, 215–221.

Martin, D. and Notelovitz, M. (1993). Effects of aerobic training on bone mineral density of postmenopausal women. *J. Bone Miner. Res.*, **8**, 931–936.

McKay, H.A., Petit, M.A., Schutz, R.W. et al. (2000). Augmented trochanteric bone mineral density after modified physical education classes: a randomized school-based exercise intervention study in prepubescent and early pubescent children. *J. Pediatr.*, **136**, 156–162.

Milgrom, C., Finestone, A., Levi, Y. et al. (2000). Do high impact exercises produce higher tibial strains than running? *Br. J. Sports Med.*, **34**, 195–199.

Morris, F.L., Naughton, G.A., Gibbs, J.L. et al. (1997). Prospective ten-month exercise intervention in premenarcheal girls: positive effects on bone and lean mass. *J. Bone Miner. Res.*, **12**, 1453–1462.

Mosekilde, L. (1993). Vertebral structure and strength in vivo and in vitro. *Calcif. Tissue Int.*, **53**, S121–S126.

Mosley, J.R. and Lanyon, L.E. (1998). Strain rate as a controlling influence on adaptive modeling in response to dynamic loading of the ulna in growing male rats. *Bone*, **23**, 313–318.

Nordin, M. and Frankel, V.H. (1989). *Basic Biomechanics of the Musculoskeletal System*, 2nd edn. Philadelphia: Lea & Febiger.

Orwoll, E.S., Ferar, J., Oviatt, S.K. et al. (1989). The relationship of swimming exercise to bone mass in men and women. *Arch. Intern. Med.*, **149**, 2197–2200.

Paganini-Hill, A., Chao, A., Ross, R.K. et al. (1991). Exercise and other factors in the prevention of hip fracture: the Leisure World study. *Epidemiology*, **2**, 16–25.

Parkkari, J., Kannus, P., Palvanen, M. et al. (1999). Majority of hip fractures occur as a result of a fall and impact on the greater trochanter of the femur: a prospective controlled hip fracture study with 206 consecutive patients. *Calcif. Tissue Int.*, **65**, 183–187.

Petersen, M.M., Jensen, N.C., Gehrchen, P.M. et al. (1996). The relation between trabecular bone strength and bone mineral density assessed by dual photon and dual energy X-ray absorptiometry in the proximal tibia. *Calcif. Tissue Int.*, **59**, 311–314.

Petit, M.A., McKay, H.A., MacKelvie, K.J. et al. (2002). A randomized school-based jumping intervention confers site and maturity-specific benefits on bone structural properties in girls: a hip structural analysis study. *J. Bone Miner. Res.*, **17**, 363–372.

Preisinger, E., Alacamlioglu, Y., Pils, K. et al. (1996). Exercise therapy for osteoporosis: results of a randomised, controlled trial. *Br. J. Sports Med.*, **30**, 209–212.

Raab-Cullen, D.M., Akhter, M.P., Kimmel, D.B. et al. (1994). Bone response to alternate-day mechanical loading of the rat tibia. *J. Bone Miner. Res.*, **9**, 203–211.

Rico, H., Revilla, M., Hernandez, E.R. et al. (1993). Bone mineral content and body composition in postpubertal cyclist boys. *Bone*, **14**, 93–95.

Riggs, B.L. and Melton, L.J.I. (1986). Involutional osteoporosis. *N. Engl. J. Med.*, **314**, 1676–1686.

Robling, A.G., Burr, D.B. and Turner, C.H. (2000). Partitioning a daily mechanical stimulus into discrete loading bouts improves the osteogenic response to loading. *J. Bone Miner. Res.*, **15**, 1596–1602.

Robling, A.G., Burr, D.B. and Turner, C.H. (2001). Recovery periods restore mechanosensitivity to dynamically loaded bone. *J. Exp. Biol.*, **204**, 3389–3399.

Robling, A.G., Hinant, F.M., Burr, D.B. et al. (2002). Shorter, more frequent mechanical loading sessions enhance bone mass. *Med. Sci. Sports Exerc.*, **34**, 196–202.

Rubin, C.T. and Lanyon, L.E. (1984). Regulation of bone formation by applied dynamic loads. *J. Bone Joint Surg.*, **66-A**, 397–402.

Rubin, C.T. and Lanyon, L.E. (1985). Regulation of bone mass by mechanical strain magnitude. *Calcif. Tissue Int.,* **37**, 411–417.

Rutherford, O.M. and Jones, D.A. (1992). The relationship of muscle and bone loss and activity levels with age in women. *Age Ageing,* **21**, 286–293.

Sinaki, M. and Mikkelsen, B.A. (1984). Postmenopausal spinal osteoporosis: flexion versus extension exercises. *Arch. Phys. Med. Rehabil.,* **65**, 593–596.

Sinaki, M., Itoi, E., Wahner, H.W. et al. (2002). Stronger back muscles reduce the incidence of vertebral fractures: a prospective 10 year follow-up of postmenopausal women. *Bone,* **30**, 836–841.

Snow-Harter, C., Bouxsein, M.L., Lewis, B.T. et al. (1992). Effects of resistance and endurance exercise on bone mineral status of young women: a randomized exercise intervention trial. *J. Bone Miner. Res.,* **7**, 761–769.

Taaffe, D.R., Snow-Harter, C., Connolly, D.A. et al. (1995). Differential effects of swimming versus weight-bearing activity on bone mineral status of eumenorrheic athletes. *J. Bone Miner. Res.,* **10**, 586–593.

Tinetti, M.E., Speechley, M. and Ginter, S.F. (1988). Risk factors for falls among elderly persons living in the community. *N. Engl. J. Med.,* **319**, 1701–1707.

Turner, C.H. (1999). Toward a mathematical description of bone biology: the principle of cellular accommodation. *Calcif. Tissue Int.,* **65**, 466–471.

Turner, C.H., Owan, I. and Takano, Y. (1995). Mechanotransduction in bone: role of strain rate. *Am. J. Physiol.,* **269**, E438–E442.

Umemura, Y., Ishiko, T., Tsujimoto, H. et al. (1995). Effects of jump training on bone hypertrophy in young and old rats. *Int. J. Sports Med.,* **16**, 364–367.

Umemura, Y., Ishiko, T., Yamauchi, T. et al. (1997). Five jumps per day increase bone mass and breaking force in rats. *J. Bone Miner. Res.,* **12**, 1480–1485.

Umemura, Y., Sogo, N. and Honda, A. (2002). Effects of intervals between jumps or bouts on osteogenic response to loading. *J. Appl. Physiol.,* **93**, 1345–1348.

Whalen, R.T., Carter, D.R. and Steele, C.R. (1988). Influence of physical activity on the regulation of bone density. *J. Biomech.,* **21**, 825–837.

WHO Study Group (1994). *Assessment of Fracture Risk and its Application to Screening for Postmenopausal Osteoporosis.* WHO Technical Report Series. Geneva: World Health Organization.

Wolff, I., van Croonenborg, J.J., Kemper, H.C.G. et al. (1999). The effect of exercise training programs on bone mass: a meta-analysis of published controlled trials in pre- and postmenopausal women. *Osteoporosis Int.,* **9**, 1–12.

Young, D., Hopper, J.L., Nowson, C.A. et al. (1995). Determinants of bone mass in 10- to 26-year-old females: a twin study. *J. Bone Miner. Res.,* **10**, 558–567.

Zmuda, J.M., Cauley, J.A. and Ferrell, R.E. (1999). Recent progress in understanding the genetic susceptibility to osteoporosis. *Genet. Epidemiol.,* **16**, 356–367.

ADAPTATIONS OF MUSCLE AND CONNECTIVE TISSUE

Akeson, W.H., Woo, S.L.-Y., Amiel, D. and Doty, D.H. (1977). Rapid recovery from contracture in rabbit hindlimb. *Clin. Orthop. Rel. Res.,* **122**, 359–365.

Akeson, W.H., Amiel, D. and Woo, S.L.-Y. (1980). Immobility effects on synovial joints. The pathomechanics of joint contracture. *Biorheology,* **17**, 95–110.

Atha, J. (1981). Strengthening muscles. *Exerc. Sports Sci. Rev.,* **9**, 1–74.

Bamman, M.M., Clarke, M.S.F., Feeback, D.L., et al. (1998). Impact of resistance exercise during bed rest on skeletal muscle sarcopenia and myosin isoform distribution. *J. Appl. Physiol.,* **84**, 157–163.

Berger, R. (1962). Effect of varied weight training programs on strength. *Res. Q. Exerc. Sport,* **33**, 168–181.

Davies, C.T.M. and Sargeant, A.J. (1975). Effects of exercise therapy on total and component tissue leg volumes of patients undergoing rehabilitation of lower limb injury. *Ann. Hum. Biol.,* **2**, 327–337.

Davies, C.T.M. and Young, K. (1983). The effects of training at 30 and 100% maximal isometric force (MVC) on the contractile properties of the triceps surae in man. *J. Physiol.,* **336**, 22–23P.

Dean, C.M., Mackey, F.H. and Katrak, P. (2000). Examination of shoulder positioning after stroke: a randomised controlled pilot trial. *Aust. J. Physiother.,* **46**, 35–40.

Duchateau, J. and Hainaut, K. (1987). Electrical and mechanical changes in immobilised human muscle. *J. Appl. Physiol.,* **62**, 2168–2173.

Duchateau, J., and Hainaut, K. (1990). Effects of immobilisation on contractile properties, recruitment and firing rates of human motor units. *J. Physiol.,* **422**, 55–65.

Dyck, P.J., Thomas, P.K., Lambert, E.H. and Bunge, R. (1984). *Peripheral Neuropathy,* vol. II. Philadelphia: W.B. Saunders.

Edgerton, V.R., Barnard, R.J., Peter, J.B., Maier, A. and Simpson, D.R. (1975). Properties of immobilised hindlimb muscles of the Galago senegalensis. *Exp. Neurol.,* **46**, 115–131.

Enoka, R.M. (1988). Muscle strength and its development. New perspectives. *Sports Med.,* **6**, 146–168.

Fox, P., Richardson, J., McInnes, B., Tait, D. and Bedard, M. (2000). Effectiveness of a bed positioning program for treating older adults with knee flexion contractures who are institutionalised. *Phys. Ther.,* **80**, 363–372.

Fukunaga, T., Roy, R.R., Shellock, F.G. et al. (1992). Physiological cross-sectional area of human leg muscles based on magnetic resonance imaging. *J. Orthop. Res.,* **10**, 926–934.

Gandevia, S.C. and McKenzie, D.K. (1988). Activation of human muscles at short muscle lengths during maximal static efforts. *J. Physiol.,* **407**, 599–613.

Gossman, M.R., Sahrmann, S.A. and Rose, S.J. (1982). Review of length-associated changes in muscle. Experimental evidence and clinical implications. *Phys. Ther.,* **62**, 1799–1808.

Guttman, L. (1976). *Spinal Cord Injuries. Comprehensive Management and Research,* 2nd edn. Oxford: Blackwell.

Hardy, M.A. (1989). The biology of scar formation. *Phys. Ther.*, **69**, 1014–1024.

Harvey, L.A., Batty, J., Crosbie, J., Poulter, S. and Herbert, R.D. (2000). A randomized trial assessing the effects of 4 weeks of daily stretching on ankle mobility in patients with spinal cord injuries. *Arch. Phys. Med. Rehabil.*, **81**, 1340–1347.

Herbert, R.D. (1988). The passive mechanical properties of muscle and their adaptations to altered patterns of use. *Aust. J. Physiother.*, **34**, 141–149.

Herbert, R. (1993a). Human strength adaptations – implications for therapy. In: *Key Issues in Musculoskeletal Physiotherapy*, ed. J. Crosbie and J. McConnell, pp. 142–171. Oxford: Butterworth-Heinemann.

Herbert, R. (1993b). Preventing and treating stiff joints. In: *Key Issues in Musculoskeletal Physiotherapy*, ed. J. Crosbie and J. McConnell, pp. 114–141. Oxford: Butterworth-Heinemann.

Herbert, R.D. and Balnave, R.J. (1993). The effect of position of immobilisation on rabbit soleus muscle resting length and stiffness. *J. Orthop. Res.*, **11**, 358–366.

Herbert, R.D. and Crosbie, J. (1997). Rest length and compliance of non-immobilised and immobilised rabbit soleus muscle and tendon. *Eur. J. Appl. Physiol.*, **76**, 472–479.

Herbert, R.D., Dean, C., and Gandevia, S.C. (1998). Effects of real and imagined training on voluntary muscle activation during maximal isometric contractions. *Acta Physiol. Scand.*, **163**, 361–368.

Heslinga, J.W. and Huijing, P.A. (1993). Muscle length–force characteristics in relation to muscle architecture: a bilateral study of gastrocnemius medialis muscles of unilaterally immobilized rats. *Eur. J. Appl. Physiol.*, **66**, 289–298.

Hughes, G.R.V. (1977). *Connective Tissue Disease*. Oxford: Blackwell.

Ingemann-Hansen, T. and Halkjaer-Kristensen, J. (1980). Computerised tomography determination of human thigh components. *Scand. J. Rehabil. Med.*, **12**, 27–31.

Jarvinen, M.K. and Lehto, M.U.K. (1993). The effects of early mobilisation and immobilisation on the healing process following muscle injuries. *Sports Med.*, **15**, 78–89.

Jones, D.A. and Rutherford, O.M. (1987). Human muscle strength training: the effects of three different regimes and the nature of the resultant changes. *J. Physiol.*, **391**, 1–11.

Jozsa, L., Kannus, P., Thoring, J., Reffy, A., Jarvinen, M. and Kvist, M. (1990). The effect of tenotomy and immobilisation on intramuscular connective tissue. *J. Bone Joint Surg.*, **72-B**, 293–297.

Khouw, W. and Herbert, R.D. (1998). Optimisation of isometric strength training intensity. *Aust. J. Physiother.*, **44**, 43–46.

Lannin, N., McCluskey, A., Herbert, R.D. and Cusick, A. (2002). Hand splinting in the functional position after brain impairment: a randomized controlled trial. *Arch. Phys. Med. Rehabil.*, **84**, 297–302.

LeBlanc, A., Gogia, P. and Schneider, V. (1988). Calf muscle area and strength changes after five weeks of horizontal bed rest. *Am. J. Sports Med.*, **16**, 624–629.

Light, K.E., Nuzick, S., Personius, W. and Barstrom, A. (1984). Low-load prolonged stretch vs. high-load brief stretch in treating knee contractures. *Phys. Ther.*, **64**, 330–333.

Mastaglia, F.L. and Walton, J. (1982). *Skeletal Muscle Pathology*. Edinburgh: Churchill Livingstone.

McDonagh, M.J.N. and Davies, C.T.M. (1984). Adaptive response of mammalian skeletal muscle to exercise with high loads. *Eur. J. Appl. Physiol.*, **52**, 139–155.

McDougall, J.D., Elder, G.C.B., Sale, D.G. et al. (1980). Effects of strength training and immobilisation on human muscle fibres. *Eur. J. Appl. Physiol.*, **43**, 25–34.

Moseley, A.M. (1997). The effect of casting combined with stretching on passive ankle dorsiflexion in adults with traumatic head injuries. *Phys. Ther.*, **77**, 248–259.

Narici, M.V., Roi, G.S., Landoni, L., Minetti, A.E. and Cerretelli, P. (1989). Changes in force, cross-sectional area and neural activation during strength training and detraining of human quadriceps. *Eur. J. Appl. Physiol.*, **59**, 310–319.

Noyes, F.R. (1977). Functional properties of knee ligaments and alterations induced by immobilisation. *Clin. Orthop. Rel. Res.*, **123**, 210–242.

O'Dwyer, N.J., Nielson, P.D. and Nash, J. (1989). Mechanisms of muscle growth related to muscle contracture in cerebral palsy. *Dev. Med. Child Neurol.*, **31**, 543–547.

Rooney, K., Herbert, R. and Balnave, R. (1994). Fatigue contributes to the strength training stimulus. *Med. Sci. Sports Exerc.*, **26**, 1160–1164.

Rutherford, O.M., Jones, D.A. and Round, J.M. (1990). Long-lasting unilateral muscle wasting and weakness following injury and immobilisation. *Scand. J. Rehabil. Med.*, **22**, 33–37.

Sale, D.G. (1988). Neural adaptation to resistance training. *Med. Sci. Sports Exerc.*, **20**, S135–S145.

Sale, D.G. (1992). Neural adaptation to strength training. In: *Strength and Power in Sport*, ed. P.V. Kuomi, pp. 249–265. Oxford: Blackwell.

St-Pierre, D. and Gardiner, P.F. (1987). The effect of immobilisation and exercise on muscle function: a review. *Physiother. Can.*, **39**, 24–36.

Steffen, T.M. and Mollinger, L.A. (1995). Low-load, prolonged stretch in the treatment of knee flexion contractures in nursing home residents. *Phys. Ther.*, **75**, 886–895.

Stillwell, D.L., McLarren, G.L. and Gersten, J.W. (1967). Atrophy of quadriceps muscle due to immobilisation of the lower extremity. *Arch. Phys. Med. Rehabil.*, **48**, 289–295.

Sunderland, S. (1991). *Nerves and Nerve Injuries*. Edinburgh: Churchill Livingstone.

Szeto, G., Strauss, G., De Demenico, G. and Lai, H.S. (1989). The effect of training intensity on voluntary isometric strength improvement. *Aust. J. Physiother.*, **35**, 210–217.

Tabary, J.C., Tabary, C., Tardieu, C. and Tardieu, G. (1972). Physiological and structural changes in the cat's soleus muscle due to immobilisation at different lengths by plaster casts. *J. Physiol.*, **224**, 231–244.

Toursel, T., Stevens, L., Granzier, H. and Mounier, Y. (2002). Passive tension of rat skeletal soleus muscle fibers: effects of unloading conditions. *J. Appl. Physiol.*, **92**, 1465–1472.

Vinken, P.J., Bruyn, G.W., Klawans, H.L. and Braakman, R. (1990). *Head Injury*. Amsterdam: Elsevier.

Walton, J.N. (1974). *Disorders of Voluntary Muscle,* 3rd edn. Edinburgh: Churchill Livingstone.

Walton, J. (1985). *Brain's Diseases of the Nervous System*, 9th edn. Oxford: Oxford University Press.

Wigerstad-Lossing, I., Grimby, G., Jonsson, T. et al. (1988). Effects of electrical muscle stimulation combined with voluntary muscle contractions after knee surgery. *Med. Sci. Sports Exerc.*, **20**, 93–98.

Williams, P.E. (1990). Use of intermittent stretch in the prevention of serial sarcomere loss in immobilised muscle. *Ann. Rheum. Dis.*, **49**, 316–317.

Williams, P.E. and Goldspink, G. (1978). Changes in sarcomere length and physiological properties in immobilised muscle. *J. Anat.*, **127**, 459–468.

Williams, P.E. and Goldspink, G. (1984). Connective tissue changes in immobilized muscle. *J. Anat.*, **138**, 343–350.

Witzmann, F.A., Kim, D.H. and Fitts, R.H. (1982a). Hindlimb immobilisation: length–tension and contractile properties of skeletal muscle. *J. Appl. Physiol.*, **53**, 335–345.

Witzmann, F.A., Kim, D.H. and Fitts, R.H. (1982b). Recovery time course in contractile function of fast and slow skeletal muscle after hindlimb immobilisation. *J. Appl. Physiol.*, **53**, 677–682.

Woo, S.L.-Y. (1986). Biomechanics of tendons and ligaments. In: *Frontiers in Biomechanics*, ed. G.W. Schmid-Schönbein, S.L.-Y. Woo and B.W. Zweifach. pp. 180–195. New York: Springer-Verlag.

Woo, S.L.-Y. and Buckwalter, J.A. (1988). *Injury and Repair of the Musculoskeletal System*. Illinois: AAOS.

Young, A., Hughes, I., Round, J.M. and Edwards, R.H.T. (1982). The effect of knee injury on the number of muscle fibres in the human quadriceps. *Clin. Sci.*, **62**, 227–234.

Yue, G. and Cole, K.J. (1992). Strength increases from the motor program: comparison of training with maximal voluntary and imagined muscle contractions. *J. Neurophysiol.*, **67**, 1114–1118.

REGAINING SKILL IN MOTOR PERFORMANCE

Agahari, I., Shepherd, R.B. and Westwood, P. (1996). A comparative evaluation of lower limb forces in two variations of the step exercise in able-bodied subjects. In: *Proceedings of the First Australasian Biomechanics Conference*, ed. M. Lee, W. Gilleard, P. Sinclair et al., pp. 94–95. Sydney, NSW, Australia: University of Sydney.

Andriacchi, T.P., Andersson, G.B.J., Fermier, R. et al. (1980). A study of lower limb mechanics during stairclimbing. *J. Bone Joint Surg.*, **62A**, 749.

Annett, J. (1971). Acquisition of skill. *Br. Med. Bull.*, **27**, 266–271.

Annett, J. and Kay, H. (1957). Knowledge of results and skilled performance. *Occup. Psychol.*, **31**, 69–79.

Arbib, M.A., Iberall, T. and Lyons, D. (1986). Coordinated control programs for movements of the hand. In: *Hand Function and the Neocortex*, ed. A.W. Goodwin and I. Darian-Smith, pp. 111–129. Berlin: Springer-Verlag.

Asmussen, E. and Bonde-Petersen, F. (1974). Storage of elastic energy in skeletal muscles in man. *Acta Physiol. Scand.*, **91**, 385–392.

Baker, P.D., Evans, D.M. and Lee, C. (1991). Treadmill gait retraining following fractured neck of femur. *Arch. Phys. Med. Rehabil.*, **72**, 649–652.

Beggs, W.D.A. and Howarth, C.I. (1972). The movement of the hand towards a target. *Q. J. Exp. Psychol.*, **24**, 448–453.

Bernstein, N.A. (1967). *The Co-ordination and Regulation of Movement*. Oxford: Pergamon Press.

Bobbert, M.F. and van Ingen Schenau, G.J. (1988). Coordination in vertical jumping. *J. Biomech.*, **21**, 249–262.

Bosco, C., Viitasalo, J.T., Komi, P.V. and Luhtanen, P. (1982). Combined effect of elastic energy and myoelectrical potentiation during stretch-shortening cycle exercise. *Acta Physiol. Scand.*, **114**, 557–565.

Buchner, M., Larson, E.B., Wagner, E.H. et al. (1996). Evidence for a non-linear relationship between leg strength and gait speed. *Age Ageing*, **25**, 386–391.

Canning, C. (1987). Training standing up following stroke – a clinical trial. In: *Proceedings of the Tenth International Congress of the World Confederation for Physical Therapy (Sydney)*, pp. 915–919.

Carr, J.H. and Gentile, A.M. (1994). The effect of arm movement on the biomechanics of standing up. *Hum. Move. Sci.*, **13**, 175–193.

Carr, J.H. and Shepherd, R.B. (1987). *A Motor Relearning Programme for Stroke*, 2nd edn. Oxford: Butterworth-Heinemann.

Carr, J.H. and Shepherd, R.B. (1998). *Neurological Rehabilitation: Optimizing Motor Performance*. Oxford: Butterworth-Heinemann.

Carr, J.H. and Shepherd, R.B. (2000). A motor learning model for rehabilitation. In: *Movement Science: Foundations for Physical Therapy in Rehabilitation*, 2nd edn, ed. J.H. Carr and R.B. Shepherd, pp. 33–110. Rockville, MD: Aspen.

Carr, J.H. and Shepherd, R.B. (2003). *Stroke Rehabilitation. Guidelines for Exercise and Training to Optimize Motor Skill*. Oxford: Butterworth-Heinemann.

Castiello, U., Bennett, K.M.B. and Stelmach, G.E. (1993). The bilateral reach to grasp movement. *Behav. Brain Res.*, **56**, 43–57.

Cordo, P.J. and Nashner, L.M. (1982). Properties of postural adjustments associated with rapid arm movements. *J. Neurophysiol.*, **47**, 287–302.

Crossman, E.R.F.W. (1959). A theory of the acquisition of speed-skill. *Ergonomics*, **2**, 153–166.

Dean, C.M., Richards, C.L. and Malouin, F. (2000). Task-related training improves performance of locomotor tasks in chronic stroke. A randomized controlled pilot study. *Arch. Phys. Med. Rehabil.*, **81**, 409–417.

Depena, J. and Chung, C.S. (1988). Vertical and radial motions of the body during the take-off phase of high jumping. *Med. Sci. Sports Exerc.*, **20**, 290.

Drabsch, T., Lovenfosse, J., Fowler, V., Adams, R. and Drabsch, P. (1998). Effects of task-specific training on walking and sit-to-stand after total hip replacement. *Aust. J. Physiother.*, **44**, 193–198.

Ellenbecker, T.S., Davies, G.J. and Rowinski, M.J. (1988). Concentric versus eccentric isokinetic strengthening of the rotator cuff: objective data versus functional test. *Am. J. Sports Med.*, **16**, 64–69.

Gelfand, I.M., Gurfinkel, V.S., Tsetlin, M.L. and Shik, M.L. (1971). Some problems in the analysis of movements. In: *Models of the Structural–Functional Organization of Certain Biological Systems*, ed. I.M. Gelfand, V.S. Gurfinkel, S.V. Fomin and M.L. Tsetlin., pp. 329–345. Cambridge: MIT Press.

Gentile, A.M. (1972). A working model of skill acquisition with applications to teaching. *Quest*, **17**, 3–23.

Gentile, A.M. (2000). Skill acquisition: action, movement, and neuromotor processes. In: *Movement Science: Foundation for Physical Therapy in Rehabilitation,* 2nd edn, ed. J.H. Carr and R.B. Shepherd, pp. 111–187. Rockville, MD: Aspen.

Gibson, J.J. (1966). *The Senses Considered as Perceptual Systems.* Boston: Houghton Mifflin.

Gibson, J.J. (1986). *The Ecological Approach to Visual Perception.* Hillsdale, NJ: Lawrence Erlbaum.

Godges, J.J., MacRae, P.G. and Engelke, K.A. (1993). Effects of exercise on hip range of motion, trunk muscle performance, and gait economy. *Phys. Ther.*, **73**, 468–477.

Gonnella, C., Hale, G., Ionta, M. and Perry, J.C. (1981). Self-instruction in a perceptual motor skill. *Phys. Ther.*, **61**, 177–184.

Gottlieb, G.L., Corcos, D.M., Jaric, S. and Agarwal, G.C. (1988). Practice improves even the simplest movements. *Exp. Brain Res.*, **73**, 436–440.

Greene, P.H. (1982). Why is it easy to control your arms? *J. Mot. Behav.*, **14**, 260–286.

Gregoire, L., Veeger, H.E., Huijing, P.A. and van Ingen Schenau G.J. (1984). Role of mono- and biarticular muscles in explosive movements. *Int. J. Sports Med.*, **5**, 301–305.

Hakkinen, K. and Komi, P.V. (1983). Electromyographic changes during strength training and detraining. *Med. Sci. Sports Exerc.*, **15**, 455–460.

Henderson, S.A., Finlay, O.E., Murphy, N. et al. (1992). Benefits of an exercise class for elderly women following hip surgery. *Ulster Med.*, **61**, 144–159.

Higgins, J.R. (1972). Movements to match environmental demands. *Res. Q.*, **43**, 312–336.

Hinrichs, R.N. (1990). Whole body movement: coordination of arms and legs in walking and running. In: *Multiple Muscle Systems*, ed. J.M. Winters and S.L.-Y. Woo, pp. 694–705. New York: Springer-Verlag.

Irrgang, J.J. (1993). Modern trends in anterior cruciate ligament rehabilitation: nonoperative and postoperative management. *Clin. Sports Med.*, **12**, 797–813.

Jacobs, R. and van Ingen Schenau, G.J. (1992). Control of an external force in leg extensions in humans. *J. Physiol.*, **457**, 611–626.

Jevsevar, D.S., Riley, P.O., Hodge, W.A. and Krebs, D.E. (1993). Knee kinematics and kinetics during locomotor activities of daily living in subjects with knee

arthroplasty and in healthy control subjects. *Phys. Ther.*, **73**, 229–239.

Johnson, P. (1984). The acquisition of skill. In: *The Psychology of Human Movement*, ed. M.M. Smyth and A.M. Wing, pp. 215–240. London: Academic Press.

Kitai, T.A. and Sale, D.G. (1989). Specificity of joint angle in isometric training. *Eur. J. Appl. Physiol.*, **58**, 744–748.

Komi, P.V. (1986). The stretch-shortening cycle and human power output. In: *Human Muscle Power*, ed. N.L. Jones, N. McCartney and A.J. McComas, pp. 27–39. Champaign, IL: Human Kinetic.

Komi, P.V. and Buskirk, E. (1972). Effect of eccentric and concentric muscle conditioning on tension and electrical activity of human muscle. *Ergonomics*, **154**, 417–434.

Kottke, F.K. (1980). From reflex to skill: the training of coordination. *Arch. Phys. Med. Rehabil.*, **61**, 551–561.

Lee, D.N. and Aronson, E. (1974). Visual proprioceptive control of standing in infants. *Percept. Psychophys.*, **15**, 529–532.

Lee, D.N. and Lishman, J.R. (1975). Visual proprioceptive control of stance. *J. Hum. Move. Stud.*, **1**, 87–95.

Leont'ev, A.N. and Zaporozhets, A.V. (1960). *Rehabilitation of Hand Function.* London: Pergamon.

Lindh, M. (1979). Increase of muscle strength from isometric quadriceps exercises at different knee angles. *Scand. J. Rehabil. Med.*, **11**, 33–36.

Magill, R.A. (2001). *Motor Learning Concepts and Applications*, 6th edn. New York: McGraw-Hill International.

Malouin, F., Potvin, M., Prevost, J., Richards, C.L. and Wood-Dauphinee, S. (1992). Use of an intensive task-oriented gait training program in a series of patients with acute cerebrovascular accidents. *Phys. Ther.*, **72**, 781–793.

Mann, R. and Hagy, J. (1980). Biomechanics of walking, running and springing. *Am. J. Sports Med.*, **8**, 345–350.

Marteniuk, R.G. (1976). *Information Processing in Motor Skills*, New York: Holt, Rinehart and Winston.

McConnell, J. (1993). Promoting effective segmental alignment. In: *Key Issues in Musculoskeletal Physiotherapy*, ed. J. Crosbie and J. McConnell, pp. 172–194. Oxford: Butterworth-Heinemann.

Morrissey, M.C., Herman, E.S. and Johnson, M.J. (1995). Resistance training modes: specificity and effectiveness. *Med. Sci. Sports Exerc.*, **27**, 648–660.

Mulder, T. (1991). A process-oriented model of human motor behavior: toward a theory-based rehabilitation approach. *Phys. Ther.*, **71**, 157–164.

Newell, K.M. (1976). Knowledge of results and motor learning. *Exerc. Sports Sci. Rev.*, **4**, 195–227.

Newell, K.M. (1981). Skill learning. In: *Human Skills,* ed. D. Holding, pp. 203–226. New York: John Wiley.

Oxendine, A. (1984). *Psychology of Motor Learning*, 2nd edn. Englewood Cliffs: Prentice-Hall.

Pai, Y. and Rogers, M.W. (1991). Segmental contribution to total body momentum in sit-to-stand. *Med. Sci. Sports Exerc.*, **23**, 225–230.

Palmitier, R.A., An, K.N., Scott, S.G. and Chao, E.Y.S. (1991). Kinetic chain exercise in knee rehabilitation. *Sports Med.*, **11**, 402–413.

Rasch, P.J. and Morehouse, C.E. (1957). Effect of static and dynamic exercises on muscular strength and hypertrophy. *J. Appl. Physiol.*, **11**, 29–34.

Rutherford, O.M. (1988). Muscular coordination and strength training implications for injury rehabilitation. *Sports Med.*, **5**, 196–202.

Rutherford, O.M. and Jones, D.A. (1986). The role of learning and coordination in strength training. *Eur. J. Appl. Physiol.*, **55**, 100–105.

Sale, D.G. (1988). Neural adaptation to resistance training. *Med. Sci. Sports Exerc.*, **20**, 135–145.

Sale, D. and MacDougall, D. (1981). Specificity in strength training: a review for the coach and athlete. *Can. J. Appl. Sports Sci.*, **6**, 87–92.

Schenkman, M., Berger, R.A., Riley, P.O., Mann, R.W. and Hodge, W.A. (1990). Whole-body movements during rising to standing from sitting. *Phys. Ther.*, **70**, 638–648.

Schmidt, R.A. (1975). A schema theory of discrete motor learning. *Psychol. Rev.*, **82**, 225–260.

Schmidt, R.A. (1988). *Motor Control and Learning: A Behavioral Emphasis*, 2nd edn. Champaign: Human Kinetics.

Scholz, J.P. (1993). Organization principles for the coordination of lifting. *Hum. Move. Sci.*, **12**, 537.

Shepherd, R.B. and Gentile, A.M. (1994). Sit-to-stand: functional relationships between upper body and lower limb. *Hum. Move. Sci.*, **13**, 817–840.

Sherrington, C. and Lord, S.R. (1997). Home exercise to improve strength and walking velocity after hip fracture: a randomized controlled trial. *Arch. Phys. Med. Rehabil.*, **78**, 208–212.

Stelmach, G.E. (1978). *Information Processing in Motor Control and Learning*. New York: Academic Press.

Thepaut-Mathieu, C., Van Hoecke, J. and Maton, B. (1985). Length specificity of strength and myoneural activation improvements following isometric training. In: *Biomechanics X-A*, ed. B. Johnson, pp. 513–517. Champaign: Human Kinetics.

Turvey, M.T., Fitch, H.L. and Tuller, B. (1982). The Bernstein perspective: 1. The problems of degrees of freedom and context-conditioned variability. In: *Human Motor Behavior: An Introduction*, ed. J.A.S. Kelso. pp. 271–282. Hillsdale: Lawrence Erlbaum.

van der Weel, F.R., van der Meer, A.L.H. and Lee, D.N. (1991). Effect of task on movement control in cerebral palsy: implications for assessment and therapy. *Dev. Med. Child Neurol.*, **33**, 419–426.

Westwood, P. (1992). *An Investigation into the Effect of Task-Specific Training on the Biomechanics of Standing up in Patients Following Total Hip Replacement*. MAppSc thesis, School of Physiotherapy, University of Sydney, Australia.

Winstein, C.J. and Knecht, H.G. (1990). Movement science and its relevance to physical therapy. *Phys. Ther.*, **70**, 759–762.

Winter, D.A. (1991). *The Biomechanics and Control of Human Gait: Normal Elderly and Pathological*. Waterloo: University of Waterloo Press.

Wise, S.P. and Desimone, R. (1988). Behavioral neurophysiology: insights into seeing and grasping. *Science*, **242**, 736–740.

Wooden, M.J., Greenfield, B., Johanson, M. et al. (1992). Effects of strength training on throwing velocity and shoulder muscle performance in teenage baseball players. *J. Sports Physiother.*, **15**, 223–228.

Young, R.P. and Marteniuk, R.G. (1995). Changes in inter-joint relationships of muscle moments and powers accompanying the acquisition of a multi-articular kicking task. *J. Biomech.*, **28**, 701–713.

Chapter **3**

Diagnostic imaging in musculoskeletal physiotherapy

G. Bigg–Wither and P. Kelly

INTRODUCTION

Successful physiotherapy management of musculoskeletal disorders depends on a thorough
physical examination. In many musculoskeletal
conditions a detailed history and physical examination may suffice, but in other cases the neglect
of radiological investigations may lead to inappropriate or harmful treatment. To make best use of
the results of these investigations, physiotherapists
need to be aware of the principles and practices
of radiology.

There are few instances in musculoskeletal disorders where radiological findings solely determine
diagnosis and management, but there are many
cases where appreciation of these findings will
have a large impact on clinical decisions regarding
treatment and prognosis. In some countries (e.g.
Australia and some states and provinces of North
America) physiotherapists act as primary contact
practitioners and may order X-rays. The subject of
radiological investigation in the practice of physiotherapy has received little attention to date. Because
of recent technological developments in the diagnosis of musculoskeletal problems this topic now
deserves more attention from the profession.

Imaging is an extension of the history and physical examination and plays a key role in helping to
arrive at an accurate diagnosis by confirming a
clinical impression, excluding unsuspected pathology and providing important prognostic information so that an appropriate treatment plan can be

instigated. It should be noted that the X-ray report should not be seen as a statement of absolute truth but rather as a specialist's opinion.

Findings should be correlated with the overall clinical picture. Even when X-rays are normal, if the physiotherapist is suspicious of underlying pathology, e.g. when the patient has intractable night pain, weight loss or the pain is not behaving in an expected musculoskeletal pattern, the physiotherapist should consult with relevant specialists, particularly radiologists, to ensure appropriate further investigation. For example, a man presents complaining of upper cervical spine pain following trauma. Physical examination findings that were inconsistent with findings in the history (e.g. severe spasm elicited on palpation of cervical spine and continuous headaches) led the physiotherapist to suspect the presence of pathology such as fracture. On the other hand, imaging findings may be entirely unrelated to the patient's symptoms, e.g. signs of intervertebral disc degeneration in an elderly patient, or a rotator cuff tear (see section on Clinical problems and their evaluation using imaging techniques, later in this chapter).

Several different modalities for imaging the musculoskeletal system are now commonly utilized in day-to-day practice, from plain film radiography to the more powerful and sophisticated ultrasound, computed tomography (CT) and magnetic resonance imaging (MRI). We need to understand what are the clinical indications, the capabilities and limitations, possible adverse effects, and, in these times of cost containment, the expense of these various imaging investigations. What specific information the clinician wishes to know, the personal preference and expertise of the radiologist and the availability of the various imaging modalities will also have a part to play in this decision process.

Careful clinical evaluation is essential before choosing any imaging test. One must always ask: 'What useful information will this test provide?' and 'Will the result affect patient management?'

It is recommended that physiotherapists utilize the services of a specialist radiology practice where there is radiologist supervision and a written report is provided by the radiologist. All requests for such investigations should have a clear clinical indication, and this should be stated on the request form. This will allow the radiologist to plan

a suitable examination and provide an informed report. It is recommended that imaging examinations other than standard X-rays are requested in consultation with a radiologist or relevant medical practitioner.

To maximize the benefit from X-ray examinations and to be able to recognize normal and abnormal findings you will need to be knowledgeable about radiographic anatomy (see Appendix in Chapter 6) and terminology utilized in radiology reports. You should also understand common disease processes, their imaging correlation and also what are significant and clinically relevant findings versus normal variants or incidental findings of little clinical significance. The only way to improve your X-ray interpretation skills is to look at as many films as possible. Most hospital radiology departments will have a film library which you should utilize.

X-ray safety

Many of the imaging techniques described in this chapter use X-ray radiation as the basis of image formation. X-rays are a form of ionizing radiation and so there is a risk of cell damage. Especially of concern is the possibility of inducing malignancy or gene mutation, which are both chance phenomena related to dose, but there is no safe dose below which these effects cannot occur. There is some uncertainty about the risks of inducing these effects with the low doses of radiation utilized in modern diagnostic radiology, but the risks are thought to be very small. The embryo and children are at greater risk. The International Commission of Radiological Protection recommends that radiological examinations should be carried out only when the information obtained will be useful for the management of the patient. There should be no such thing as a routine X-ray examination; there should always be a clear clinical indication. A person, for example, who has severe pain arising from the cervical region following trauma will require imaging to exclude fracture or disturbance of alignment. The person who is suffering from a mild strain of the gastrocnemius does not routinely require an X-ray examination because diagnosis can be made satisfactorily on clinical examination. Sometimes the physiotherapist may not order an X-ray for a person with a minor musculoskeletal dysfunction on the first consultation but if the problem is not responding in the normal predictable manner, X-rays may be required to provide more information regarding the underlying pathology or to exclude unsuspected pathologies. Repeated examinations, particularly when they involve the radiosensitive organs (thyroid, bone marrow, female breast and gonads) should be avoided (i.e. spine and pelvic examinations), especially in close succession.

All X-ray examinations are avoided throughout pregnancy, especially during the first trimester, and generally will not be performed at all when a woman has missed a period and early pregnancy is possible.

In the remainder of this chapter the basic physical principles involved in image formation with the different imaging modalities will be discussed along with their advantages and disadvantages and a current evaluation of their role in musculoskeletal imaging.

IMAGING TECHNIQUES, THEIR ROLE IN DIAGNOSIS AND THE ADVANTAGES AND DISADVANTAGES IN THEIR USE

Some imaging techniques have specific clinical indications for their use (e.g. ultrasound, CT, MRI) and each examination is tailored to answer a specific clinical question. Other techniques (e.g. plain film radiography) are used for more general imaging purposes.

Plain film radiography

X-rays generated in an X-ray tube pass through the body region of interest to form an image on photographic film with contrast in the image reflecting differential absorption of the X-ray beam by the various tissues in the path of the beam (depending primarily upon atomic number and density of the tissues).

Role

Plain films are almost always the initial form of imaging. They are able to document the majority of fractures and other structural bony abnormalities such as arthritis, tumour, infection, metabolic bone disease (e.g. osteoporosis and Paget's disease) and

developmental anomalies. In many instances no further imaging will be required. However, when there are no relevant plain film findings and there is clinical suspicion of abnormality (e.g. stress fracture) or the plain films are not suitable to evaluate fully a suspected abnormality (e.g. disc herniation or rotator cuff tear), further evaluation can be provided with other more sensitive and sophisticated imaging modalities.

Advantages

- Very good spatial resolution. The structure of bone is well demonstrated, as are soft-tissue calcifications
- Good overall evaluation of the anatomy and alignment of the entire region
- Relatively cheap and widely available.

Disadvantages

- Poor resolution of the soft-tissue structures – at best, can only differentiate fat from all the other soft tissues and so are very limited in the evaluation of the articular and periarticular soft-tissue structures apart from demonstrating soft-tissue calcification. However, soft-tissue swelling and joint effusions can often be appreciated.

- Planar images – superimpose all the structures in the body in the path of the X-ray beam and so difficulties may arise in evaluating abnormalities in regions with complex anatomy (e.g. pelvis). In general, a plain film examination of a region should always include two views at right angles to each other.

- Utilize ionizing radiation. Examinations of the spine and pelvis require the highest radiation doses.

Cross-sectional imaging

Being able to image only a selected thin slice of the body without the superimposition of other structures can have significant advantages in visualizing the various bony and soft-tissue structures and their interfaces and to localize abnormalities accurately.

Ultrasound, CT and MRI are all relatively new modalities which utilize state-of-the-art technology to produce cross-sectional (tomographic) images with superb detail. Their introduction has allowed musculoskeletal imaging to reach a very sophisticated level with the added benefit of decreasing the need for more invasive investigations such as myelography.

Because cross-sectional images view only a small area of the anatomy in one plane at a time, multiple images (scans) are required to evaluate a region of interest. In addition, images may be required in multiple planes as well (e.g. axial, sagittal, coronal or oblique) depending upon the orientation of the structure or abnormality in question.

Conventional tomography

This technique utilizes conventional X-ray tubes and image receptors which are capable of moving relative to each other so as to blur out all structures except those in a chosen focal plane. However, there is usually some unwanted blurring of the focal plane structures as well. Images can be obtained in multiple planes, including the sagittal and coronal planes. The radiation dose is moderately high, depending upon the number of scans required.

Before the widespread introduction of CT and MRI, this technique was frequently employed in bone imaging (e.g. tibial plateau and vertebral column fractures, evaluation of the sternoclavicular and temporomandibular joints and in the assessment of chronic osteomyelitis searching for a sequestrum and/or cortical disruption). Nowadays, tomography has been largely superseded by CT and MRI as they can provide images of superior detail, especially in regard to the soft tissues, and utilize less or no ionizing radiation.

However, tomography can still be useful in certain circumstances, mainly in the spine where tomograms can evaluate multiple segments in the sagittal plane on one image (e.g. to visualize better the craniocervical junction and upper cervical spine, and the lower cervical and upper thoracic spine). Tomography is also useful when artefacts from metal implants preclude useful CT or MRI imaging or there is a contraindication to an MRI examination.

Ultrasound

Ultra-high-frequency sound waves (ultrasound) are propagated into the tissues via a probe (transducer) placed upon the skin surface. The sound waves are both reflected and transmitted at interfaces between the different tissues, and by calculating the time it takes an echo to return to the transducer the depth of a structure can be determined and an image formed. Each individual tissue has a characteristic echotexture which relates to its own unique internal structure.

Musculoskeletal imaging is performed with a high-resolution (5–10 MHz) probe and images can be obtained of the various soft-tissue structures, including tendons, ligaments, bursae and muscles.

Role Diagnostic ultrasound is now well established in musculoskeletal imaging and clinical applications include:

1. Evaluation of:
   (a) tendons:
       - tendinopathy
       - tenosynovitis
       - tendon rupture (e.g. rotator cuff, Achilles tendon, patellar tendon, tibialis posterior tendon)
       - tendon dislocation (e.g. long head of biceps, flexor and extensor tendons of the hand)
       - tendon impingement (e.g. impingement of the rotator cuff tendons beneath the coracoacromial arch with shoulder abduction)
   (b) ligaments (e.g. rupture of collateral ligaments of the knee)
   (c) muscles (e.g. tear, haematoma)
2. Characterizing the location and nature (e.g. solid or cystic) of palpable soft-tissue masses (e.g. popliteal (Baker's) cyst, ganglion). Neoplastic soft-tissue masses are better evaluated with MRI
3. Identifying joint and bursal effusions (e.g. transient synovitis of the hip, subacromial bursitis)
4. Assessing congenital hip dislocation in infants.

Good results require considerable experience in a practice where a special interest is taken in this particular branch of ultrasonic imaging.

Advantages

- Very good image detail (can visualize the fibrillar structure of tendons)

- Cross-sectional images in a variety of planes
- Real-time (dynamic) imaging – structures can be visualized as they move through their physiologic range of motion
- Interactive – any area of tenderness or a palpable mass can be precisely localized with the transducer
- Side-to-side comparison – facilitates detection of any abnormality
- No harmful biological effects have been identified to date (does not utilize ionizing radiation)
- Low to moderate cost
- Widely available.

Disadvantages

- Ultrasound cannot penetrate bone and so unable to image:
  - **(1)** the internal structure of bone, although the surface contour of bone can be seen
  - **(2)** structures covered by bone (e.g. cruciate ligaments)
- Limited depth penetration – cannot image deep structures
- Small field of view
- Contrast resolution is limited
- Alterations in echogenicity may lack specificity
- Images may be difficult to interpret by the novice
- Difficult learning curve – quality of images is operator-dependent. It is important that the radiologist has correlated his or her results with surgical findings to enhance accuracy of diagnosis.

Computed tomography

Initially, a scout image (digital radiograph) is obtained to plan where the scans will be taken. Cross-sectional images are produced by rotating a thin X-ray beam and detector array around the outside of the body through the region of interest. The X-ray transmission data are digitized and then reconstructed with high-speed computers into a two-dimensional image of the internal body structures. As this is a digital imaging process, contrast in the image can be manipulated to emphasize bony or soft-tissue structures. Section thickness can be as small as 1.0 mm when high-resolution detail of the bone or joints is required.

Role CT is now frequently utilized in musculo-skeletal imaging. Clinical applications include evaluation of:

1. Intervertebral disc herniation, spinal stenosis and associated compression of neural structures. In the lumbar spine a modern CT scanner is usually able to discriminate disc, bone, nerve roots and thecal sac and has a high accuracy in visualizing disc herniations and also the cause(s) and severity of spinal stenosis. CT is less reliable in the cervical spine without intrathecal contrast. Thin-section axial scans are obtained at the clinically involved level(s) and the adjacent levels both above and below.
2. Complex fractures and dislocations, especially when they involve joints (e.g. acetabulum, vertebral column, tibial plateau, calcaneus, proximal humerus, radial head, distal radius, ankle, carpus and tarsus) where CT is very helpful in determining the need for surgical intervention. Subluxation or dislocation of the sternoclavicular and distal radioulnar joints is best assessed with CT as plain X-rays may be unreliable.
3. Shoulder instability – performed in conjunction with arthrography.
4. Suspected fractures with negative plain films (e.g. femoral neck, hook of the hamate and stress fractures of the sacrum and navicular) and evaluation of fracture union (e.g. scaphoid).
5. Evaluation of joint problems (e.g. subtalar joints when tarsal coalition is suspected, osteochondral lesions and loose bodies of the ankle, knee and elbow joints).
6. Evaluation of patellofemoral alignment and tracking with knee flexion.
7. Measurement of true leg-length discrepancy (determined from scout images).
8. Osteonecrosis – useful in staging (but not early detection) of osteonecrosis of the femoral head.
9. Assessment of bone tumours.
10. Evaluation of chronic osteomyelitis (searching for a sequestrum and/or cortical disruption).

Advantages

- Excellent detail of bony architecture. Occasionally, three-dimensional reconstruction

can be helpful in allowing a single image to show the entire region (e.g. fractures of the acetabulum)
- Good resolution of soft-tissue structures
- Non-invasive
- Fairly widely available.

Disadvantages

- Limited scanning planes. Depending on the region of the body, anatomical restrictions may limit scanning to only the axial plane (e.g. spine and shoulder). However, newer multidetector spiral CT scanners can very quickly scan large areas with thin sections and provide multiplanar reconstructions of similar quality to the direct scanning plane.

- Artifact sensitivity – streak artifacts may be caused by metal implants or superficial bony structures (e.g. shoulders when scanning the lower cervical segments), which may preclude any useful imaging of that region. Plaster casts do not degrade images.

- Soft-tissue resolution is degraded in obese persons (e.g. when evaluating possible disc herniation). This is especially a problem with older model scanners.

- Utilize ionizing radiation. However, the dose is less than conventional tomography but CT doses are generally higher than an equivalent plain film examination of the same region.

- Cost – moderately expensive.

Magnetic resonance imaging

This is based upon the rather complex principle of nuclear magnetic resonance. The hydrogen nucleus (a single proton), the large majority of which are contained in tissue water molecules, is utilized for imaging. The body is placed in a very-high-strength magnetic field ($0.5–1.5\,T$), which magnetizes the hydrogen protons, and coils around the body part emit a sequence of radiofrequency waves which excite the hydrogen protons to a resonance state. When the hydrogen protons return to the ground state an MR signal is emitted (echo), the intensity of which reflects the proton density and relaxation properties of the hydrogen protons in a particular tissue. Different sequences are utilized to emphasize

anatomic detail (T_1-weighted) or contrast between normal and abnormal soft tissues (T_2-weighted).

Role MRI can offer an accurate and comprehensive non-invasive evaluation of many musculoskeletal problems, including:

1. Intervertebral disc degeneration, disc displacements, spinal stenosis, infective spondylodiscitis and any associated compression of the neural structures. The high intrinsic contrast resolution of MRI allows direct visualization of the thecal sac, spinal cord, nerve roots, discs, bone and bone marrow. Disc degeneration can be assessed by the reduced water content (dehydration) of the nucleus pulposus. A modern MRI unit utilizing dedicated surface coils and the ability to produce high-resolution thin sections has a very high degree of accuracy in the assessment of disc herniations and spinal stenosis in both the cervical and lumbar regions. MRI is currently the only reliable imaging method that can differentiate postoperative scarring from recurrent disc herniation in the failed back syndrome. This is achieved with intravenous gadolinium (a paramagnetic contrast agent), which will enhance fibrosis but not avascular disc material.
2. Intrinsic spinal cord disease, including spinal cord injury.
3. Knee:
   (a) trauma – meniscal and ligamentous tears, osteochondral lesions and trabecular microfractures (bone 'bruises'). Accuracy is as good as arthroscopy.
   (b) patellofemoral tracking.
4. Shoulder – impingement, rotator cuff tear and instability.
5. Osteonecrosis – very sensitive and specific in the early detection of osteonecrosis. MRI is very important in the assessment of possible osteonecrosis of the hip in being able to detect osteonecrosis prior to femoral head collapse and also showing the size and position of any osteonecrotic segment. Surgical intervention may be considered in the early stages to help prevent articular collapse.
6. Ankle – osteochondral lesions. Tendon (e.g. Achilles and tibialis posterior) and ligament injuries.

7. Wrist – tears of the triangular fibrocartilage complex and intercarpal ligaments. Evaluation of the carpal tunnel. Assessment of osteonecrosis of the lunate.
8. Temporomandibular joints – evaluation of internal disc derangements. MRI is considered to be the current procedure of choice to image the temporomandibular joint.
9. Occult fractures (e.g. femoral neck stress fractures).
10. Evaluation of bony and soft-tissue tumours and marrow infiltrating disorders. Very important in the staging of bone tumours.

The very high cost of this technology has limited the widespread use of MRI.

MRI competes with arthroscopy in the evaluation of internal derangements of the joints, especially the knee, and to a lesser extent the shoulder. Arthroscopy is invasive and requires a general anaesthetic but has the potential advantage of being able to perform certain therapeutic procedures (e.g. repair of a torn knee meniscus) at the same time.

Advantages

- Superb anatomic detail because of the high intrinsic contrast resolution, especially of soft-tissue structures allowing visualization of all the articular and periarticular structures such as cartilage, tendons, ligaments and bone marrow as well as the spinal cord and nerve roots. MRI has the best overall soft-tissue resolution of any imaging modality.
- Very sensitive in the detection of disease.
- Can image directly in any plane (multiplanar). Sagittal images are very useful in the spine.
- Non-invasive.
- No known harmful biological effect (does not utilize ionizing radiation).

Disadvantages

- High cost
- Limited availability at present
- Bony abnormality and small areas of calcification are not as well shown as with plain films or CT
- Abnormalities may lack specificity for a particular disease process (e.g. tendinosis versus a partial tendon tear)

- Metallic objects in the body may present a hazard, e.g.:
  (1) clips on a cerebral aneurysm (may twist off)
  (2) cardiac pacemakers
  (3) metallic foreign bodies in the eyes
  The metal implants used in orthopaedics (e.g. prosthetic joints and internal fixation devices) are generally safe as they are solidly fixed to bone – they cause focal signal loss, but generally less artifact than with CT
- Claustrophobia – the person has to lie in a narrow tunnel
- Clinicians may be unfamiliar with MRI images and radiologist expertise may be limited as MRI is a relatively new imaging modality.

Myelography

Myelography involves injecting water-soluble contrast into the subarachnoid space via a spinal puncture (lumbar or cervical). Contrast fills the subarachnoid space of the thecal sac and nerve root sleeves and so outlines the contour of the thecal sac, nerve roots and spinal cord. Standard radiographs are then taken and any displacement or compression of these neural structures can be assessed. Compressed nerve roots often appear swollen.

Advantages

- Moderately high accuracy in diagnosis of compression of the spinal cord and/or nerve roots. However, the accuracy of lumbosacral disc herniation is not as good as at other levels as the nerve roots may be separated from the disc by plentiful epidural fat.
- Very good spatial resolution, and a single image covers the entire region, showing all of the neural structures at once, facilitating comparison.
- Image format is familiar to clinicians and the images are usually straightforward to interpret.

Disadvantages

- Invasive procedure. With modern contrast agents and fine-gauge needles, significant adverse reactions such as headache, nausea, vomiting, seizures and arachnoiditis are rare.

- Lacks some specificity. It can be difficult to tell the exact nature of a compressing structure (e.g. disc or bone). Postmyelography CT is often utilized to make this distinction. Also, following back surgery, it is difficult to differentiate epidural fibrosis versus recurrent disc herniation. MRI (with gadolinium) is very helpful in these circumstances.

- Nerve root sleeves may not fill with contrast (e.g. arachnoiditis following prior surgery) and so assessment of nerve root compression is very difficult. CT and MRI are useful in these circumstances.

- Far lateral disc herniations are not usually shown. These make up approximately 12% of disc herniations. Nerve root compression occurs at the exit foramen or just beyond and as the nerve root sleeve does not extend out this far, myelography often fails to demonstrate these foraminal disc herniations. However, they are well demonstrated by CT and MRI.

To improve the diagnostic accuracy of myelography, CT is frequently performed shortly after the myelogram.

Discography

This invasive procedure uses X-ray guidance to place a needle directly into the nucleus pulposus of the intervertebral disc and then a small volume of contrast is injected directly into the disc. Usually two or three discs are evaluated. There are two parts to the examination:

1. an image (plain film or CT) of the disc architecture to show (a) any disruption of the nucleus pulposus or (b) ruptures of the annulus fibrosis where disc herniations can occur
2. provocative – to see if the person's usual symptoms are reproduced when the disc volume is increased by the contrast injection.

With the advent of non-invasive methods to assess disc degeneration and herniation such as MRI and CT, discography is only infrequently performed now, although the procedure has a small but enthusiastic following, mainly for the value of the provocative part of the study. Discography can be helpful in localizing the symptomatic disc

herniation prior to surgery when there is herniation at more than one level.

Radionuclide bone scan

This involves an intravenous injection of a radio-actively tagged substance (tracer) which localizes in bony and joint tissue (usually 99 m-technetium-labelled methyldiphosphonate (MDP)). The scan detects altered physiology by concentrating in areas of increased vascularity and areas of increased bone turnover. The emitted radiation is recorded by a gamma-camera adjacent to the body. The whole body is imaged with spot views of the regions of interest. Cross-sectional images (SPECT – single-photon emission computed tomography) are possible with a special rotating gamma-camera device. This allows more exact localization of abnormalities in the bone (e.g. vertebral pedicle (suggests malignancy) versus facet joint (suggests degenerative disease) versus pars defect (suggests symptomatic spondylolysis)).

The modern technique, which improves specificity, involves a triple phase study with: (1) images immediately following injection showing blood flow; (2) blood pool images at 10 min detecting areas of abnormal vascularity in the soft tissues; and (3) delayed images (2–3 h after injection) demonstrating areas of increased bone uptake ('hot') or occasionally areas of decreased bone uptake ('cold') when a lesion fails to stimulate osteoblastic activity (e.g. myeloma) or the blood supply is compromised (e.g. osteonecrosis).

Role

Clinical applications include:

1. Evaluation of bone pain when plain films are normal (e.g. stress fractures, shin splints, infection, tumour)
2. Infection:
   (a) to detect early osteomyelitis – plain films may take up to 10 days to show any abnormality
   (b) cellulitis versus osteomyelitis – delayed images do not show increased bony uptake with cellulitis alone
   (c) reactivation of chronic osteomyelitis.
3. To screen for bony metastases – can demonstrate metastases before any plain film

changes. Unreliable in multiple myeloma as the lesions may not stimulate osteoblastic activity.

4. To help characterize bone tumours. A lesion without increased uptake is usually considered benign. However, some benign lesions can show increased uptake.
5. Evaluation of the painful joint prosthesis – helping to differentiate mechanical loosening from infective loosening. Indium-labelled leukocytes or gallium may be used in addition to MDP as they are more specific for infection.
6. To assess the activity and distribution of arthritis (e.g. rheumatoid arthritis) and metabolic bone disease (e.g. Paget's disease).
7. Assessment of osteonecrosis – useful in early detection to help identify areas of vascular compromise ('cold'). However, MRI is superior in this respect. Increased tracer uptake occurs in the repair and revascularization stages.

Advantages

- High sensitivity – will detect bony abnormalities before any plain film changes
- Whole body imaged
- Widely available
- Low to moderate cost

Disadvantages

- Relatively non-specific. The bone scan is good for localizing an abnormality but further imaging is usually required to define the exact nature of the abnormality
- Spatial resolution not as good as other modalities
- May be difficult to detect abnormalities in regions with a normally high bone turnover (e.g. growing epiphyses, sacroiliac joints)
- Moderate radiation dose.

Arthrography

This specialized procedure evaluates internal derangements of joints by injecting a contrast agent into a joint followed by a radiographic examination. The contrast may be: (1) positive (water-soluble iodine containing compound); (2) negative (air); or, more commonly; (3) a combination of both (double contrast). Using X-ray guidance (fluoroscopy) a needle is placed into the joint followed by injection

of the contrast agent(s). In experienced hands the procedure is relatively straightforward and minimally invasive with few adverse effects. The most common complaint is aggravation of joint pain.

The radiographic examination to follow can involve plain films, CT or digital subtraction techniques. Currently, MR arthrography is being evaluated, especially in the shoulder. The MR contrast agent gadolinium is injected into the joint followed by an MRI examination. Its role is yet to be fully defined, but the multiplanar capability and superb soft-tissue resolution may be distinct advantages.

With the introduction of sophisticated non-invasive and radiation-free imaging techniques such as ultrasound and MRI, and the widespread use of arthroscopy (especially in the knee), there has been a substantial decrease in the utilization of arthrography. However, arthrography still has a place in certain clinical situations and is often the 'gold standard' against which the accuracy of other imaging techniques is measured.

Role

Clinical indications could include:

Shoulder

- Evaluation of instability (performed in conjunction with CT)
- Rotator cuff tears
- Adhesive capsulitis (frozen shoulder).

Knee

- Meniscal tears. High accuracy in the diagnosis of meniscal tears but now has been largely replaced by MRI and arthroscopy which are able to make a more comprehensive evaluation of the knee joint
- Cystic masses about the knee – to determine if they communicate with the knee joint (e.g. popliteal (Baker's) cyst)
- Osteochondral lesions and intra-articular loose bodies
- To evaluate possible loosening of a knee joint arthroplasty.

Wrist

- To evaluate tears of the triangular fibrocartilage and intercarpal and capsular ligaments.

Hip

- Evaluation of a painful prosthesis for possible loosening. When loose, contrast may track down in the interface between the prosthesis or cement and the bone (subtraction technique required)
- Congential hip dislocation. To show the exact position of the unossified femoral head within the acetabulum and whether the limbus is everted, preventing reduction. Largely replaced by ultrasound now.

Ankle

- Osteochondral lesions
- Loose bodies within the joint cavity
- Ligamentous tears.

Elbow

- Osteochondral lesions
- Intra-articular loose bodies (often in conjunction with CT).

Temporomandibular joints

- To evaluate disc dysfunction (e.g. dislocating disc). Dynamic assessment of disc dysfunction with opening and closing of the mouth can be provided with videofluorography.

EXAMINATION BY PLAIN FILM RADIOGRAPHY – STANDARD AND SUPPLEMENTARY VIEWS

We will now discuss the plain film examination of the spine, pelvis and peripheral joints. The various projections included in a standard radiographic examination of each region will be discussed. The standard views will provide an adequate evaluation in the large majority of cases. Supplementary views are also discussed which are performed only on request to evaluate a specific clinical problem.

Cervical spine

Standard views

Frontal (anteroposterior: AP)

- demonstrates C3–C7: C1 and C2 are obscured by overlying structures. Shows the vertebral bodies, disc spaces, uncovertebral joints, spinous

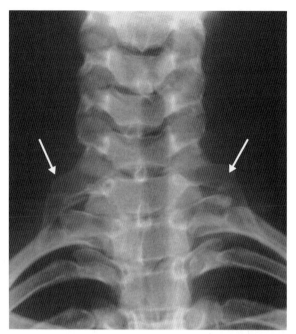

Figure 3.1 Cervical ribs. Cervical spine: frontal view. The transverse processes of C7 are elongated and shaped like miniature ribs (arrows). They may compress the neurovascular structures of the thoracic outlet.

processes (in profile), any supernumerary (cervical) rib (Fig. 3.1) and frontal alignment.

Lateral (neutral position)

- Shows the vertebral bodies, disc spaces, spinal canal, spinous processes and lateral alignment (normally a mild lordosis is present). The cervicothoracic junction may not be adequately seen due to the overlapping shoulders.

Oblique (left and right at 45°)

- The intervertebral foramina (where the nerve roots exit) are profiled. The articular pillars, facet joints and pedicles are well shown. Note: The labelling of oblique films refers only to the side of the body. The neuroforamina in profile are the same as the side of the occiput.

Supplementary views

Flexion and extension (lateral)

- to assess motion between the segments. Useful when instability is suspected (e.g. following trauma or in rheumatoid arthritis

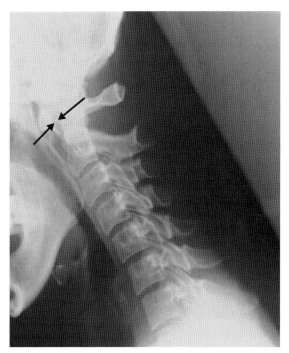

Figure 3.2 Atlantoaxial subluxation (rheumatoid arthritis). Lateral view of the cervical spine with flexion shows an abnormally widened pre-dens space (arrows). This narrows the spinal canal and cord compression may occur.

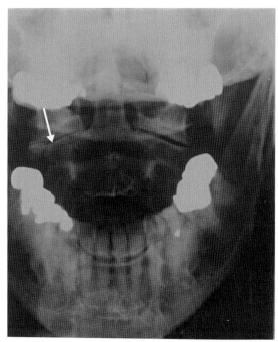

Figure 3.3 Osteoarthritis: atlantoaxial joint (arrow). Frontal view of C1 and C2 ('peg' view) showing loss of joint space, subchondral sclerosis and marginal osteophytes.

where important atlantoaxial subluxation may occur; Fig. 3.2). The space between the back of the anterior arch of the atlas and the front of the dens (pre-dens space) on the lateral view should not be greater than 2.5 mm. Any subluxation will be accentuated on the flexion view.

Odontoid ('peg') view

- frontal view of C1 and C2 with the mouth open. Utilized mainly in trauma to show any fracture of the odontoid process (dens) of C2 and to assess alignment between the lateral masses of C1 and C2 (Fig. 3.3).

'Swimmer's' view

- to show the cervicothoracic junction when this is not adequately demonstrated on the standard lateral view.

Note: The atlanto-occipital joint is not ideally shown with plain films due to overlapping structures. When specific evaluation of this joint is

required MRI, CT or conventional tomography may be utilized.

Thoracic spine

Standard views

Frontal (AP)

- Shows the vertebral bodies, disc spaces and frontal alignment. The pedicles and spinous processes are shown in profile.

Lateral

- Shows the vertebral bodies, disc spaces, posterior elements and lateral alignment (normally a mild kyphosis is present). The cervicothoracic junction and upper thoracic vertebrae are usually not well shown due to the overlying shoulders. When assessment of this area is required, a 'swimmer's' view or conventional tomography may be utilized. If the thoracolumbar junction is of particular interest (e.g. ankylosing spondylitis), frontal and lateral views centred to this region are helpful.

Lumbosacral spine

Standard views

Frontal (AP)

● Shows the vertebral bodies, disc spaces, transverse processes and frontal alignment. The pedicles, spinous processes and often the facet joints are all shown in profile.

Lateral

● Shows the disc spaces, vertebral bodies, spinal canal, spinous processes and lateral alignment (normally a mild lordosis is present). In addition, a coned view of the lumbosacral junction is performed.

Oblique (left and right at 45°)

● To optimize the evaluation of the posterior elements, especially the pars regions and facet joints.

Supplementary views

Functional views (standing) To demonstrate abnormal spinal movement (e.g. segmental instability as may occur with degenerative disease of the spine).

1. Lateral views with flexion and extension. Checked for:
   (a) forward or backward displacement of one vertebra upon another
   (b) abrupt change in the length of the pedicles
   (c) foraminal narrowing
   (d) loss of disc height
2. Optional – frontal views with lateral bending to the left and then to the right. Checked for:
   (a) asymmetry in bending
   (b) loss of normal vertebral rotation and tilt
   (c) abnormal opening or closure of disc spaces
   (d) lateral translation
   (e) malalignment of spinous processes and pedicles.

There is some controversy regarding the clinical utility of these views. They should be ordered with discretion as the radiation dose is moderate.

Note: Plain films of the spinal region may be performed either recumbent or erect. Spinal curvatures should be assessed with erect views.

Pelvis

Standard view

Frontal (AP)

● centred to include the lumbosacral junction and hip joints.

Supplementary view

'Flamingo' views for instability

● to demonstrate ligamentous instability of the symphysis pubis–sacroiliac joint complex, as can occur in athletes. Frontal views are obtained while standing on one leg, then the other leg. A difference in the height between the superior pubic rami of greater than 2 mm or widening of the symphysis beyond 10 mm is considered abnormal (Fig. 3.4a, b).

Sacrum and coccyx

Standard views

Frontal (angulated)

● the sacrum may not be ideally visualized on a frontal view of the pelvis and a coned angled view is useful when the sacrum is of clinical interest.

Lateral

● provides a lateral view of the sacrum and coccyx.

Sacroiliac joints

Standard views

Frontal pelvis – as described above.

Frontal pelvis (AP with angulation)

● X-ray beam is angulated 30° towards the head which provides a better profile of the joints. Both joints are included on a single view to facilitate comparison.

Note: Oblique views of the sacroiliac joints are not recommended as they are technically difficult to perform and are usually non-contributory to an assessment of sacroiliitis.

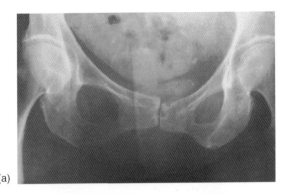

(a)

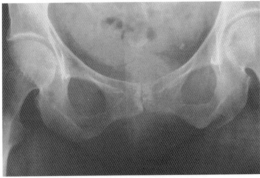

(b)

Figure 3.4a,b Osteitis pubis: 'flamingo' views. (a) standing on right leg and (b) standing on left leg. There is subchondral erosion and sclerosis of the symphysis pubis. Instability is demonstrated when standing on the right leg, where there is a greater than 2 mm difference in height between the superior pubic rami.

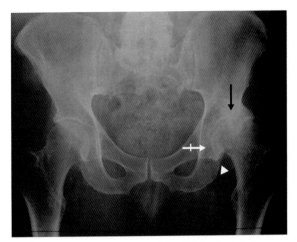

Figure 3.5 Osteoarthritis: hip joint. Pelvis: frontal view. The left hip joint shows complete loss of joint space in the weight-bearing superolateral portion of the joint with subchondral sclerosis and subchondral cyst formation (black arrow). There are prominent osteophytes at the joint margins superiorly. In addition, there is a large central osteophyte arising from the femoral head (hatched arrow) – these can form when there is lateral subluxation of the femoral head. Note also the buttressing of the medial cortex of the femoral neck (arrowhead).

Hip

Standard views

Frontal pelvis (AP)

- allows comparison with opposite hip (Fig. 3.5).

Lateral hip ('frog leg' position)

- provides a true lateral view of the femoral head and neck, but not of the acetabulum. In trauma, when the hip cannot be comfortably moved, a true lateral view (cross-table) of the femoral head and acetabulum is performed.

Supplementary views

Orthopaedic pelvis

- prior to and following hip joint replacement a low-centred frontal view of the pelvis is performed so that the entire prosthesis is included on a single film. An assessment of any leg-length discrepancy can also be made.

Oblique (anterior and posterior at 45° – 'Judet')

- these visualize the bony columns of the pelvis and the anterior and posterior acetabular rims. These views may be useful following fracture/dislocation of the acetabulum, although CT is superior in this respect.

Knee

Standard views

Frontal (AP with knee fully extended)

- shows the distal femur, patella, proximal tibia, joint space in the lateral and medial compartments and femorotibial alignment.

Lateral (20–35° of knee flexion)

- assesses patellar height and shows any joint effusions. A cross-table (decubitus) lateral view is performed in acute trauma to show the presence of any fat-fluid level which would suggest intra-articular fracture.

Patella (axial view – 'skyline')

- profiles the patellofemoral joint. Shows the morphology of the joint surfaces and patellar alignment. The preferred technique is that of Merchant with 40° of knee flexion. Skyline views of the patellofemoral joint with 30°, 60° and 90° of knee flexion for assessment of patellar tracking are not recommended as most abnormalities occur with knee flexion of 30° or less. CT and MRI are far superior in the assessment of patellar tracking.

Supplementary views

Frontal (weight-bearing)

- utilized in the evaluation of osteoarthritis of the femorotibial compartments of the knee joint. Weight-bearing on the affected side allows a more accurate assessment of the loss of cartilage space and resulting angular (usually varus) deformity (Fig. 3.6). Alternatively, a long film with weight-bearing which includes the hip and ankle joints may be utilized to allow measurement of the angular deformity along the mechanical axis of the leg as part of the preoperative work-up prior to osteotomy or total knee joint arthroplasty.

Oblique (left and right at 45°)

- useful in trauma when the standard views are normal and a joint effusion is present, to help show subtle fractures of the tibial plateaus and femoral condyles. Also allows evaluation of the proximal fibula and superior tibiofibular joint.

Intercondylar ('tunnel') view

- to show the intercondylar notch. Gives a better view of the joint surfaces of the femoral condyles, tibial plateaus and the tibial spines. Useful in demonstrating osteochondral lesions of femoral condyles and cruciate avulsion fractures.

Stress views

- infrequently utilized. Can demonstrate ligamentous instability – medial, lateral, anterior or posterior – by applying manual stress in the appropriate direction.

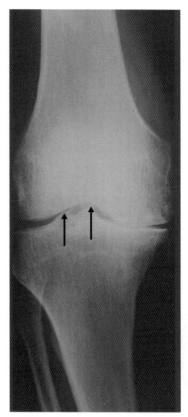

Figure 3.6 Osteoarthritis: knee joint. Frontal view weight-bearing. The weight-bearing medial femorotibial compartment demonstrates almost complete loss of articular space, subchondral sclerosis and osteophytic enlargement of the tibial spines (arrows). There is mild loss of bone stock of the medial tibial plateau and a mild varus deformity.

Ankle

Standard views

Frontal (AP)

- shows the joint surfaces (tibial plafond and talar dome), joint spaces and the malleoli.

Oblique ('mortise' view – with 15–20° of internal rotation of the foot)

- opens up the joint space to give a better profile of the ankle joint, especially medially, the inferior tibiofibular syndesmosis and the inferior tip of the lateral malleolus.

Lateral

- to show the distal tibia, talus, calcaneus and Achilles tendon. Allows assessment of any joint effusion.

Supplementary views

Stress views

- with acute twisting injuries of the ankle when plain films have excluded a fracture and ligament or tendon injury is suspected, stress views may help to demonstrate instability. Stress views may also be helpful in cases of chronic instability. Comparison is made between the injured and normal sides as the degree of ankle joint laxity is variable. For medial (deltoid) and lateral ligament injuries frontal views are taken with manually applied eversion or inversion stress respectively. Any abnormal widening (greater than 5°) of the ankle joint mortise (talar tilt) compared to the normal side suggests instability. Stress views are contraindicated in children with open growth plates.

Axial view of calcaneus

- useful in suspected calcaneal fractures.

CT is utilized for the assessment of intra-articular calcaneal fractures.

Subtalar joints

- Not ideally assessed by plain film radiography

Note: These joints are best assessed with coronal CT (e.g. tarsal coalition).

Shoulder

Standard views

Frontal (external and internal rotation)

- to evaluate the glenohumeral and acromioclavicular joints. The external rotation view is performed obliquely so as to give a true frontal profile of the glenohumeral joint and a true frontal view of the scapula. This view also profiles the greater tuberosity and is useful for detecting calcification in the supraspinatus tendon (Fig. 3.7). The internal rotation view is useful for detecting

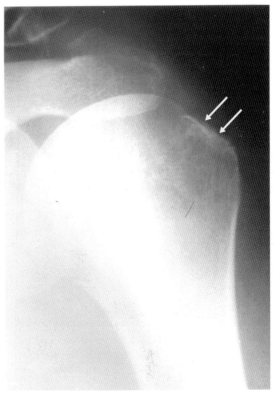

Figure 3.7 Calcific tendinitis. Shoulder: frontal view with external rotation. Calcification is present in the distal portion of the supraspinatus tendon (arrows) adjacent to the greater tuberosity of the humerus.

calcification in the remaining cuff tendons and viewing the acromioclavicular joint.

Lateral (transscapular Y-view)

- to assess alignment of the humeral head in the glenoid fossa and so is important in trauma. Does not profile the glenohumeral joint but demonstrates the coracoacromial arch.

Lateral (axillary projection)

- gives a true lateral view of the glenohumeral joint and shows glenohumeral alignment, but is difficult to obtain with acute trauma as some shoulder abduction is required.

Supplementary views

Supplementary views are generally indicated to identify anterior instability or impingement/ rotator cuff problems.

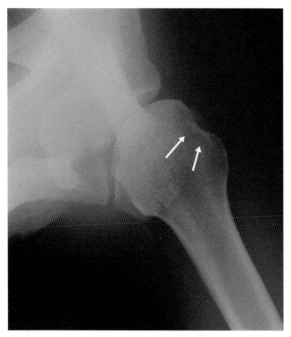

Figure 3.8 Hill–Sachs lesion. Shoulder: Stryker notch view. There is a large osteochondral defect from the posterolateral aspect of the humeral head (arrows) – proof of prior anterior dislocation.

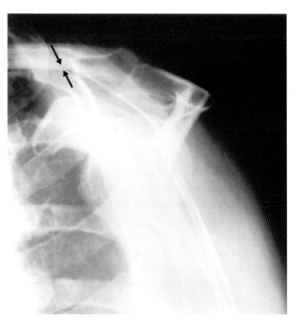

Figure 3.9 Subacromial impingement. Frontal view with caudal angulation and supraspinatus outlet view. There is a traction spur (arrows) arising from the undersurface of the anterior acromion which can impinge upon the rotator cuff leading to tendinitis and cuff tear. The greater tuberosity of the humerus is flattened and sclerotic as a result of mechanical impaction with the acromion when the shoulder is abducted.

Views used in anterior instability:

1. Two traumatic chondro-osseous lesions which are not reliably shown on standard views are a marker for anterior instability.
   (a) *Stryker notch view* gives the best view of a Hill–Sachs lesion – an osteochondral impaction fracture of the posterolateral humeral head (Fig. 3.8).
   (b) *West Point axillary view* gives the best view of a Bankart lesion (osseous type) – an osteochondral fracture or periostitis of the anteroinferior glenoid rim.

2. Views used in impingement and rotator cuff problems to demonstrate anterior subacromial and acromioclavicular joint spurs.
   (a) *Supraspinatus outlet view* – profiles the coracoacromial arch (Y-view with 20° caudal angulation and weight-bearing) showing the morphology and the presence of any spurs of the anterior undersurface of the acromion (Fig. 3.9).

   (b) *Frontal view with 30° caudal angulation* – to show spurs projecting inferiorly from the undersurface of the anterior acromion and acromioclavicular joint.

Acromioclavicular joint

Standard views

Frontal (angulated)

- the standard frontal view of the shoulder shows the acromioclavicular joint, but a better profile of the joint is obtained with the X-ray beam angulated 15° towards the head.

Supplementary views

Stress views (weight-bearing)

- these may be necessary to diagnose and grade traumatic separation of the acromioclavicular–coracoclavicular complex when the standard view is normal. Weights are hung from both wrists (not held in the hands) and a single film is taken to demonstrate both joints to facilitate comparison. Assessment is made of (1) the width of the acromioclavicular joint and (2) the distance between the upper tip of the coracoid process and the adjacent undersurface of the clavicle which is indicative of coracoclavicular ligament disruption when there is a 5 mm or greater increase in coracoclavicular distance.

Sternoclavicular joints

- adequate plain film views are difficult to obtain and they are often non-diagnostic. CT is the preferred examination to assess subluxation, dislocation, erosion and hyperostosis.

Elbow

Standard views

Frontal (AP with the elbow joint extended and the hand in full supination)

- shows the distal humerus including the epicondyles, proximal radius and ulna, and the joint spaces.

Lateral (90° of elbow flexion)

- provides a lateral view of the distal humerus and proximal forearm. The olecranon process is well shown. Joint effusion can be assessed by displacement of fat pads.

Supplementary views

1. In the case of trauma when a joint effusion is demonstrated but no fracture is seen on the stand-ard views, the following views may be helpful to show minimally displaced fractures of the radial head, capitellum and coranoid process:
   (a) *oblique (lateral and medial)*
   (b) *radial head – capitellum view* – eliminates overlap of the humeroulnar and humeroradial joints (radial head is projected anterior to coronoid process)

2. Further views may be helpful in showing osteophytes from the humeroulnar joint, loose

bodies in the space between the olecranon process and capitellum and periarticular calcifications:
   (a) *axial view* (elbow flexed 45°) provides an axial view of the olecranon process and profiles the epicondyles.

Wrist

Standard views

Frontal (PA)

- shows the radiocarpal and intercarpal joints, carpal arcs (proximal and distal rows of carpal bones) and any ulnar variance (ulna shorter or longer than the radius).

Lateral (neutral position)

- important in assessing axial alignment for various instability patterns that can follow ligamentous injury.

Oblique (semipronated and semisupinated)

- to show the ulnar and radial aspects of the carpus respectively.

Supplementary views

Scaphoid views

- to enhance fracture detection.

Stress views

- may be useful when carpal instability is suspected following ligamentous injury (e.g. scapholunate dissociation, dorsal and volar instability, or ulnar translocation of the carpus):
   1. Frontal views with ulnar and radial deviation
   2. Lateral views with palmarflexion and dorsiflexion
   3. Frontal view with a clenched fist (gripview) – accentuates potential scapholunate dissociation by loading the capitate on to the proximal carpal row.

Carpal tunnel view

- to demonstrate the osseous structures of the carpal tunnel, including the hook of the hamate.

Note: The soft-tissue structures of the carpal tunnel are much better evaluated with ultrasound or MRI.

Distal radioulnar joint

- Subluxation or dislocation of this joint is not reliably demonstrated on plain films and, when indicated, CT should be used to assess alignment or instability of this joint.

CLINICAL PROBLEMS AND THEIR EVALUATION USING IMAGING TECHNIQUES

We have chosen topics to discuss which are both common and likely to be of interest to the physiotherapist. The clinical background is presented along with the various imaging modalities that may be utilized, a description of the imaging findings and, finally, clinical correlation of signs and symptoms.

Spinal and pelvic problems

The taking of spinal and pelvic radiographs using the views described is only one aspect of a clinical examination. In isolation, standard radiographs are rarely indicative of appropriate management. They do, however, serve a very useful role in excluding unsuspected important disease and mechanical deformity. Most persons attending for physiotherapy for spinal pain have normal films or ones that show degenerative disease of the spine. It is important for the practitioner to have an appreciation of some of the more common abnormalities of the axial skeleton seen on imaging studies.

Degenerative disease of the spine

Also referred to as osteoarthritis and spondylosis, degenerative disease of the spine encompasses a variety of distinct and separate disease processes of the spine. Most commonly it is primary (or idiopathic), but it may be secondary to trauma, an underlying arthritis (e.g. rheumatoid arthritis) or infection.

Degeneration of the intervertebral disc This involves two separate entities:

1. Intervertebral osteochondrosis – where the chondromucoid elements of the nucleus pulposus decrease, with resultant dehydration and

loss of viscoelasticity of the disc. The radiographic changes include (Fig. 3.10):
   (a) loss of disc height
   (b) gas within the disc space – the so-called vacuum phenomenon – due to gas (approximately 90% nitrogen) collecting within the clefts of a degenerating disc (Fig. 3.11)
   (c) sclerosis of the vertebral body endplates adjacent to the disc
   (d) loss of the normal cervical or lumbar lordosis
   (e) disc calcification – usually localized to one or two discs in the mid thoracic and upper lumbar spine.

2. Spondylosis deformans – the formation of bony outgrowths (osteophytes) from the vertebral body margin at the site of the ligamentous attachment of the disc. This is thought to result from the breakdown of the outer fibres of the annulus fibrosus which allows disc material to stress the ligamentous attachment. Radiographically, the osteophytes first appear horizontally from the vertebral body margin and then tend to curve vertically and may eventually bridge the disc space in an attempt to stabilize the spine. In the cervical spine osteophytes from the posterior vertebral margin can form an osteophytic bar which may compress the adjacent spinal cord.

Osteoarthritis of the zygapophyseal (facet) joints This is often a sequela of degeneration of the disc which allows excessive stress of these joints but, occasionally, osteoarthritis can predominate in these joints with little or no radiographic change in the discs. Clinical features of facet joint disease include local pain on palpation over the facet joint and back pain which may radiate and mimic sciatica. Radiographic features include (Figs 3.10 and 3.11):

1. joint space narrowing
2. subchondral sclerosis
3. osteophytosis.

The osteophytes may be of clinical importance as they may:

1. hypertrophy the facet joints and contribute to stenosis in the spinal canal (Fig. 3.11)
2. project into the nerve root canals (lateral recess (Fig. 3.12) or exit foramen (Fig. 3.13)) where they may impinge upon nerve roots

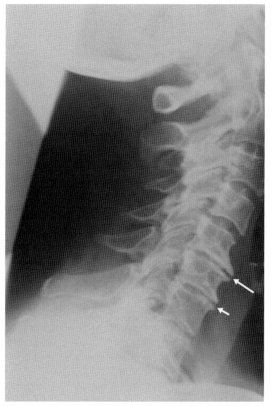 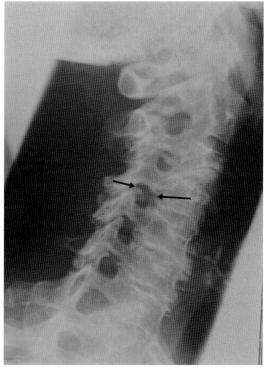

(a)   (b)

Figure 3.10a,b Degenerative disease of the cervical spine. Cervical spine: (a) lateral and (b) oblique views. The C5–C6 (long arrow in (a)) and C6–C7 (short arrow in (a)) discovertebral joints are narrowed with subchondral sclerosis and osteophytes at the vertebral body margin. There is also involvement of the facet joints and uncovertebral joints. The oblique view shows osteophytes (arrows) projecting into the neuroforamina where they may cause nerve root compression.

3. project into the foramen transversarium (cervical spine only) where they may impinge upon the vertebral artery. This is rare.

Uncovertebral (neurocentral) joint arthrosis These are small synovial joints located at the posterolateral margins of the vertebral bodies C3–C7 which commonly degenerate when they are impacted with the loss of disc height that occurs with disc degeneration. X-rays show (Fig. 3.14):

1. rounding off of the uncinate process
2. narrowing of joint space
3. osteophytes which may project into the neuroforamina and cause nerve root compression (assessed on the oblique views). It is thought that the neuroforamina need to

be narrowed by at least 50% to be clinically significant.

Complications of degenerative spinal disease
Alterations of vertebral alignment

1. Segmental instability – see discussion under Functional views of lumbosacral spine, above
2. Degenerative spondylolisthesis.

Slippage of one vertebra upon another (spondylolisthesis) is commonly seen in the degenerative spine. It is due to subluxation of osteoarthritic facet joints and is most commonly seen in the mobile segments of the cervical and lumbar spine (e.g. C5–C6, C6–C7, L3–L4, L4–L5). Two patterns occur: (1) anterolisthesis, due to anterior slippage of the upper vertebra (Fig. 3.15); or (2) retrolisthesis, due

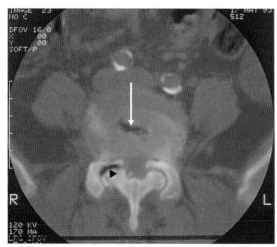

Figure 3.11 Degenerative spinal stenosis. Axial computed tomography scan through the L4–L5 disc space. The central spinal canal is narrowed as a result of a bulging disc, osteophytic facet joint hypertrophy and ligamenta flava hypertrophy. Compression of the nerve roots lying within the thecal sac may occur. Note the gas (vacuum phenomenon) in the degenerative disc (arrow) and right facet joint (arrowhead).

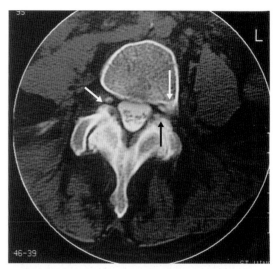

Figure 3.13 Foraminal stenosis. Computed tomography myelogram: axial scan below the pedicles of L4. Osteophytes from the posterior vertebral body margin (long white arrow) and the facet joint (black arrow) narrow the left L4 exit foramen and nerve root compression (short white arrow) may occur.

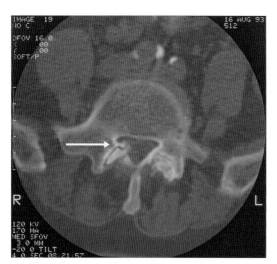

Figure 3.12 Lateral recess stenosis. Computed tomography axial scan through the pedicles of L5. Osteophytes from the facet joint project into the lateral recess where they may compress the right L5 nerve root (arrow).

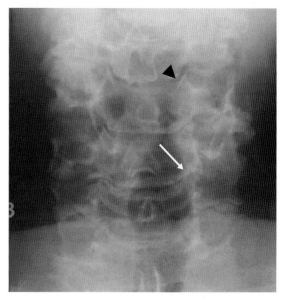

Figure 3.14 Uncovertebral joint osteoarthrosis. There is loss of joint space, rounding off and osteophytic enlargement of the uncovertebral joints (arrow). A normal joint (arrowhead) is shown for comparison.

to posterior slippage of the upper vertebra. In both instances the spinal canal is narrowed as a result, contributing to spinal stenosis, but the slip may be asymptomatic. This is to be contrasted with the situation of spondylolisthesis associated with pars defects (lytic spondylolisthesis) where the spinal canal is widened and stretching of the nerve roots can occur.

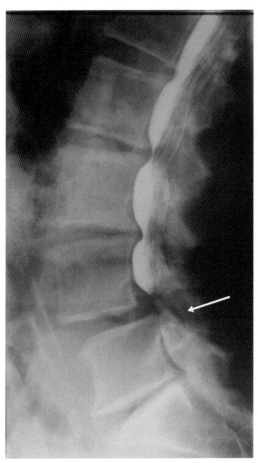

Figure 3.15 Degenerative spinal stenosis. Myelogram: lateral view. (For frontal view, see Fig. 3.18.) There is multilevel spinal stenosis compressing the thecal sac. This is most marked at the L4–L5 level where a degenerative spondylolisthesis further narrows the spinal canal (arrow).

Intervertebral disc herniation and spinal stenosis
Plain films cannot directly show the spinal cord, cerebrospinal fluid, thecal sac, nerve roots or herniated discs (except in the rare instance of a calcified disc herniation). Due to the very close anatomical relationships disc herniation and spinal stenosis may cause spinal cord compression (myelopathy) or nerve root compression (radiculopathy) and when this is suspected clinically on the basis of symptoms and objective neurological findings other imaging modalities such as CT (Fig. 3.16), MRI (Fig. 3.17) and myelography (Fig. 3.18) are utilized. Surgical intervention may be considered in these patients and accurate radiological diagnosis is mandatory.

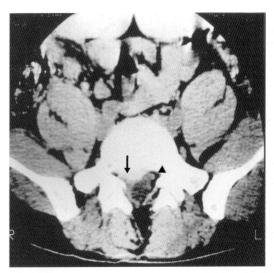

Figure 3.16 Intervertebral disc herniation. Axial computed tomography scan through the L4–L5 disc shows focal left-sided paracentral herniation which can compress the left L5 nerve root as it leaves the thecal sac (arrow). There is also degenerative facet joint hypertrophy. The normal right side is shown (arrowhead).

Intervertebral disc herniation   Disc material which is displaced posteriorly, posterolaterally or laterally can be very important clinically due to potential compression of the spinal cord and/or nerve roots. The extent of the disc displacement is described by the following terms:

1. Bulging annulus – here the annular fibres remain intact but protrude in a diffuse pattern into the spinal canal.

2. Disc protrusion (or prolapse) – the nucleus pulposus protrudes focally through some of the fibres of the annulus fibrosus but is still contained by intact outer fibres.

3. Disc extrusion – when the nucleus pulposus extrudes through all the fibres of the annulus fibrosus, but remains confined by the posterior longitudinal ligament.

4. Disc sequestration – where the herniated disc material penetrates the posterior longitudinal ligament and lies free in the epidural space, or a separated disc fragment migrates superiorly or inferiorly beyond the disc space beneath the posterior longitudinal ligament.

Figure 3.17 Lumbar disc herniation. Magnetic resonance imaging scan: sagittal section. T_1-weighted (left) and T_2-weighted (right) images. There is a paracentral herniation of the L4–L5 disc (arrows) compressing the L5 nerve root as it leaves the thecal sac. The loss of signal in the L4–L5 disc on the T_2 image reflects the dehydration seen with disc degeneration.

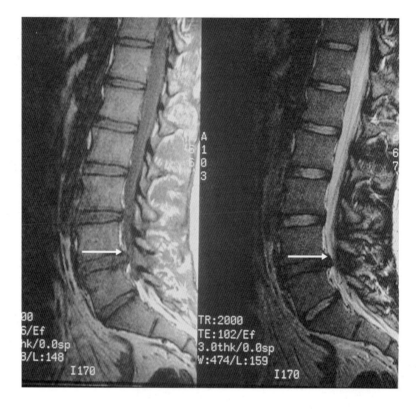

Disc protrusion, extrusion and sequestration are all types of herniation of the nucleus pulposus. Imaging cannot usually distinguish disc protrusion versus extrusion. Posterolateral (or paracentral) disc herniation is the most common pattern (Fig. 3.16) which is thought to be due to the fewer and weaker annular fibres in this region. Less commonly, nerve root compression may occur at the exit foramen (foraminal disc herniation) when a far lateral disc herniation migrates upwards (Fig. 3.19). A combination of paracentral and lateral disc can compress two separate nerve roots.

Spinal stenosis   Stenosis in the central spinal canal is due to a combination of bony and soft-tissue factors such as disc bulging, osteophytes from the posterior vertebral body margin, facet joint and ligamentum flavum hypertrophy and spondylolisthesis (Figs 3.11 and 3.15), often on a background of a developmentally small canal. It often occurs at multiple levels and can produce significant compression of the thecal sac and its contents. In the lumbar spine, spinal stenosis can produce the clinical syndrome of intermittent neurogenic claudication (activity-related pain and weakness in the legs) whereas in the cervical spine limb weakness and hyperreflexia may occur.

Stenosis may also occur in: (1) the lateral recess (Fig. 3.12) or exit foramen (Fig. 3.13) of the nerve root canals of the lumbar spine, usually due to adjacent facet joint osteophytes; or (2) the nerve root canal in the cervical spine, usually due to uncovertebral joint osteophytes (Figs 3.10 and 3.14). In both instances compression or entrapment of the nerve roots may occur.

Degenerative disease of the spine predominates in the weight-bearing mid and lower segments of the cervical, thoracic and lumbar spine. Degenerative changes in the thoracic segments are seldom of clinical significance as compression of the neural structures at this site is unusual.

The diagnostic accuracy of MRI and CT and myelography for disc herniation and spinal stenosis is about equal. Individual practice will vary with the preference and experience of the radiologist and the availability of MRI. Most patients with suspected disc herniation or spinal stenosis will be screened non-invasively with CT or MRI. When

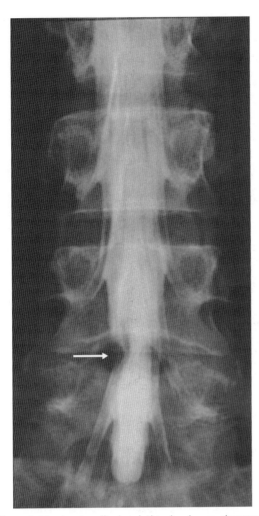

Figure 3.18 Lumbar disc herniation. Lumbar myelogram: frontal view. There is an extradural defect on the thecal sac in a left paracentral location due to disc herniation (arrow). The left L5 nerve root is compressed as it leaves the thecal sac with abrupt cut-off ('amputation') in contrast filling the nerve root sleeve.

surgery is being considered, myelography with or without postmyelography CT may be performed as an additional means to support the diagnosis and to help plan the surgical approach.

Clinical correlation   The radiographic demonstration of degenerative changes in the spine is age-related – commonly seen after the age of 40, rising to 70% of people greater than 70 years of age – and equally present in both asymptomatic and symptomatic persons. Therefore, the clinical severity of

degenerative disease correlates poorly with the severity of radiographic changes. The main role of plain films is to confirm degenerative disease in symptomatic persons and to exclude unsuspected pathology.

In addition, asymptomatic disc herniation and spinal stenosis are not uncommon, so any imaging abnormality must be carefully correlated with the person's symptoms and findings on clinical examination. If a person on clinical examination has clear findings of nerve root compression and a demonstrable disc herniation on imaging, physiotherapy treatment may still be given but the extent of the herniation and the severity or chronicity of the symptoms will all affect treatment outcome and raise the possibility of surgical intervention. The majority of persons who have disc herniation settle with conservative management.

Persons who have severe intermittent neurogenic claudication and clear radiological evidence of canal stenosis usually respond poorly to physiotherapeutic measures. Conservative management involves rest, anti-inflammatory drugs and facet joint or epidural injection. The aim of the conservative therapy is to reduce the inflammatory response in neural tissue as one cannot affect the bony entrapment. If this fails and the patient is severely disabled, surgical decompression is required and is usually successful in relieving the claudicant symptoms.

Anatomical anomalies of the vertebral column
Anomalies of the bony configuration of the spine are commonly seen. Minor asymmetries and even malformations are frequently seen, especially in the cervical and lumbar spine on plain films. Most of these anomalies are of no clinical significance and they are no more prevalent in persons with spinal pain. However, spondylolysis, spondylolisthesis or a transitional vertebra may render a spine more vulnerable to back pain.

Spondylolysis and spondylolisthesis   Spondylolysis (pars defect) is a bony defect in the pars interarticularis (the part between the superior and inferior articular process) of a vertebra. This is a fairly common entity which may be unilateral or bilateral. The usual site of involvement is a mid or lower lumbar vertebra, especially L5 (Fig. 3.20). Spondylolysis may cause back and/or radicular

Figure 3.19 Foraminal disc herniation. Axial computed tomography scans show a right-sided far lateral herniation of the L4–L5 intervertebral disc (arrow) which has migrated upwards into the exit foramen where it displaces the exiting L4 nerve root.

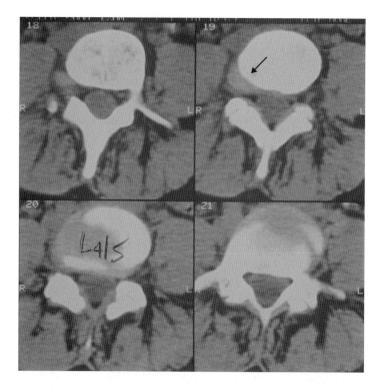

pain, but it is often asymptomatic. The aetiology of this condition is thought to be an acquired fracture occurring in infancy or early adult life. Most often this is a stress-type fracture following repeated trauma. These defects tend to persist and, unlike other stress fractures, tend to heal with fibrous union (pseudoarthrosis) and little periosteal callus. The nerve roots run adjacent to the pars defect and may get caught up in the fibrosis around a pars defect.

Spondylolysis, when bilateral, may be associated with displacement of one vertebral body on to the adjacent one (spondylolisthesis), the vertebra with the pars defect slipping forward on the vertebra below (Fig. 3.20). This is referred to as a lytic spondylolisthesis and should be distinguished from the more commonly seen degenerative spondylolisthesis. The magnitude of the slip is usually small (less than 1 cm) and progression is not usually seen beyond skeletal maturity. The slip may not be symptomatic.

Radiographic features of spondylolysis A lucent line is demonstrated through the pars region. This is often visible on the lateral view (Fig. 3.20), but is seen to best advantage on the oblique view (as a

break through the neck of the 'scottie dog'). If there is any doubt, CT can provide further evaluation. If there is a unilateral pars defect, hypertrophy and reactive sclerosis of contralateral pedicle may be seen.

Radiographic features of spondylolisthesis Spondylolisthesis when present is measured. There may be tilt as well as translation. The vertebra can tilt forward and narrow the neuroforamina and this may allow entrapment of nerve roots at the exit foramen. A radionuclide bone scan may be helpful in detecting early defects when plain films are normal, and to ascertain whether a discovered defect is symptomatic.

Clinical correlation Spondylolisthesis is a good example where radiographs will greatly help in the diagnosis and management of spinal pain. If on clinical grounds the therapist feels that the person's pain is related to a radiographically demonstrated slip then this pain may be due to instability at the defect or entrapment of a nerve root. Careful evaluation of the signs and symptoms will establish what structures are involved and the appropriate management.

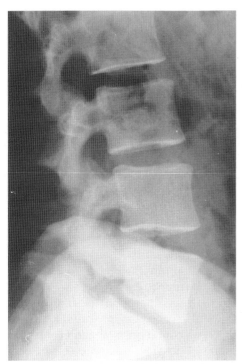

Figure 3.20   Lytic spondylolisthesis. Lumbar spine: lateral view. There are lytic defects through the pars interarticularis of L5. There is an associated minor forward slip of L5 on S1.

Transitional vertebrae at the lumbosacral junction
It is not uncommon to find congenital transitional vertebrae at the lumbosacral junction. A wide variety of patterns exist, including sacralization of L5 and lumbarization of S1, which may be complete or incomplete. A true joint may exist between an enlarged transverse process of L5 and the adjacent ala of the sacrum, which can be unilateral (Fig. 3.21) or bilateral. Degenerative changes can occur in these joints due to the altered mechanics and this may progress to bony ankylosis. There is also an increased incidence of pars defects. The relationship between low back pain and transitional vertebrae at the lumbosacral junction is debated. It has been suggested that a unilateral joint between the transverse process of L5 and the sacrum is more likely to be symptomatic.

Cartilaginous nodes   Also commonly known as Schmorl's nodes, cartilaginous nodes represent disc material that has been displaced either superiorly or inferiorly through the cartilaginous and vertebral body endplates into the spongy bone of

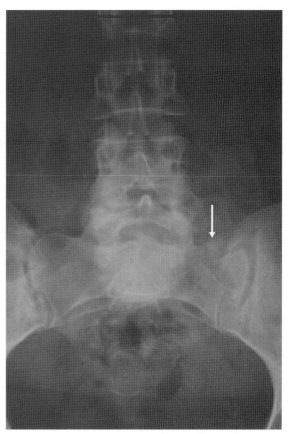

Figure 3.21   Transitional vertebra. Lumbosacral frontal view. An enlarged right-sided transverse process of L5 (arrow) forms a true joint with the ala of the sacrum.

the vertebral body. They occur in a variety of conditions that can weaken the cartilaginous endplate of the disc or the subchondral bone plate of the vertebral body including trauma, disc degeneration and rheumatoid arthritis and Scheuermann's disease (juvenile kyphosis). Cartilaginous nodes are not synonymous with Scheuermann's disease.

Radiographic features of cartilaginous nodes are characteristic – a rounded radiolucent area of variable size with the vertebral body, immediately adjacent to the endplate, surrounded by a cap of sclerosis. Mild endplate irregularity and cartilaginous node formation are frequently seen around the thoracolumbar junction, without kyphosis. These findings are not likely to be symptomatic and are of doubtful clinical significance.

Avulsion of the ring apophysis   A related condition is avulsion of the ring apophysis. This occurs in

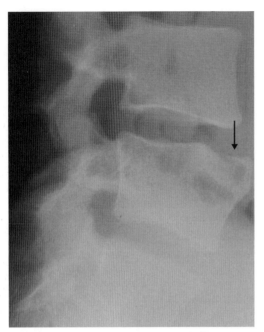

Figure 3.22 Avulsion of the ring apophysis (limbus vertebrae). Lumbar spine: lateral view. A triangular fragment of bone (arrow) is separated from the anterosuperior aspect of the L5 vertebral body.

the skeletally immature before apophyseal fusion when the cartilaginous growth plate is a point of weakness. Disc material may herniate through this area isolating a small wedge-shaped segment of the apophysis. This usually occurs at the anterosuperior corner of a lumbar vertebral body (limbus vertebrae; Fig. 3.22). However, the avulsed ring apophysis can occasionally occur from the posterior corner of the vertebral body when it could potentially compress neural structures in the spinal canal.

Spinal alignment Slight malalignments of spinal curvature on erect radiographs are quite common and are mainly asymptomatic. Some practitioners place great emphasis on these findings but any abnormal finding must be carefully correlated with the person's symptoms and objective clinical findings. Two common alignment problems in the spine are scoliosis and kyphosis.

Scoliosis The cause of scoliosis may be structural, postural or protective, and imaging can clearly help in this differentiation. Many scolioses cause no trouble for years but as age advances symptoms

are thought to develop because of increased mechanical strains on joints and soft tissues. Some people develop a scoliosis in response to a short leg. The scoliosis develops as a compensatory mechanism and usually the convexity in the lumbar area is on the side of the short leg.

Idiopathic scoliosis in adolescents and young adults is a common finding. However, symptoms are rare and if back pain is present, it is likely to be unrelated. The large majority of persons with a postural scoliosis do not have any underlying structural abnormality and do not require an X-ray examination. If there is significant back pain associated with scoliosis a radiological work-up using special long films with the person standing and bending in various directions may be indicated, but this should only be requested by a specialist orthopaedic surgeon.

Scoliosis may appear in the lumbar spine of elderly persons and may progress. It is uncertain whether this condition is a significant source of symptoms or not. The exact cause is unclear but it is not usually the result of degenerative disease of the spine. However, complicating degenerative change can occur and this is most marked along the concavity of the curve.

Thoracic kyphosis In the younger person increased thoracic kyphosis can be postural or structural, and if the latter, the likely cause is Scheuermann's disease. Although definitions vary, the essential feature of Scheuermann's disease is a fixed lower thoracic kyphosis in an adolescent person. Cartilaginous node formation, endplate irregularity and anterior wedging of the vertebral bodies are seen involving at least three contiguous vertebrae. It is thought to be the result of trauma during the vulnerable stage of rapid growth on a background of congenital endplate weakness.

An exaggerated thoracic kyphosis is common in elderly patients. This can result from one of two processes or, more commonly, a combination of both:

1. Osteoporotic kyphosis – the osteoporotic vertebrae collapse anteriorly (insufficiency fracture) and so become wedge-shaped. Involvement predominates in the weight-bearing middle and lower thoracic segments, especially T6 and T7.

2. Senile kyphosis – related to degeneration of the anterior aspect of the discs. Radiographs show narrowing of the disc space, endplate sclerosis and osteophytes in the anterior aspect of the disc. Eventually, bony ankylosis occurs at this site.

Diffuse idiopathic skeletal hyperostosis (DISH) The essential feature of this skeletal disorder is an excessive bone-forming tendency at entheses (where the ligaments and tendons attach to bone) which are sites of stress. This is a fairly common entity seen in middle-aged and older persons, is more frequent in males and the cause is unknown. The radiographic changes are often quite striking with exuberant new bone formation and large irregular bony outgrowths. The majority of patients have symptoms, but these are generally mild.

Spinal manifestations of DISH Radiographic changes are most commonly seen in the middle and lower thoracic segments where there is flowing ossification along the anterolateral aspect of the vertebral bodies in the anterior longitudinal ligament and annulus fibrosus, which is often quite thick and often has an undulating contour. There are often lucent gaps where it crosses the disc spaces (Fig. 3.23a).

It is not unusual to see progressive involvement into the upper lumbar and mid and lower cervical segments. The most common symptoms are spinal stiffness and mild non-radiating back or neck pain. In the cervical spine the ossification may also occur at the posterior vertebral body margin and so may cause spinal stenosis.

DISH in the spine is differentiated from degenerative disc disease by the absence of: (1) loss of disc height; (2) vacuum phenomena; and (3) subchondral sclerosis, from ankylosing spondylitis by the absence of: (1) vertebral body erosion; and (2) ankylosis of the facet joints, and from acromegaly by the absence of soft-tissue thickening.

Extraspinal manifestations of DISH Extraspinal manifestations are also frequent and distinctive. Radiographic changes include:

1. Pelvis:
   (a) well-defined bony proliferation, without erosion, at the iliac crest, ischial tuberosity and trochanters. This often has a 'whiskering' configuration.
   (b) ligamentous ossification (e.g. iliolumbar (Fig. 3.23b) and sacrotuberous).
   (c) para-articular osteophytes in relation to the inferior aspect of the sacroiliac joints and acetabulum which may progress to para-articular osseous bridging (Fig. 3.23b).

2. Heel and elbow – well-defined spurs which are often quite large arising from the superior (Achilles tendon attachment) or inferior surface (plantar fascia attachment) of the calcaneal tuberosity (Fig. 3.24), or the olecranon process (triceps tendon attachment). Clinically, there may be non-inflammatory tendinosis and palpable spurs.

3. Knee – cortical thickening of the anterior surface of the patella and large bony spurs arising from the inferior and superior margins of the patella, extending into the adjacent ligaments.

Osteitis pubis

This clinical entity is a potential cause of pubic pain in athletes (e.g. soccer players and runners) and can also be seen in women following childbirth or pelvic operations. The exact cause in athletes is not clear but it is thought to result from repetitive minor trauma during activities that excessively stress the symphysis and sacroiliac joint complex (e.g. running, jumping and kicking). Tension from the hip adductors and rectus abdominis muscles may also be a factor.

Clinical features include localized pubic pain and tenderness, muscle spasm and an antalgic limp which can mimic adductor muscle strain, and muscle stretching will aggravate the pain. In addition, a clicking sensation may be present, indicating instability.

Radiographic features include:

1. symmetrical bony resorption at the medial ends of the pubic bones with cortical irregularity and sclerosis (Fig. 3.4)
2. widening of the symphysis pubis
3. stress sclerosis on the iliac side of the sacroiliac joints. This is usually triangular in shape, localized to the inferior aspect of the joint and symmetrical (osteitis condensans ilii)
4. instability of the symphysis pubis–sacroiliac joint complex (demonstrated on 'flamingo' views; Fig. 3.4).

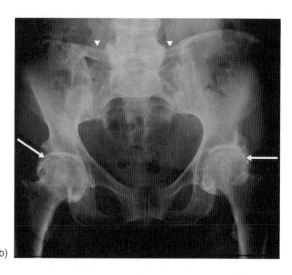

(b)

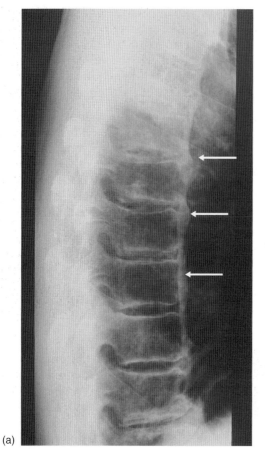

(a)

Figure 3.23a,b Diffuse idiopathic skeletal hyperostosis (DISH). (a) Thoracic spine: lateral view. There is thick-flowing ossification adjacent to the anterior vertebral body margin (arrows). The discovertebral joints are normal. (b) Pelvis: frontal view. Prominent para-articular ossification of the hip joints (joint space is normal) which effectively ankyloses the hip joints (arrows). In addition, there is ossification of the iliolumbar ligaments (arrowheads).

PERIPHERAL JOINT PROBLEMS

Three musculoskeletal syndromes have been chosen to illustrate the application of modern imaging technology in the evaluation of bony and soft-tissue problems of the shoulder and knee. These syndromes are: impingement and rotator cuff tears, glenohumeral instability and disorders of patellofemoral alignment and tracking. Newer imaging modalities can detect soft-tissue lesions with increased accuracy. It may be argued that a careful clinical examination can accurately assess the state of the soft-tissues but imaging technology can be utilized when necessary to confirm a clinical impression and to document more accurately soft-tissue abnormalities.

Physiotherapists occasionally treat persons who have shoulder pain which is resistant to all forms of therapy and detailed imaging can be of great assistance in further management. The requesting of these investigations is best performed by the person's primary care medical practitioner or a specialist.

Impingement and rotator cuff tears

The impingement (painful arc) syndrome is a common shoulder complaint that relates to obstruction to gliding of the subacromial tissues under the coracoacromial arch. It is associated with bursitis, rotator cuff tendinitis and tear, and also bicipital tendinitis. The large majority of cuff tears are

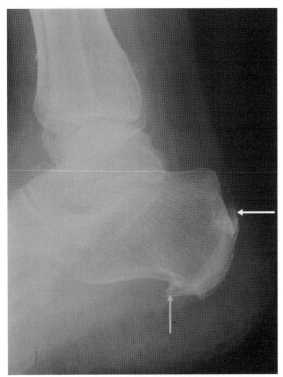

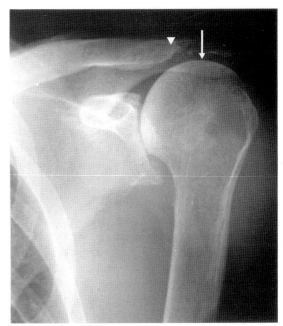

Figure 3.25 Cuff tear arthropathy. A full-thickness tear of the rotator cuff can allow upward subluxation of the humeral head with erosion of the undersurface of the acromion (arrow) and outer end of the clavicle (arrowhead). There is secondary osteoarthritis of the glenohumeral joint (loss of joint space and subchondral sclerosis).

Figure 3.24 Calcaneal traction spurs. There are well-defined bony spurs at the attachment of the plantar fascia (grey arrow) and Achilles tendon (white arrow) to the calcaneal tuberosity.

thought to be primarily the result of chronic impingement, although tears may occur in older persons without impingement due to age-related degeneration of the tendons and also as a result of a single episode of acute trauma. Impingement most commonly occurs at the site between the anterior third of the acromion and the underlying cuff tendons (supraspinatus outlet impingement).

Evaluation of impingement by imaging techniques

Impingement is primarily a clinical diagnosis but there are anatomical findings that can contribute to impingement and subsequent cuff disease. Various imaging modalities are used, including plain films, ultrasound and MRI.

Plain films   The following findings can be identified on plain films:

1. Anterior subacromial spurs (traction spur resulting from stressing of the coracoacromial ligament; Fig. 3.9)

2. Hooked configuration of the undersurface of the anterior acromion (developmental in nature)
3. Arthrosis of the acromioclavicular joint producing inferiorly pointing osteophytic spurs and/or joint hypertrophy.

The two supplementary impingement views (supraspinatus outlet view and frontal view with caudal angulation) are useful in documenting impingement anatomy as acromioplasty may be considered. Acromioplasty, ideally, should be performed at a stage before a full-thickness cuff tear develops.

Later findings of impingement observed on plain films include:

1. A greater tuberosity which shows flattening, sclerosis and cystic change (the result of mechanical impaction; Fig. 3.25) and this is usually associated with insertional damage to the cuff tendon.

2. A decrease in acromiohumeral space (between the top of the humeral head and inferior surface of the acromion). The acromiohumeral space is

largely occupied by the supraspinatus tendon and should normally measure greater than 7 mm. At this stage there is usually a full-thickness cuff tear.

3. Subacromial erosion – eventually this process may progress to allow the humeral head to migrate proximally and articulate upon the undersurface of the acromion where it produces a concave pressure erosion. At this stage a massive retracted cuff tear is usually present. Secondary osteoarthritis can then occur in the glenohumeral joint and this endstage of impingement is known as 'cuff tear arthropathy' (Fig. 3.25).

Ultrasound   Ultrasonic visualization in real time of the cuff tendons gliding under the coracoacromial arch is valuable in the assessment of impingement. Any buckling or hesitancy of the cuff beneath the arch which corresponds with the person's pain is highly suggestive of clinically relevant impingement.

MRI   MRI can provide an accurate and comprehensive evaluation of impingement. The osseous, bursal and tendinous manifestations of mechanical impingement can all be detected simultaneously.

Calcification may be associated with impingement syndromes. The calcification is usually the result of inflammation and subsequent degeneration of the rotator cuff tendons from chronic impingement and can be acutely painful. Periarticular calcification is identified on plain films and may be deposited in:

1. The rotator cuff tendons – most commonly adjacent to the greater tuberosity in the supraspinatus tendon (Fig. 3.7)
2. The subacromial–subdeltoid bursa. Often this is the result of tendon calcification rupturing into the adjacent bursa.

Evaluation of rotator cuff tears by imaging techniques

Cuff tears can be accurately diagnosed with ultrasound, arthrography and MRI. The majority of cuff tears occur in the supraspinatus tendon about 2 cm proximal to its insertion on the greater tuberosity where the impingement process most commonly occurs. Determining whether a full-thickness cuff tear is present may be useful in management as surgical repair may be considered.

Ultrasound   In experienced hands ultrasound has a high accuracy in the diagnosis of cuff tears, especially full-thickness tears. Full-thickness tears appear as a localized area of focal thinning in the cuff with an associated contour abnormality of the adjacent deep surface of the deltoid muscle (Fig. 3.26). With large tears there is complete absence of the cuff as the torn edge is retracted under the acromion. Assessment can also be made of the status of the cuff muscles, the biceps tendon in both its intra- and extra-articular portions, and the presence of any bursal or biceps tendon sheath effusions. Fluid in the biceps tendon sheath is a non-specific finding that is most commonly seen with cuff tears but can also be seen with the impingement syndrome, adhesive capsulitis, labral tears and primary biceps tendinitis.

Arthrography   This minimally invasive technique has a high accuracy for the diagnosis of full-thickness cuff tears and partial-thickness tears involving the humeral side of the cuff. Contrast enters the subacromial bursa from the joint capsule through the defect in the torn cuff. Evaluation of the characteristics of the tear is limited. Arthrography is a useful alternative where ultrasonic expertise is not available.

MRI   As well as a high accuracy in the demonstration of cuff tears, MRI can provide an evaluation superior to ultrasound or arthrography in estimating the size and position of a tear, degree of proximal retraction, whether there are degenerative changes in the torn edges and the degree of atrophy of the cuff muscles. Some clinicians find this extra information useful to help identify cases where surgical repair is less likely to be successful. MR arthrography can offer improved accuracy in the diagnosis of cuff tears.

Correlation of imaging results of rotator cuff tears with signs and symptoms

Cuff tears are one cause of pain and/or weakness of the shoulder. However, cuff tears may be asymptomatic, especially in the elderly population.

Glenohumeral instability

This clinical entity is usually seen in the younger athletic population with recurrent subluxation or

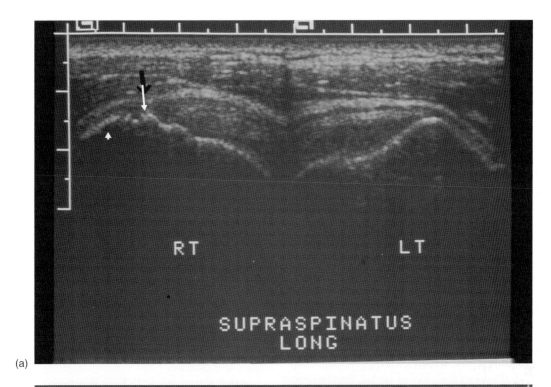

(a)

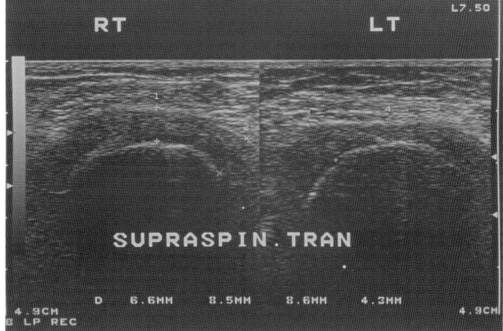

(b)

Figure 3.26a,b   Rotator cuff tear. Ultrasound images showing the distal portion of supraspinatus tendon (arrows) in (a) longitudinal and (b) transverse sections. There is focal thinning and flattening of the upper surface of the left supraspinatus tendon a short distance before it inserts onto the greater tuberosity of the humerus. A normal right-sided tendon is shown for comparison.

dislocation of the shoulder and may present as an impingement syndrome. Imaging is useful in confirming a clinical impression of instability, documenting the direction of the instability (anterior, posterior or multidirectional) and helping to decide the need for and type of surgery (e.g. open versus arthroscopic).

The soft-tissue abnormalities associated with instability include:

1. Tears and detachment of the glenohumeral ligament–labral complex (Fig. 3.26). When this occurs at the glenoid insertion, it is known as a Bankart lesion
2. Capsular redundancy (intrasubstance ligament failure)
3. Capsular stripping from the scapular neck (Fig. 3.27).

The bony lesions associated with instability (Hill–Sachs lesion and bony Bankart lesion) can be shown with instability views.

CT arthrography, which distends the joint capsule and allows evaluation of labral, ligamentous and capsular attachments, is an accurate imaging means to document these lesions of instability (Fig. 3.27). The role of MR arthrography is currently under investigation with benefits of multiplanar imaging and better visualization of the glenohumeral ligaments and labro–biceps complex.

Disorders of patellofemoral alignment and tracking

CT and MRI are very useful in the evaluation of disorders of patellar alignment and tracking. A kinematic study is performed by taking axial scans through the mid-portion of both patellae with the knee in different degrees of flexion throughout the range 5–40° (Fig. 3.28).

Assessment is made of the morphology and congruence of the articular facets of the patella and the apposing femoral trochlear groove. For example, a dominant lateral facet of the patella, small lateral femoral trochlea and a shallow femoral trochlear groove all tend to be associated with patellar malalignment and subluxation (Fig. 3.29), as are patellae which are positioned too high (patella alta) or too low (patella baja) in the trochlear groove.

Patellar tracking with knee flexion is then evaluated. Normally during knee flexion the ridge between the lateral and medial patellar facets should travel in a vertical plane centred in the trochlear groove without transverse displacement or tilt of the patella.

The common malalignment syndromes are:

1. Lateral subluxation of the patella – the ridge of the patella is displaced laterally relative to the trochlear groove. The subluxation tends to improve with increasing knee flexion with the patella normally centred by 40° of knee flexion. Lateral subluxation may be combined with lateral tilting of the patella, usually when the lateral femoral trochlea is hypoplastic (Fig. 3.29). In addition, cartilage damage is often seen at the point of impact between the lateral patellar facet and lateral femoral trochlea.

   Deficient medial stabilizers are thought to be responsible and a redundant lateral patellar retinaculum is often seen.

2. Excessive lateral pressure syndrome (ELPS) – this clinicoradiological entity is characterized by lateral tilting of the patella without significant lateral subluxation. The tilt tends to increase with increasing knee flexion. The lateral

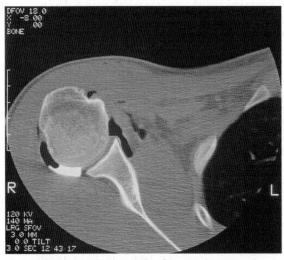

Figure 3.27 Anterior instability. Computed tomography arthrogram: axial section at the level of the subscapularis tendon. The anterior glenoid labrum is detached from the glenoid rim (compare with normal posterior labrum). In addition, there is capsular stripping along the anterior scapular neck.

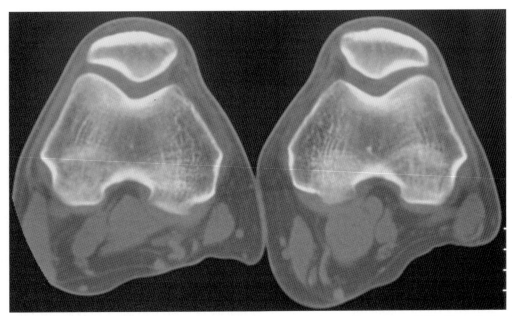

Figure 3.28   Patellofemoral computed tomography. Axial section through the patellar equator at 30° of knee flexion. Normal examination showing normal morphology of the joint surfaces and normal alignment with the medial patellar ridge centred in the femoral trochlear groove.

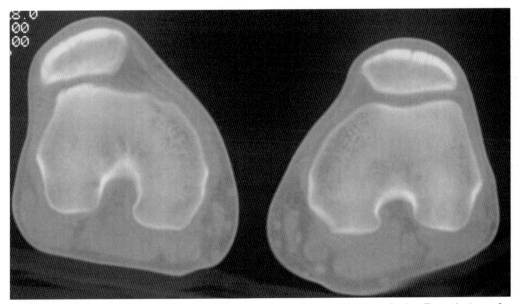

Figure 3.29   Patellofemoral dysplasia. Axial computed tomography section at 40° of knee flexion. The articular surfaces of the patellae show dominant lateral facets which are flat with a poorly developed interfacetal ridge. The femoral trochlear groove is very shallow with hypoplastic lateral trochleas. On the left there is malalignment – the patella is laterally subluxed with tilt and there is irregularity and sclerosis of the lateral bony joint surfaces from mechanical impaction.

patellar facet is usually dominant and will often show stress-related change with a thickened subchrondral bone plate and a traction spur at its lateral margin. Excessively taut lateral structures are thought to be responsible and a tight, shortened lateral retinaculum is usually shown.

CT and MRI are helpful in confirming patello-femoral malalignment, characterizing its type and severity and also in planning corrective treatment.

MRI of the ankle

MRI of the ankle is one of the most frequently performed musculoskeletal MRI examinations in our practice. Most frequently, the clinical setting is chronic posttraumatic ankle pain which has not responded in the expected fashion.

The ankle joint and its supporting ligaments and tendons are anatomically very complex and it can be difficult clinically to be certain of the origin of pain and multiple pathologies may coexist. MRI can offer an improved diagnosis rate over the clinical examination.

Causes of chronic ankle pain that can be reliably depicted with MRI include:

1. Anterolateral impingement – synovial hypertrophy with or without fibrotic scarring may form in the anterolateral gutter and become entrapped within the joint during dorsiflexion. Typically, this appears as a wedge-shaped meniscoid lesion in the anterolateral gutter and is amenable to surgical excision.
2. Osteochondral lesions of the talar dome occur at the lateral and medial corners of the talar dome and are thought to result from impaction injuries. They are not reliably shown on plain films.

    The size, location and stability of the lesion and the status of the overlying cartilage can be assessed with MRI and are important in directing management.
3. Stress fractures may not show on plain films but are accurately detected with MRI.
4. Posterior tibial tendon injury – see discussion that follows.
5. Peroneal tendon tears or dislocation.

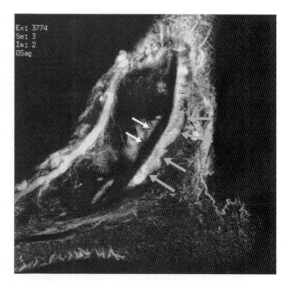

Figure 3.30 Posterior tibial tendon: partial-thickness chronic tear. Sagittal magnetic resonance imaging shows fusiform swelling of the tendon (grey arrows) with longitudinal splits and high signal fluid distension of the synovial sheath (white arrows).

Posterior tibial tendon tears

The posterior tibial tendon maintains the longitudinal arch of the foot, inverts the hindfoot and plantarflexes the ankle and is the main dynamic stabilizer of the hindfoot against valgus or eversion stresses. Typically, chronic tears of this tendon occur in middle-aged to elderly women following overuse or minor trauma. In the later stages there is a painful planovalgus hindfoot deformity.

MRI can accurately depict the type (partial- or full-thickness), location (often behind the medial malleolus where the tendon acutely angulates) and the extent of the tear, which will be important in directing appropriate management.

We have chosen to illustrate a low-grade partial-thickness chronic tear (Figs 3.30 and 3.31) which is characterized by:

1. fusiform swelling of the tendon
2. longitudinal splits in the tendon (high signal foci within the tendon substance)
3. fluid and synovial bands in the enveloping tendon sheath
4. medial malleolar spur.

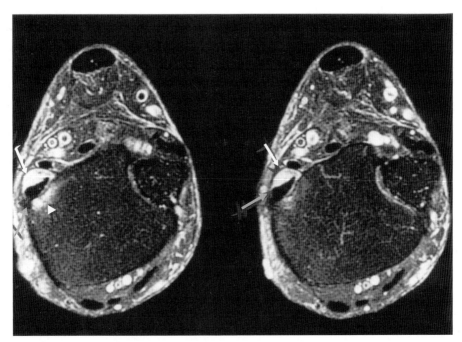

Figure 3.31   Posterior tibial tendon: partial thickness chronic tear. Axial magnetic resonance imaging shows enlarged tendon lying in the retromalleolar groove (grey arrows) with high signal fluid distension of the synovial sheath (white arrows) and a medial malleolar spur (arrowhead) containing high signal bone marrow oedema.

CONCLUSIONS

A plain film radiographic examination will be the initial and often the only form of imaging investigation required with many musculoskeletal problems. When imaging beyond plain films is considered necessary, there is a wide and often confusing range of more sophisticated imaging modalities available, each with its own individual advantages and disadvantages. Many factors are involved in selecting the appropriate modality, including what particular information the clinician desires, the preference and expertise of the radiologist, availability, cost and whether the investigation is invasive or utilizes ionizing radiation. Arthroscopy is a competing force in the evaluation of internal derangements

of joints, especially the knee. Imaging pathways are in a constant state of flux as further advances in imaging technology become available.

It has not been the aim of this chapter to cover any one particular area of diagnostic imaging in depth or to review recent radiological literature, but rather to stimulate and interest the physiotherapist in this area. For this reason further suggested reading has been included. The physiotherapist has an important part to play in the diagnosis of musculoskeletal pain and dysfunction. In some countries the responsibility of ordering imaging investigations has been accepted both at a professional and government level, and it serves the physiotherapist well to keep abreast of current imaging practices to ensure optimum patient care.

FURTHER READING

NORMAL ANATOMY
Agur, A. and Lee, M. (1991). *Grant's Atlas of Anatomy*, 9th edn. London: Williams & Wilkins.
An atlas with imaging correlation.

Johnson, W.H. and Kennedy, J.A. (1982). *Radiographic Skeletal Anatomy*, 2nd edn. London: Churchill Livingstone.
Labelled standard radiographs with anatomic correlation.

IMAGING OF MUSCULOSKELETAL DISORDERS

Resnick, D. (1989). *Bone and Joint Imaging*. London: W.B. Saunders.

A condensed single-volume version of the next reference. Highly recommended as reference.

Resnick, D. and Niwayama, G. (1988). *Diagnosis of Bone and Joint Disorders*, 2nd edn. London: W.B. Saunders.

A standard reference book (six volumes, superbly illustrated, and excellent radiologic–pathologic correlation).

Stoller, D. (1997). *Magnetic Resonance Imaging in Orthopaedics and Sports Medicine*. Philadelphia: J.B. Lippincott.

A comprehensive text of musculoskeletal MRI with excellent illustrations, including normal MRI anatomy.

ORTHOPAEDIC PHYSICAL ASSESSMENT

Magee, D.J. (1987). *Orthopedic Physical Assessment*. London: W.B. Saunders.

Chapter 4

Principles of examination and measurement

E.M. Gass

CHAPTER CONTENTS

The role of the physiotherapist has changed significantly since early in the twentieth century when members of groups such as the Australian Massage Society and the Chartered Society of Massage and Medical Gymnastics in the UK began working with medical practitioners in physical rehabilitation. Of critical importance to the present role definition is the way physiotherapists examine patients, decide a clinical diagnosis and, in combination with the patient's needs and goals, implement an effective dose of appropriate treatment to cause a favourable adaptation or outcome. The process of diagnosis in physiotherapy has been the subject of several articles in professional journals (Rose, 1988; Sahrmann, 1988; Jette, 1989; Guccione, 1991; Di Fabio, 1999). There is no consensus yet on what constitutes a diagnosis made by physiotherapists; however, it is generally agreed that this diagnosis will be complementary to the diagnosis of the medical practitioner (Rose, 1988; Sahrmann, 1988). The traditional idea of diagnosis related to identifying a disease or pathogen resulted in a direct path from diagnosis to treatment. A contemporary view of diagnosis by a physiotherapist would include identification of specific dysfunction related to the diagnostic label, with interrelationships between dysfunction and diagnosis forming the basis for treatment (Di Fabio, 1999).

As Di Fabio (1999) suggests, physiotherapists need to 'come out of the closet' and be explicit about the methods of clinical reasoning that underpin conclusions about diagnosis and dysfunction and hence guidelines for management.

Despite some lack of consensus about the parameters of the diagnosis made by physiotherapists, it is evident that as direct-access physiotherapy practice has increased, so has the expectation that a diagnosis will be made. In 1984 the House of Delegates of the American Physical Therapy Association (APTA) passed a motion which stated that physical therapists may establish a diagnosis within the scope of their knowledge, experience and expertise (APTA, 1984). The current Australian Physiotherapy Competency Standards (ACOPRA, 2002) include several performance criteria relating to assessment and diagnosis.

Changes in diagnostic inclusion in medical referrals to an outpatient physiotherapy department of a large teaching hospital in a major city of Australia have been analysed (Wong et al., 1994). Using randomly selected medical referral forms from 1982 and 1989 these authors were able to categorize diagnostic inclusion and referral mode. The majority of referrals in both years included a formal diagnosis, but significantly more in 1982. In 1989 the medical referrals were less likely to specify the type of physiotherapy treatment, rather asking for physiotherapy in general as a treatment and indicating expected patient outcomes. This study concluded that the differences in medical referral in 1982 and 1989 suggested a trend toward an expectation by medical practitioners of greater autonomy by physiotherapists in making decisions in clinical practice. A decline in prescriptive referral to physiotherapists in the UK has previously been reported (Williams, 1983), but 74% of referring physicians in North America are reported to have indicated a preference for prescriptive referral (Uili et al., 1984). These latter findings are of some concern because it has also been established that medical practitioners are familiar with traditional technical physiotherapy procedures or modalities, and less familiar with the current approach of prescribing a variety of management strategies based upon a sound examination (Uili et al., 1984; Stanton et al., 1985).

In a study investigating decisions made by physiotherapists (Dennis, 1987), patient referrals to physiotherapists from medical practitioners accounted for 67% of the total, 19% presented with no referral, 12% presented at the recommendation of a lay person and 2% were referred by other health professionals. Some form of treatment was prescribed in 45% of the referrals from medical practitioners and other health professionals, with electrotherapy being the most frequently requested modality. Overall this study provided evidence that prescriptive referral occurred in less than 25% of all referrals, and that most referrals left the management decisions to the physiotherapist (Dennis, 1987). This study supported the assertion that medical practitioners are, on the whole, unaware of the range and extent of current physiotherapy practice (Twomey, 1983; Uili et al., 1984). These findings reinforce the necessity for physiotherapists to make a full clinical diagnosis to enable treatment selection and progress evaluation.

PURPOSE AND AIMS OF EXAMINATION

The physiotherapist must be clear about the purpose of the clinical examination in order to collect the most relevant information. If the physiotherapist is unclear about the purpose and aims of the examination, then the procedures and tests selected, and subsequent interpretation made from the information gathered during the clinical examination, are likely to be muddled and inconclusive.

The aims of the physiotherapy examination of a patient with a musculoskeletal disorder are to:

1. establish a sound therapeutic relationship with the patient
2. make a clinical diagnosis
3. identify the goals or outcome of physiotherapy management
4. establish a set of baseline data and measurement procedures that can be used to judge treatment outcome
5. establish the presence of any contraindications or precautions to treatment
6. identify the most appropriate intervention strategy to achieve the goals
7. decide upon the dose of the specific strategies or treatments that will be effective in achieving the goals or outcomes.

To achieve these aims the clinical examination must include all procedures necessary to collect data relevant to the patient's presenting clinical picture. The methods of acquiring the data should be reliable and valid. Data interpretation and treatment selection will involve analysis of the collected data using the clinician's theoretical knowledge and previous clinical experience.

It is important to remember that the physiotherapy examination involves at least two key participants – the physiotherapist and the patient. On some occasions other health care professionals or friends or relatives of the patient are involved. The clinical examination process is an interactive one with possibilities for error and misinterpretation of information from all the participants. The examination is usually the first interaction between the patient and the physiotherapist and sets the scene for the therapeutic relationship that is to follow. In order to maximize reliability and validity of information collected, and to establish an appropriate therapeutic relationship, the physiotherapist must be sensitive and empathic to the patient, and his or her needs and goals of treatment. The physiotherapist must also instil a sense of trust in the patient, especially concerning confidentiality and privacy.

WHAT IS MEANT BY A CLINICAL DIAGNOSIS?

The term 'diagnosis' is commonly used by many health professionals. It can be defined as the process of determining, by examination of the patient, the nature and identity of a disease condition or the decision reached from such an examination (Delbridge, 1988). A medical dictionary suggests diagnosis is the term denoting the name of the disease a person has or is believed to have and the value of establishing a diagnosis is to provide a logical basis for treatment and prognosis (Taber, 1970). Such medical definitions often describe different types of diagnosis, namely cytological, differential, pathological and clinical. These different terms denote the method by which the diagnosis was made (Taber, 1970). A more straightforward definition is that 'a diagnosis is the label given to a disease on the basis of its clinical picture' (Jamison, 1999).

In the medical model, distinction is usually made between a pathological and a clinical diagnosis. Feinstein (1967) suggests that the main diagnostic taxonomy used by medical practitioners is that of pathological diagnosis based upon the nomenclature of morbid anatomy used by pathologists.

Examples of pathological diagnoses are myocardial infarction, duodenal ulcer, multiple sclerosis and nephritis. None of these diagnoses represent any entity that is seen, heard or touched in the observations made by the average clinician. These disorders are abnormalities of internal anatomic structure accessible in the main only to pathologists, hence the term 'pathological diagnosis'.

This type of diagnosis is inadequate; instead the medical clinician should classify the patient's abnormalities in physiological, biomechanical and clinical function in addition to naming the structural or pathological disorder (Feinstein, 1967). This point can be illustrated with the example of myocardial infarction – a clinician will infer or clinically diagnose myocardial infarction by observation of clinical signs and symptoms such as presence or absence of chest pain, shock, dyspnoea and arrhythmias. The clinician may see an abnormal electrocardiograph or results of other laboratory tests, but only the pathologist or surgeon will see the myocardial infarction. The pathologist would make the diagnosis of myocardial infarction by examining the heart. The major ingredients of clinical diagnosis are recognition of the clinical features of the illness, and the personal and environmental features of the patient, as well as the pathological diagnosis of the disease. A clinical diagnosis could be defined as the set of history, symptoms and signs which clearly and distinctly identify an individual patient. It may be possible to arrive at a pathological or structural diagnosis on the basis of the clinical diagnosis; however, successful treatment will usually be based upon the clinical diagnosis, not the pathological diagnosis. The pathological diagnosis is an important subset of the clinical diagnosis. The former provides the framework, prognosis and guidance for treatment, whereas the latter is usually the basis for the specific treatment and dose of treatment used.

In medicine there are two types of clinical decisions – explicatory and interventional. Explicatory decisions relate to the intellectual process of giving a name, cause or mechanism to the patient's signs and symptoms. Interventional decisions relate to choice of treatment to remedy or prevent the signs and symptoms (Feinstein, 1975). The explicatory decisions are traditionally regarded as the science of medicine whereas the interventional decisions are often regarded as the art. Unfortunately, along with this convention goes the thinking that there is no scientific challenge in the clinical management of the patient. A flaw in this thinking is that choice of treatment depends on diagnostic naming. Of course diagnosis is an important step; however, scientific selection and evaluation of the clinical intervention require much more intricate analysis of the data than simply identifying a diagnosis (Feinstein, 1975).

In physiotherapy there has traditionally been less emphasis on the diagnosis (or the science) and more emphasis on the treatment (or the art) than in medicine. Physiotherapists have a major role in delivering treatment and initiating prevention strategies, therefore care must be taken to structure the type of diagnosis that best suits physiotherapy practice and not to stereotype unthinkingly 'science' and 'art'. When Maitland (1986) separated the term diagnosis from the history, symptoms and signs with the brick-wall analogy, he implied that the history, symptoms and signs were different from a pathological diagnosis. History, symptoms and signs cannot reliably provide an uncontestable pathological diagnosis but conversely the pathological diagnosis cannot provide history, symptoms and signs. The clinical diagnosis is the basis for specific treatment and outcome decisions in most musculoskeletal disorders seen by physiotherapists. In some circumstances the pathological diagnosis does direct treatment, for example when a bone is fractured or when a ligament is ruptured. In other instances the pathological diagnosis provides guidance regarding prognosis and the overall treatment strategy, for example, a compressed spinal nerve/nerve root or gross spondylosis of the cervical spine. In such situations, however, the clinical diagnosis will direct aims of treatment, treatment strategies and choice of outcome measures. In other situations a pathological or structural diagnosis is not possible, and the clinical diagnosis will direct treatment and prognosis. Identification of both pathological and clinical diagnoses, in combination with referral to a sound theory base and appropriate referral to other health professionals, should ensure the most effective treatment prescription for each patient.

The concept of clinical diagnosis is important to current physiotherapy practice. With growing autonomy and accountability comes a need to justify procedures and process in physiotherapy. The community, health professional colleagues and the variety of bodies who pay for physiotherapy services expect that a physiotherapy service will include a diagnosis. The recognition that one of the responsibilities of a physiotherapist is to make a clinical diagnosis encourages focused physiotherapy examination procedures and evaluative clinical decision-making. It should also be remembered that diagnosis is not an end in itself, rather a 'mental resting place for prognostic considerations and therapeutic decisions' (Wulff, 1976). The parameters of the clinical diagnosis need careful thought and definition. Physiotherapists have moved from the stage of hypothesis-oriented algorithms (Rothstein and Echternach, 1986) and models of evaluation and dysfunction (Schenkman and Butler, 1989) to the challenge of specific diagnosis and diagnostic classification or taxonomy (Rose, 1988; Sahrmann, 1988; Jette, 1989). These challenges need urgent attention, not only because of the autonomy of physiotherapists but because it will remain difficult to investigate the effectiveness of physiotherapy intervention if conditions being treated cannot be clearly delineated. It would indeed lead to a unifying paradigm of musculoskeletal physiotherapy (Guccione, 1991) if diagnostic classification or the taxonomy of musculoskeletal disorders could be developed and validated.

HOW DO PHYSIOTHERAPISTS MAKE A CLINICAL DIAGNOSIS?

When the patient presents to the physiotherapist with a probable musculoskeletal disorder, the physiotherapist must systematically gather the information that will be the basis for the clinical diagnosis. First the physiotherapist asks the patient a series of questions. The responses to these questions, integrated with any other information available from laboratory tests or the medical practitioner, will provide the physiotherapist with a number of likely and unlikely possible or provisional diagnoses. The physiotherapist will refer to the knowledge base to decide which tests should be carried out in the physical examination to clarify the clinical diagnosis. Some of these tests will aim to gain more information to enable a complete clinical diagnosis, while other tests will check that apparently unlikely diagnoses identified from the history are, indeed, unlikely. The clinical diagnosis is made after thorough data-gathering and an analysis of these data. Reference to the existing knowledge base and previous clinical experience is necessary to allow formulation of the clinical diagnosis. The process by which the data are gathered is the physiotherapy examination. The important concepts underlying this examination and the commonly used components are described in detail in Chapters 5 and 6.

It has been said of the diagnostic process that it has no set starting point, no rules of evidence, information is often gained in an unorganized way and the clinician has the difficult task of translating the patient's language to clinical concepts (Grant, 1989). To make it more difficult, there are no preprepared pathways to take, nor does one necessarily know when one has finished (Grant, 1989). It could be suggested that the clinical examination provides the pathways and helps determine the endpoint. Some of the difficulties arise because of the complexity and confused nature of the information about how clinicians reason. Grant (1989) has suggested that diagnostic skill can be best improved by helping clinicians and students develop self-awareness and self-monitoring of their thinking rather than by teachers imposing forms of diagnosis. This suggestion is based upon the four key features identified in diagnostic thinking:

1. organization of clinical memory
2. individuality of thinking
3. ways of gaining access to memory
4. response to clinical information (Grant, 1989).

These concepts should be considered when planning the most effective way to examine a patient and make a clinical diagnosis. Teaching and learning in this area often concentrate on retaining large amounts of knowledge. However, it is important to organize this knowledge in a way that is clinically important and speedily retrievable. If this is done, the physiotherapist will be able to plan an appropriate examination confidently and achieve the desired aims, one of which is to make a clinical diagnosis.

PRINCIPLES OF MEASUREMENT IN PHYSIOTHERAPY PRACTICE

To make a diagnosis to provide a sound basis and justification for treatment selection, and to be able to demonstrate clinical efficacy, it is imperative that physiotherapists confront the issue of measurement in clinical practice. The importance of measurement in research, and the importance of research for professional growth, are acknowledged by most. The role of measurement in clinical practice is increasingly being recognized. Without sound measurement practices it is difficult to demonstrate the outcome of treatment. If the outcome cannot be demonstrated, then effective treatments may be ignored and ineffective treatments continued.

Outcome can be thought of as the result or visible effect of a certain event. In the context of health, outcome is often defined in terms of achievement or of failure to achieve certain goals. Outcome and need are related terms and the same instrument can usually be used to measure both. In physiotherapy practice we are increasingly concerned with outcome following our intervention. When attempting to measure outcome we need to be aware of a number of issues that can affect this variable, in addition to the treatment strategy. These include the natural history and progress of the disorder; the objectives or goals against which the outcome will be measured; a clear recognition and description of any inputs which can affect the outcome; and the desirability of specifying the hypothesized relationship between input and outcome. These issues are of more obvious importance in research but also need consideration in clinical practice to help maximize applicability and generalizability of outcome measures.

Knowledge of the natural history of a disorder is important because if one knows the time course of the problem without intervention, then this can provide a baseline against which outcomes are measured. In musculoskeletal physiotherapy there are some disorders where the natural history may be known, for example, a sprained ankle or acute low back disorder, but there are many disorders for which natural history is unknown. The best strategy under these circumstances is to use the history of the disorder under the existing pattern of physiotherapy treatment as a baseline.

New treatment strategies can then be evaluated against the outcomes associated with the existing pattern.

Definition of the objectives or aims of physiotherapy intervention can occur at a number of levels. Global objectives such as restoration of function or increased functional capacity are not particularly helpful when evaluating the short-term effectiveness of a specific treatment. There is an advantage in having specific aims such as the ability to walk up two flights of stairs with even weight-bearing or the ability to hang out one load of washing. Sometimes the objectives and aims are assumed and not stated after a physiotherapy examination, or, if formulated, the objectives only reflect the priorities of the physiotherapist. Involvement of the patient, and where appropriate family, friends and other health professionals, may result in more relevant and encompassing objectives. This in turn means more realistic and valid outcome measures.

It is almost impossible to describe outcomes unless there is careful definition of inputs. It is, however, not easy to account for all inputs in the therapeutic setting. Some recognition of the majority of inputs is necessary, however, before the physiotherapist can assume a favourable outcome is a consequence of particular clinical intervention.

If physiotherapists wish to learn from and build upon outcomes of clinical practice, then it is also important to specify the relationship between inputs and outcomes. A favourable outcome or result from treatment should not be assumed to have been caused only by the treatment. A positive outcome can be related to other factors such as the attention being received, opportunity for social interaction or the patient wishing to please the physiotherapist.

It is neither straightforward nor desirable to control for all variables in clinical practice, as elements such as social interaction and the patient feeling the centre of attention are often important components of the therapeutic experience. The physiotherapist can refer to or carry out well-designed research studies that can form the basis for interpretation of the relationship between treatment and outcome.

Basic to these issues concerning input and outcome and definition and achievement of objectives is the concept of measurement.

WHAT DO WE MEAN BY MEASUREMENT?

Measurement is the process by which one can obtain answers to questions such as 'how many?' and 'how much?' Measurement has been linked to the belief that, if something is measured, it must be scientific (Feinstein, 1967). It is reported (Feinstein, 1967) that Kelvin stated that measurement was a prerequisite to science, setting the scene for biologists and other scientists to try to measure, and for clinicians to feel lost. Medical clinicians could measure height, blood pressure and cardiac output but were unable to measure headache, angina pectoris, dyspnoea or anxiety. As science clearly depends on dimensional measurement, then this logic would suggest a clinician could never attain science because so much of the information gathered at the bedside has no dimensional expression (Feinstein, 1967). An interesting solution to this dilemma was proposed by suggesting that there are two types of measurement – mensuration and enumeration (Feinstein, 1967). Mensuration is the use of a scale to determine a dimension that represents the amount of some substance whereas enumeration is the counting of a group of entities that have been categorized as single units. A counted number is a sum of individual units whereas a dimensional number is a proportional amount of some unit demarcated on a scale. A dimensional number answers the question 'how much?' whereas a counted number will answer the question 'how many?'

In dimensional measurement the item must first be identified or extracted in some way from a collection of items and then this item is given dimension by comparing its value on a calibrated scale. In enumerational measurement the item to be tested is already a unit and the measurement consists of finding a particular category in which the unit can be counted. Mensurated variables are isolated and related to a calibrated scale whereas enumerated variables are observed and classified according to criteria. Reliability is assured if the isolation and calibration are adequate and if the observation and criteria for classification are accurate. It is worth noting that there is no ordinary method of dimensionally measuring the locations, qualities and other characteristics of the different types of pain produced by toothache, migraine, pleurisy, abdominal cramps or angina pectoris yet each of these pains can be uniquely characterized by verbal description (Feinstein, 1967).

It has been suggested (Wilkin et al., 1992) that measurement can be divided into three broad categories: discrimination, prediction and evaluation. Discrimination involves measurement of differences between groups or individuals and is necessary if differences in health experience or areas of need are to be described. Prediction, or measurement as a basis for foretelling, is useful in health because individuals who may have a certain condition or outcome in the future can be identified. If predictive measures are sound then preventive strategies or intervention can be instituted at an early stage. Evaluation involves ascertaining the amount of something, appraising or assessing. Increasingly researchers, clinicians and policy-makers are using measurement to evaluate or monitor the impact of health phenomena. Measures are needed to pick up changes between groups of patients. These changes or outcomes can then be attributed to certain interventions or treatments.

The level of precision of these categories of measurement will depend upon the context of use. The physiotherapy clinician is usually interested in differences within an individual and thus needs measures that can do this. Researchers may require a lower level of precision as they are examining differences in groups of individuals. Another factor that influences the level of precision is knowledge of the expected magnitude of the differences. If the magnitude of clinically important differences is small, then the measure chosen needs to be quite precise.

MEASUREMENT AND RELATED TERMS

Certain terms are integral to an understanding of measurement, in particular methods, reliability, validity, sensitivity and specificity. An understanding of these terms will enable the physiotherapist to design and implement sound measurement procedures in their clinical practice.

Methods

Methods is a term with which most physiotherapists will be familiar, particularly from reading research papers. Methods is the section where all procedures to be used are explained. This practice is based on the premise that in order to measure any particular item it is first necessary to describe and define exactly what it is that is to be measured. Rothstein when writing about measurement in clinical practice (Rothstein, 1985) suggests the use of the term 'operational definition' instead of methods, noting that this term means specification of the procedures or operations to be used in taking the measurement. Further, he suggests that for an operational definition to have value in clinical practice it must have some generalized applicability and sound theoretical assumptions. This term is useful because it specifies its purpose; however, it seems redundant to use a different term, operational definition, from that commonly used in the scientific community, methods. The issue at point is that whenever a physiotherapist wishes to measure something the measurement procedure should be carefully described. Succinct definition or description of the variable to be measured is essential. Such a definition or description should be acceptable to most physiotherapists and should reflect current theoretical knowledge.

In physiotherapy practice there is widespread usage of descriptive terms such as muscle weakness, muscle tightness, decreased movement and joint stiffness. When speaking with colleagues and when reading or writing clinical notes we tend to assume that the definitions of such terms are obvious and that all physiotherapists will quantify or measure these clinical phenomena in the same way. Observation for a short time would make it obvious that there is great variety in the way physiotherapists evaluate or measure such variables. This variation is based partly on an inadequate knowledge base and partly on the unwillingness of physiotherapists to access and integrate such knowledge into their clinical practice even when it is available.

Whenever clinical measurements are made the methodology must be clearly documented. This could be by written description, a diagram or photograph or a videotape. The exact definition of the variable to be measured should be provided, e.g. muscle strength might be defined as the absolute force produced during one maximal contraction, or it might be the highest step a person can climb. It is important that justification can be provided for any definition of the variable being measured and that the definition is stated clearly. Physiotherapists should feel confident in deciding on a definition.

Reliability

Reliability is a term commonly encountered in scientific literature. Definitions of the term abound, with a useful definition stating that the reliability of a measure is the extent to which it yields the same results in repeated applications on an unchanged population or phenomenon (Wilkin et al., 1992). Thus the reliability of a measurement or observation is its repeatability, i.e. providing all conditions remain the same, if the test or observation is repeated, the likelihood that the same result will be obtained. Reliability is related to terms such as stability, dependability, predictability and accuracy or the amount of measurement error (Kerlinger, 1964). One of the aims of any measurement should be to reduce random and non-random error. The more reliable a measure is, the lower the element of random error, i.e. error which follows no systematic pattern (Wilkin et al., 1992). Non-random error or bias is assessed by testing validity.

The concept of reliability depends on whether one is operating from the basis of classical measurement or generalizability theory. The former theory suggests that every measurement will consist of a true score and an error component whereas generalizability theory recognizes that there are different sources of variability for any measurement made. Under this latter theory measurement error can be divided into sources of variability of interest to the measurer. The advantage of the generalizability approach is that it provides a way to quantify many sources of variability, a common situation in physiotherapy clinical practice (Roebroek et al., 1993). For a review of measurement theory in general and these concepts in particular the reader is directed towards Domholdt (2000).

If a measurement procedure is not reliable and will not give similar results when repeated under similar conditions, or if the reliability is unknown, then it becomes difficult to interpret the results obtained by such a measure. If it were to be established that a certain clinical test, when repeated

under identical conditions, gave a result that varied by 10% in either a positive or negative direction, then the physiotherapist using this test would need to demonstrate changes of more than 10% to be able to have confidence that there had been a change in the measured variable. There are many factors that can affect the reliability of a measure, particularly the clinician, the instrument and the patient. Texts commonly discuss instrument, intrarater (in the same individual), interrater (between individuals) and intrasubject (within the same subject) reliability. Of course, even if there is high interobserver and/or intraobserver reliability, this does not necessarily imply that the observations or measurements are accurate – observers or raters can be reliably wrong!

Intrarater reliability can be defined as the consistency with which a rater assigns scores to a single set of scores on two occasions (Waltz et al., 1984). This is sometimes difficult to ascertain as the subject being repeatedly measured can change, this change being difficult to distinguish from an error on the part of the rater.

Interrater reliability is defined as consistency between different observers or users of the instrument (Wilkin et al., 1992). This is easier to ascertain as multiple raters can measure a subject at the same or closely related time. If measurements are not possible at the same time then the same difficulty of partitioning out subject variability arises as did with testing intrarater reliability.

Instrument reliability is sometimes known as test–retest reliability. Given that such testing occurs on two different occasions, the issue as to whether the subject being tested has changed or the instrument has changed is still present. (For more discussion on the types of instruments used by physiotherapists and methods to measure their reliability, see Domholdt (2000).)

Intrasubject reliability is difficult to estimate. If one were confident that both tester and instrument were perfectly reliable, then measuring the subject on two occasions could provide intrasubject reliability.

Measurement of reliability

It is possible to quantify reliability either by examining the relationship between two or more sets of repeated measures (relative reliability), or by examining the variability of the scores from measurement to measurement (absolute reliability). (For discussion on this point, see Kerlinger (1964) or Domholdt (2000).) Relative reliability is usually calculated by the use of procedures such as Pearson product-moment correlation coefficient, intraclass correlation coefficient, Cohen's kappa or the coefficient of variation. Each of these analyses gives slightly different information. It is important to remember that these correlations describe relationships between variables and cannot be used to ascribe causality. Absolute reliability is a measure of the extent to which a score varies on repeated measurement and the statistic used to measure absolute reliability is standard error of the measurement (Domholdt, 2000). The advantage of calculating and reporting the standard error of the measurement is that information is available about how much of the variability in the scores could be expected because of measurement error alone.

To decide that a real change or adaptation has occurred, it is important to know the magnitude of change that needs to be measured in a patient to reflect true change and not a measurement error. This issue is of importance in both clinical practice and research. It is tempting, particularly when one has access to measuring devices that give results in numbers, to assume that such numbers are always true. The issue of reliability relates to how confident the physiotherapist can be that the numbers have meaning and can be used to monitor progress and prescribe treatment. Physiotherapists should be aware of the basic principles of operation of these instruments and be able to go back to 'first principles' to check the numbers being generated. Manufacturers of instruments such as goniometers, tape measures or force transducers normally provide information about the accuracy of the instrument, for example 5° for a goniometer or 0.1% for a force transducer. Instruments should be calibrated against a known standard at regular intervals to ascertain the degree of accuracy. If drift of the instrument has occurred, then, depending on the instrument, adjustments can often be made to reset the instrument according to the known standard. When physiotherapists evaluate or purchase measuring or therapeutic equipment it is good practice to read

the specifications of the equipment carefully in order to be sure the accuracy is appropriate to the task to be performed.

The issue of reliability is an important one for physiotherapy for, unless reliable measurements are possible, the correct diagnosis, treatment selection and evaluation of treatment effects become difficult. In order to demonstrate clinical efficacy and respond to challenges of role definition for physiotherapy, reliable measurement must be the cornerstone of clinical practice.

Validity

Validity is a more complex concept than reliability. Validity is a term sometimes confused with reliability because it has a related, but quite different, meaning. Simply stated, a valid measurement is one that actually measures what it is supposed to measure. The validity of an instrument relates to the non-random or systematic error (Wilkin et al., 1992). A valid measurement procedure therefore allows legitimate judgement or inference (Rothstein, 1985). One of the reasons validity is a more complex concept than reliability is that validity usually necessitates some inquiry into the nature and meaning of the variables (Kerlinger, 1964). For example, a thermometer is routinely used to measure temperature. It has been pointed out that the reason a patient's temperature is measured is not to infer something about the kinetic energy of molecules, rather, on the basis that an elevated temperature can infer presence of infection, or the presence of disorder or disease (Rothstein, 1985). Another example is the use of the test of bending forwards trying to reach fingertips to the floor. It is valid to infer something about the person's flexibility through flexion from this test; however, it would not be valid to infer the amount of lumbar flexion as so many other factors such as range of hip movement and length of hamstrings muscles can contribute to the forward flexion range.

A number of different types of validity have been identified, most importantly content, concurrent, predictive and construct validity (Cronbach and Meehl, 1955; Domholdt, 2000).

Content validity is concerned with how representative the content of the measure is of the universe of content of the property being measured. To ascertain content validity one could ask whether the choice of, and relative importance given to, each component of the index is appropriate for the domains they are supposed to measure (Wilkin et al., 1992). An example is functional ability, a broad term with a large number of subsets such as activities of daily living, grooming activities, mobility activities, leisure activities and work activities. A test high in content validity would theoretically be a representative subset of the universe of functional ability. In reality, however, the universe of content only exists as a theoretical concept. To decide whether a test has sufficient content validity, a judgement is made by deciding how representative the tests to be used are of the item under consideration. Careful definition and description of test items are necessary to allow the judgement to be made. Content validity is particularly relevant to questionnaire or observational measuring instruments. The Functional Status Index (FSI) test, for example, was designed to measure the degree of dependence, pain and difficulty experienced by people with arthritis living in the community (Wilkin et al., 1992), and it has been tested for interobserver and test–retest reliability with satisfactory results (Harris et al., 1986). Content validity is claimed to be better with this instrument than other measures of function; however, comparisons between FSI scores, patient self-ratings and staff ratings have produced varied results (Denniston and Jette, 1980). When designing such measuring instruments it is useful to evaluate the content validity or spend time researching the content validity of existing similar instruments. Content validity should be evaluated by both experts in the area and representatives of the community to be measured.

Concurrent and predictive validity are similar to each other as both relate to prediction against an outside criterion, and both are characterized by checking the measuring instrument against some outcome (Kerlinger, 1964). The term 'criterion validity' is sometimes used to encompass the two terms (Domholdt, 2000). When a measurement tool, such as manual ligament testing of the ankle, is compared with a measurement standard, such

as arthroscopy or radiological testing, then concurrent validity is being determined. Predictive validity is more concerned with tests that measure performance in a certain way and predict what the status will be in the future. Many health-screening programmes are based on predictive validity.

Construct validity is concerned with the underlying explanation or meaning of the test. This type of validity is different from the others because there is a preoccupation with theory, the theoretical constructs and testing of hypothesized relations (Kerlinger, 1964). The question that defines construct validity is: do the results obtained confirm the expected pattern of relationships or hypotheses derived from the theoretical constructs on which the measure is based (Wilkin et al., 1992)?

Construct validation and empirical scientific inquiry are closely allied. In order to determine construct validity, Cronbach (1960) has suggested three key steps:

1. identifying any constructs that might account for test performance
2. deriving hypotheses from the theory involving the construct
3. testing the hypotheses empirically.

Strength is a poorly delineated construct in physiotherapy literature (Domholdt, 2000). The term 'strength' can mean a variety of things and, before construct validity can be maximized, the basic concepts underlying the measures must be very clear. First one must decide, for example, whether the underlying construct is isometric, functional or eccentric strength. Once this decision is made, the construct must be clearly defined and delineated to allow measurement. Careful definition or delineation will not only help ensure construct validity but other physiotherapists are then able to evaluate such definitions and form their own opinion of the construct (Domholdt, 2000). Ultimately this process will provide a strong basis for refinement and improvement of testing procedures. Clear and careful definition of constructs in physiotherapy in the public domain is the first step towards a coherent research effort and outcome-oriented clinical practice.

The accuracy of diagnostic tests

R. Herbert

Diagnosis involves classifying people into groups that do and do not have a particular condition. The decision to classify a person as having or not having a particular diagnosis is based on the findings of diagnostic tests. Some diagnostic tests simply involve asking questions of the patient (for example, we might ask whether people get morning stiffness to determine the presence of inflammatory disease). Others involve complex manual manoeuvres (such as the pivot shift test for anterior cruciate ligament rupture) or technologically complex procedures (such as magnetic resonance imaging).

We say that a test is positive when its findings are indicative of the presence of the condition, and we say the test is negative when its findings are indicative of the absence of the condition. However, most tests are imperfect. Thus even good clinical tests will sometimes be negative when the condition being tested for is present (false-negative), or positive when the condition being tested for is absent (false-positive). Thus the process of applying and interpreting diagnostic tests is probabilistic – the findings of a test often increase or decrease suspicion of a particular diagnosis but, because most tests are imperfect, it is rare that a single test clearly rules in or rules out a diagnosis. Good diagnostic tests have sufficient accuracy that positive findings greatly increase suspicion of the diagnosis and negative tests greatly reduce suspicion of the diagnosis.

We can learn about the accuracy of diagnostic tests from clinical studies in which a group of patients is subjected both to the test of interest and a test which is believed to be highly accurate (the 'reference standard' or 'gold standard' test). For example, the accuracy of Lachman's test for rupture of the anterior cruciate ligament can be determined by testing patients suspected of anterior cruciate ligament injury with both Lachman's test and arthroscopy. In this case arthroscopy is the reference standard. It is a simple matter to assess the degree of concordance between the findings of the test of interest and the reference standard. If the level of concordance is high, the test is accurate.

The most common way of describing the accuracy of diagnostic tests (i.e. the concordance of the findings of the test and the reference standard) is in terms of sensitivity and specificity. Sensitivity is the probability that people who truly have the condition (as determined by testing with the reference standard) will test positive. It is estimated from the proportion (or percentage) of people who truly have the condition that test positive. Specificity is the probability that people who do not have the condition (again, as determined by testing with the reference standard) will test negative. It is estimated from the proportion (or percentage) of people who truly have the condition that test positive. Clearly, it is desirable that sensitivity and specificity are as high as possible – that is, it is desirable that sensitivity and specificity are close to 100%.

Though widely used, there is one major limitation to the use of sensitivity and specificity as indexes of the accuracy of diagnostic tests. Fundamentally, sensitivity and specificity are quantities that we do not need to know about. Sensitivity tells us the probability that a person who has the condition will test positive. Yet when we test patients in the course of clinical practice we *know* if the test was positive or negative so we don't need to know the probability of a positive test occurring. Moreover, we *don't know*, when we apply the test in clinical practice, if the person actually has the condition (if we did, there would be no point in carrying out the test). There is no practical value in knowing the probability that the test is positive when the condition is present. Instead, we need to know the probability of the person having the condition if the test is positive. There is a similar problem with specificities – we don't need to know the probability of a person testing negative when he or she does not have the condition, but we do need to know the probability of the person having the condition when he or she tests negative.

LIKELIHOOD RATIOS

Likelihood ratios provide an alternative way to describe the accuracy of diagnostic tests (Sackett et al., 1985). Importantly, likelihood ratios can be used to determine what we really need to know about. With a little numerical jiggery-pokery, likelihood ratios can be used to determine the probability that a person with a particular test finding (positive or negative) has the condition that is being tested for. The likelihood ratio tells us how much more likely a particular test result is in people who have the condition than it is in people who don't have the condition. As most tests have two outcomes (positive or negative), this means we can talk about two likelihood ratios – one for positive test outcomes (we call this the positive likelihood ratio) and one for negative test outcomes (we call this the negative likelihood ratio).

The positive likelihood ratio tells us how much more likely a positive test finding is in people who have the condition than in those who don't. Obviously it is desirable for tests to be positive more often in people who have the condition than those who don't, so consequently it is desirable to have positive likelihood ratios with values greater than 1. In practice positive likelihood ratios with values greater than about 3 become useful and positive likelihood ratios with values greater than 10 become very useful.

The negative likelihood ratio tells us how much more likely a negative test finding is in people who have the condition than those who don't. This means that is desirable for tests to have negative likelihood ratios of less than 1. The smallest value negative likelihood ratios can have is zero. In practice, negative likelihood ratios with values less than about a third (0.33) become useful and negative likelihood ratios with values less than about one-tenth (0.10) become very useful.

Many studies of diagnostic tests only report the sensitivity or the specificity of the tests, but not likelihood ratios. Fortunately it is an easy matter to calculate likelihood ratios from sensitivity and specificity:

$$LR+ = \text{sensitivity}/(1 - \text{specificity})$$
$$LR- = (1 - \text{sensitivity})/\text{specificity}$$

where $LR+$ is the positive likelihood ratio and $LR-$ is the negative likelihood ratio. (Alternatively, if sensitivity and specificity are calculated as percentages, you can insert 100 instead of 1 in the equations.)

Therefore, if sensitivity is 90% and specificity is 80%, the positive likelihood ratio is 4.5 (i.e. $90/(100 - 80)$) and the negative likelihood ratio is 0.125 (i.e. $(100 - 90)/80$). In this example the positive likelihood ratio is big enough to be quite useful and the negative likelihood ratio is small enough to be very useful.

USING LIKELIHOOD RATIOS TO CALCULATE THE PROBABILITY THAT A PERSON HAS A PARTICULAR DIAGNOSIS

From the moment a person presents for a physiotherapy consultation most physiotherapists will begin to make guesses about the person's probable diagnosis. For example, a young adult male may attend physiotherapy and begin to describe an ankle injury incurred the previous weekend. Even before he describes the injury, the physiotherapist may have arrived at a provisional diagnosis. It may be obvious from the way in which the patient walks into the room that he or she has an injury of the ankle. Most commonly, injuries to the ankle are ankle sprains or ankle fractures. But it is rare that someone can walk soon after an ankle fracture, so the physiotherapist's suspicion is naturally directed towards an ankle sprain, or perhaps a muscle tear. This simple scenario provides an important insight into the process of diagnosis: physiotherapists usually develop hypotheses about the likely diagnosis very early in the examination. Thereafter most of the examination is directed towards confirming or refuting those diagnoses. Additional pieces of information are accrued with the aim of proving or disproving diagnosis. Thus we can think of the examination as a process of progressive refinement of the probability of a diagnosis. The real value of likelihood ratios is that they tell us how much to change our estimates of the probability of a diagnosis on the basis of a particular test's finding.

If we want to use likelihood ratios to refine our estimates of the probability of a diagnosis, we need first to be able to quantify probabilities. Probabilities can lie on a scale from 0 (no possibility) to 1 (definite), or, more conveniently, from 0% to 100%. Consider the following case scenario:

Case 1

A 23-year-old male reports that 3 weeks ago he twisted his knee during an awkward tackle while playing soccer. Although he experienced only moderate pain at the time, the knee swelled immediately. In the 3 weeks since the injury, the swelling has only partly subsided. The knee feels unstable and there have been several occasions of giving way.

What probability would you assign to the diagnosis of a torn anterior cruciate ligament? Most physiotherapists would assign a high probability, perhaps between 70% and 90%, implying that between 7/10 and 9/10 of patients presenting like this are subsequently found to have a tear of the anterior cruciate ligament. For now, let us assign a probability of 80%. Because we have not yet formally tested the hypothesis that this patient has a torn anterior cruciate ligament, we will call this the *pretest* probability (Sox et al., 1988). That is, we estimate that the pretest probability that this patient has a torn anterior cruciate ligament is 80%.

It appears likely that this patient has a torn anterior cruciate ligament, but the diagnosis is not yet sufficiently likely that we can act as if that diagnosis is certain. The usual course of action would be to test this diagnostic hypothesis, probably with an anterior draw test, or Lachman's test or the pivot shift test (Magee, 1997). Clearly if these tests are positive, we should be more inclined to believe the diagnosis of anterior cruciate ligament tear, and if the tests are negative we should be less inclined to believe that diagnosis. The question is, if the test is positive, *how much* more inclined

should we be to believe the diagnosis? And if the test is negative, *how much* less inclined should we be to believe the diagnosis? Likelihood ratios provide a measure of how much more or how much less we should believe a particular diagnosis on the basis of particular test findings (Go, 1998).

A recent systematic review of diagnostic tests for injuries of the knee (Solomon et al., 2001) concluded that the positive likelihood ratio for the anterior draw test was 3.8 (this is higher than 1, which is necessary for the test to be of any use at all, and high enough to make it diagnostically useful). The negative likelihood ratio was 0.3 (this is less than 1, which is necessary for the test to be of any use, and low enough to be useful).

Now we need to combine three pieces of information: our estimate of the pretest probability, our test finding (whether or not the test was positive), and information about the diagnostic accuracy of the test (the positive or negative likelihood ratio depending upon whether the test was positive or negative). The easiest way to combine these three pieces of information is with a likelihood ratio nomogram, such as the one reproduced in Figure 4.1 (Fagan, 1975; Davidson, 2002). The nomogram contains three columns. Reading from left to right, the first is the pretest probability, the second is the likelihood ratio for the test, and the third is what we want to know: the probability that the person has the diagnosis (the posttest probability). All we need do is draw a line from the point on the first column that is our estimate of the pretest probability through the second column at the likelihood ratio for the test (we use the positive likelihood ratio if the test was positive and the negative likelihood ratio if the test was negative). When we extrapolate the line to the right-most column it intersects that column at the posttest probability. We have estimated the probability that the person has the condition on the basis of our estimate of the pretest probability, the test result (positive or negative) and what we know about the properties of the test (expressed in terms of its likelihood ratios).

Returning to our example, we find that the young man with the suspected anterior cruciate ligament tear tests positive with the anterior draw test. By using the nomogram, we can estimate a revised (posttest) probability of anterior cruciate ligament lesion given the positive test finding.

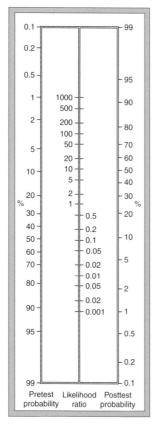

Figure 4.1 A nomogram for determining the posttest probability of a diagnosis. (Reproduced from Davidson (2002), with permission.)

The posttest probability is 94%. If the test had been negative we would use the negative likelihood ratio in the nomogram, and we would conclude that this man's posttest probability of having an anterior cruciate ligament tear is 55%.

This illustrates a central concept in diagnosis. The proper interpretation of a diagnostic test can only be made after consideration of pretest probabilities. Theoretically these pretest probabilities could be evidence-based (for example, they could be based on epidemiological data about the prevalence of the condition being tested for in the population to whom the test is applied).

However, such information is rarely available. More often pretest probabilities are based on clinical intuition and experience – the therapist estimates the pretest probability based on the proportion of people with such a presentation who, in his or her experience, have subsequently been found to have

this diagnosis. Thus rational diagnosis is inherently subjective and experience-based.

Many therapists feel suspicious about the inherent subjectivity of this approach to diagnosis. (The approach is sometimes called a Bayesian approach.) Subjectivity, where it produces variation in practice, is probably undesirable. However, the alternatives (such as ignoring what intuition says about pretest probabilities and making uniform assumptions about pretest probabilities like 'all pretest probabilities are 50%') are likely to produce much less accurate diagnoses. So, for the foreseeable future, diagnosis will remain as much an art as a science.

Viewed in this way, the process of diagnosis is one in which intuition-based estimates of the probability of a diagnosis are replaced with progressively more objective estimates based on test findings. Indeed if, after conducting a test, the diagnosis remains uncertain, the posttest probability can be used as a refined estimate of the next pretest probability, and sequential testing can proceed in this way (the posttest probability of one test becoming the pretest probability of the next test) until a diagnosis is confirmed or rejected. We say that a diagnosis is confirmed once the posttest probability has become very high, and we say that the diagnosis is rejected once the posttest probability has become very low.

A consequence is that a given test finding should be interpreted quite differently when applied to different people, because different people will present with different pretest probabilities. To illustrate this point, consider a second case:

Case 2

A 32-year-old netball player reports that she twisted her knee in a game 3 weeks ago. At the time her knee locked and she was unable to straighten it fully. She does not recall significant swelling, and reports no instability. However, in the 3 weeks since her injury, there have been several occasions when the knee locked again. Between locking episodes the knee appears to function near-normally.

This is not a classic presentation of an anterior cruciate ligament lesion. A more likely explanation of this woman's knee symptoms is that she has a meniscal tear. We might estimate the pretest probability of an anterior cruciate ligament lesion for this woman to be 15%. If this woman tests positive to the anterior draw test, we would obtain a posttest probability of 40%. (Try it and see if you get the same answer.) In other words there is a 60% probability (100 − 40%) that she does *not* have an anterior cruciate ligament lesion, even though she tested positive with the anterior draw test. This illustrates that a positive anterior draw test should be considered to be much less indicative of an anterior cruciate ligament lesion when the pretest probability is low. Perhaps that is not clever statistics, just common sense!

If we had used a more accurate test (of which the Lachman test may be an example – one study estimated that its positive likelihood ratio was 42; Solomon et al., 2001) then we should have expected to modify our estimates of the probability of the diagnosis more. With a positive likelihood ratio of 42 and pretest probability of 15%, a positive Lachman test gives a posttest probability of 88%.

Weighting of clinical information

E.M. Gass

The process of arriving at a clinical diagnosis relies heavily on how we weight the importance of the data gathered. The weight attached to a piece of information refers to the significance assigned to this piece of information by the clinician. This in turn will affect the decisions made by the clinician. Likelihood ratios may be very helpful, as just illustrated in the previous section. However, it may still be difficult for clinicians to state explicitly what weighting was assigned to different pieces of information gathered during the examination, even though intuitively they know that different weights are being assigned.

The physiotherapist must assess the significance or importance of information as it is acquired, as a basis for the decisions that are made in order to weight according to importance. The significance of the presence and the absence of clinical features needs to be known. Importance of data gathered may vary depending on what other symptoms or signs are present (or absent) in the patient.

Research in medical literature would suggest that different speciality groups attach different weights to the same information (Balla, 1982). Cardiologists, neurologists and medical students were provided with brief case histories in one study (Balla, 1982). One patient had olfactory sensations and déjà vu, both strong cues for epilepsy, but all other signs and symptoms of epilepsy were noted as being absent. Most of the participants diagnosed epilepsy; however, preference for this diagnosis increased with expertise. When additional information was provided that this patient had been drinking and felt ill before he collapsed then the students and cardiologists diagnosed this as an epileptic fit but the neurologists did not. This seemed to suggest that this additional information had more weight for the experts than those less experienced in neurological diagnosis.

Another point about weighting of information is that the same symptoms and signs in different settings can have different weights. For example, a study was conducted with medical students, cardiologists and neurologists (Balla, 1982). Brief case histories of three patients were presented. All patients had typical fainting spells. Patient A was a young girl who 'blacked out' in church, patient B was a much older person who fainted and no information about age or sex was provided about patient C. All respondents were confident to diagnose that patient A was experiencing vasovagal episodes because of their knowledge that such a cause is common in young females. The respondents were much less confident about a vasovagal diagnosis for patient B because this is a much less common cause in older people. No accurate diagnosis was possible for patient C. This study showed how the same signs and symptoms in three different settings had completely different weighting and how this was related to prior knowledge. Interestingly, it has been shown that negative information is difficult to handle, even if it contains critical information.

Negative information is frequently ignored by inexperienced clinicians, although experts may regard it highly. If a young male has headaches there are many possible diagnoses. Given that temporal arteritis and polymyalgia rheumatica are diseases of the elderly (Balla, 1985) then, as this information is absent or negative in this example, these diagnoses should be unlikely. Similarly a blackout in a child could be caused by petit mal but if the patient is 50 years old and suffers his first blackout, then it cannot be petit mal (Balla, 1985).

Other chapters in this book (Chs 5 and 6) will discuss specific aspects of making a clinical diagnosis. In general, however, in order to make a diagnosis and make clinical decisions, the physiotherapist must collect and process information. This process involves both the patient and the physiotherapist receiving, providing and interpreting information in relation to their own experience and knowledge. Related concepts important in the context of information gathering include reliability, validity, specificity, sensitivity, prevalence and likelihood ratios. These concepts need to be applied in order that the physiotherapist can make a sound judgement about the data being gathered, and be reasonably certain about the diagnosis made and plan of action proposed.

It is important to recognize explicitly that one of the purposes of the physiotherapy examination procedure for those with musculoskeletal disorders is to diagnose. This recognition will help physiotherapists structure and interpret the examination and may lead to the development of a taxonomy or classification of musculoskeletal clinical diagnoses. This would improve patient management and form the basis for continued questioning, discussion and research.

RELIABILITY AND VALIDITY WHEN TAKING A HISTORY AND PERFORMING THE PHYSICAL EXAMINATION

Identification of the clinical diagnosis and selection of treatment depend on gathering reliable and valid data in the clinical examination. Whenever evaluating reliability the physiotherapist should know the normal response to a test so that responses outside the normal range can be analysed systematically for their clinical relevance. This could involve measurement of many people of different ages and characteristics, possibly outside the usual clinical setting. The data obtained in the physical examination should correlate with the data obtained in the history. This correlation is often difficult for students to recognize because their main concern is to complete the history or the physical examination without missing out relevant procedures. Repetition with patients and practice with colleagues will help overcome this problem so that the more important concept of internal consistency of the examination can be mastered. Internal consistency means that the data collected are homogenous and accurate. If one were to intercorrelate samples of the data there would be high reliability. If inconsistent data appear then either the information gathering and testing procedures need modification, or alternative diagnoses need to be entertained, or both.

Laboratory and radiographic investigations are all too often assumed to be highly reliable. Reading of X-rays and electrocardiographs shows large individual variations, and errors also occur with laboratory investigations. Such test results should be seen as part of the information gathering towards the clinical diagnosis proposed by the physiotherapist. Physiotherapists need to be aware of sensitivity and specificity of laboratory and radiography tests and to have some idea whether the test results are useful for confirming a diagnosis (sensitivity) or excluding a diagnosis (specificity). Such information can be found in textbooks describing laboratory and radiographic tests or can be ascertained by enquiry to the laboratory or medical practitioner concerned. This information is important to be able to weight information appropriately.

Reliability of information collected during the history-taking can be affected by the source of the data and the method of collection of the data. When questioned, patients must interpret their own signs and symptoms and convey this interpretation to the physiotherapist. This can be a source of confusion and possibly error. The patient may have inadequate verbal skills to describe symptoms in any detail, simply stating he or she feels unwell and has great pain. The history of any precipitating incident and subsequent development of symptoms often provides strong evidence for a particular diagnosis yet the patient's memory can be unreliable and hence provide inaccurate or conflicting information.

The skill of the physiotherapist comes from recognizing that this information is unreliable, despite trying different questioning strategies and manoeuvres, and then putting less weight on this information when it comes to making a diagnosis. The physiotherapist needs to be aware that bias can be a source of reasoning error (Norman et al., 1992). Specifically reasoning error can be due to faulty perception or elicitation of cues, incomplete factual knowledge or misapplication of known facts to a particular situation (Scott, 1995). Inaccurate history-taking on the part of the physiotherapist can also lead to unreliable data. Balla and Iansek (1979) suggest that the major problem is lack of data clarification whereby instead of being absolutely sure of the detail of what the patient is reporting, the physiotherapist may assume he or she knows what is meant and not seek to establish the actual details.

REFERENCES

American Physical Therapy Association (1984). *House of Delegates Policies*, p. 19. Alexandria, Virginia: American Physical Therapy Association.

Australian Council of Physiotherapy Regulating Authorities Inc (ACOPRA) (2002). Australia: Australian Physiotherapy Competency Standards.

Balla, J.L. (1982). The use of critical cues and prior probability in decision making. *Methods of Information in Medicine*, **19**, 88–92.

Balla, J.L. (1985). *The Diagnostic Process*. Cambridge: Cambridge University Press.

Balla, J.L. and Iansek, R. (1979). The neurological diagnostic process. In: *Proceedings of the 5th Asian and Oceanic Congress of Neurology*, ed. G.L. Gamez. Manila Excerpta Medica.

Cronbach, L. (1960). *Essentials of Psychological Testing*, 2nd edn, p. 12. New York: Harper and Row.

Cronbach, L. and Meehl, P. (1955). Construct validity of psychological tests. *Psychol. Bull.*, **LII**, 281–302.

Davidson, M. (2002). The interpretation of diagnostic tests: a primer for physiotherapists. *Aust. J. Physiother.*, **48**, 227–233.

Delbridge, A. (ed.) (1988). *The Macquarie Dictionary*, 2nd edn. Sydney, Australia: Macquarie Library.

Dennis, J.K. (1987). Decisions made by physiotherapists: a study of private practitioners in Australia. *Aust. J. Physiother.*, **33**, 181–191.

Denniston, O.L. and Jette, A.M. (1980). A functional status assessment instrument: validation in an elderly population. *Health Services Research*, **15**, 21–34. In: *Measures of Need and Outcome for Primary Health*

Care (1992), eds D. Wilkin, L. Hallam, and M.A. Dogget, pp. 56–57. Oxford: Oxford University Press.

Di Fabio, R.P. (1999). Secrets of diagnosis. *J. Orthop. Sports Phys. Ther.*, **29**, 504.

Domholdt, E. (2000). *Physical Therapy Research – Principles and Applications*. Philadelphia: W.B. Saunders.

Fagan, T.J. (1975). Nomogram for Bayes theorem. *N. Eng. J. Med.*, **293**, 257.

Feinstein, A.R. (1967). *Clinical Judgement*. New York: Robert Ekrieger.

Feinstein, A.R. (1975). Science, clinical medicine and the spectrum of disease. In: *Textbook of Medicine*, ed. P.B. Beeson and W. McDermott, pp. 3–6. Philadelphia: W.B. Saunders.

Go, A.S. (1998). Refining probability: an introduction. In: *Evidence-Based Medicine: A Framework For Clinical Practice*, ed. D.J. Friedland, A.S. Go, J.B. Davoren, et al., pp. 11–33. Stamford, CT: Appleton & Lange.

Grant, J. (1989). Clinical decision making – rational principles, clinical intuition or clinical thinking? In: *Learning in Medical School*, ed. J.L. Balla, p. 83. Hong Kong: Hong Kong University Press.

Guccione, A. (1991). Physical therapy diagnosis and the relationship between impairments and function. *Phys. Ther.*, **71**, 499–503.

Harris, B.A., Jette, A.M., Campion, E.W. and Cleary, P.D. (1986). Validity of self report measures of functional disability. *Topics in Geriatric Rehabilitation* **1**, 31–41. In: *Measures of Need and Outcome for Primary Health Care* (1992), ed. D. Wilkin, L. Hallam and M.A. Doggett, pp. 56–57. Oxford: Oxford University Press.

Jamison, J.R. (1999). *Differential Diagnosis for Primary Practice.* Edinburgh: Churchill Livingstone.

Jette, A.M. (1989). Diagnosis and classification by physical therapists: a special communication. *Phys. Ther.,* **69**, 87–89.

Kerlinger, F.N. (1964). *Foundations of Behavioural Research,* pp. 429–453. New York: Holt, Rinehart and Winston.

Magee, D.J. (1997). *Orthopedic Physical Assessment*, 3rd edn. Philadelphia: W.B. Saunders.

Maitland, G.D. (1986). *Vertebral Manipulation,* 5th edn, pp. 6–7. London: Butterworths.

Norman, G.R., Brooks, L.R., Coblentz, C.L., Babcock, C.J. (1992). The correlation of feature identification and category judgements in diagnostic radiology. *Memory and Cognition,* **20**, 344–355.

Roebroek, M.E., Harlaar, J. and Lankhorst, G.J. (1993). The application of generalisability theory to reliability assessment: an illustration using isometric force measurements. *Phys. Ther.,* **73**, 386–395.

Rose, S.J. (1988). Musing on diagnosis – editorial. *Phys. Ther.,* **68**, 1665.

Rothstein, J.M. (1985). Measurement and clinical practice: theory and application. In: *Measurement in Physical Therapy,* ed. J.M. Rothstein, pp. 3, 16. New York: Churchill Livingstone.

Rothstein, J.M. and Echternach, J.L. (1986). Hypothesis-oriented algorithm for clinicians. *Phys. Ther.,* **66**, 1388–1394.

Sackett, D.L., Haynes, R.B. and Tugwell, P. (1985). *Clinical Epidemiology: A Basic Science For Clinical Medicine.* Boston: Little and Brown.

Sahrmann, S.A. (1988). Diagnosis by the physical therapist – prerequisite for treatment. *Phys. Ther.,* **68**, 1703–1706.

Schenkman, M. and Butler, R.B. (1989). A model for multisystem evaluation, interpretation and treatment of individuals with neurologic dysfunction. *Phys. Ther.,* **65**, 27–30.

Scott, I. (1995). Teaching clinical reasoning: a case-based approach. In: *Clinical Reasoning in the Health Professions,* ed. J. Higgs and M. Jones, pp. 290–297. Oxford: Butterworth-Heinemann.

Solomon, D.H., Simel, D.L., Bates, D.W., Katz, J.N. and Schaffer, J.L. (2001). Does this patient have a torn meniscus or ligament of the knee? Value of the physical examination. *J. A. M. A.,* **286**, 1610–1620.

Sox, H.C., Blatt, M.A., Higgins, M.C. and Marton, K.I. (1988). *Medical Decision Making.* Boston, MA: Butterworths.

Stanton, P.E., Fox, K., Frangos, K.M., Hoover, D.H. and Spilecki, M. (1985). Assessment of resident physicians knowledge of physical therapy. *Phys. Ther.,* **65**, 27–30.

Taber, C.W. (ed.) (1970). *Taber's Cyclopaedic Medical Dictionary.* Philadelphia, PA: F.A. Davis.

Twomey, L.T. (1983). The physiotherapist. *Med. J. Aust.,* **1**, 422–424.

Uili, R.M., Shepard, K. and Savinar, E. (1984). Physician knowledge and utilization of physical therapy procedures. *Phys. Ther.,* **64**, 1523–1530.

Waltz, C.F., Strickland, O.L. and Lenz, E.R. (1984). *Measurement in Nursing Research,* p. 17. Philadelphia, PA.

Wilkin, D., Hallam, L. and Doggett, M.-A. (1992). *Measures of Need and Outcome for Primary Health Care,* pp. 56–57. Oxford: Oxford University Press.

Williams, J.L. (1983). The three times a week syndrome. *Physiotherapy,* **69**, 235–237.

Wong, W.P., Galley, P. and Sheehan, M. (1994). Changes in medical referrals to an outpatient physiotherapy department. *Aust. J. Physiother.,* **40**, 9–14.

Wulff, H.R. (1976). *Rational Diagnosis and Treatment.* Oxford: Blackwell Scientific.

Chapter 5

The history

K.M. Refshauge, J. Latimer, and C.G. Maher

The history is arguably the most important part of the whole examination because it is from the history that we decide the nature of the patient's problem, and the possible treatments that might consequently be used. From the history we develop hypotheses about the probable location and type of pathology, the clinical symptoms to be treated, possible strategies to manage the problem, contraindications or precautions to examination and treatment procedures, and likely prognosis. We rarely gain completely new ideas from the physical examination, rather we test the hypotheses we derived from the history, confirming some and rejecting others.

For patients suffering low back or neck pain the first decisions to make are:

- Are there any red flags, i.e. is there any serious pathology?
- Is the pain coming from the back or neck?
- Is the condition simple low back or neck pain?
- Is physiotherapy appropriate for the condition or should we refer the patient for some other type of investigation or treatment?

For patients with musculoskeletal conditions not including the spine, a similar triage is performed:

- Are there any red flags, i.e. is there any serious pathology?
- What is the source of the symptoms?
- Is physiotherapy appropriate for the condition or should we refer the patient for some other type of investigation or treatment?

In addition to diagnostic decisions, further important decisions made from the history include:

- What procedures should be performed in the physical examination?
- Are there any contraindications or precautions to examination or treatment?
- What management strategies are likely to help the most?
- How long is it going to take the patient to get better (prognosis)?
- What is the patient expecting from treatment?

The patient's expectations of treatment should be established during the first visit. The physiotherapist should discuss these expectations with the patient rather than make assumptions, and ensure that expectations are realistic and achievable. In this way the patient and the physiotherapist work together to maximize the benefit from treatment. This avoids the scenario where a patient is disappointed because return to work or sport, for example, is not yet possible, but the physiotherapist believes that the patient is progressing satisfactorily because a small increase in range of movement has been achieved. If a patient believes that the treatment is ineffective or misdirected, compliance with treatment and home programmes is likely to be reduced.

Maitland (1964) first described several categories of information that should form the basis for questions routinely asked by physiotherapists treating patients with musculoskeletal conditions. It is a tribute to his thorough approach that the categories of questions he encouraged physiotherapists to enquire about have changed little since his original description.

Generally, the structure of the history consists of seven categories, each category relating to one aspect of the problem. These are:

1. area of symptoms
2. current history
3. behaviour of symptoms over a 24-h period
4. irritability of symptoms (how easily symptoms are aggravated)
5. past history
6. questions to determine contraindications and precautions to examination and treatment ('special questions')
7. 'social' history.

Some information about all decisions (pathological and clinical diagnoses, physical examination procedures, treatment, precautions and contraindications to treatment, and prognosis) will be obtained from each of the above categories. Thus, ideas are formed about several types of decisions simultaneously, comparing new information with existing hypotheses. The use of information gained from these categories is summarized in Table 5.1.

Judgements about each of the above types of decisions are made by comparing several different pieces of information. There is rarely a single piece of information that is definitive. However, rather than asking all questions relating to one type of decision, such as diagnosis or prognosis, questions in one category that relate to one aspect of the problem are usually grouped together, so that, for example, information about the type and location of symptoms is gained before progressing to other aspects of the problem, such as when and how the injury occurred. This method increases both the efficiency and effectiveness of the interview process. The use of a routine set of questions has been developed to ensure that relevant information is gathered efficiently (Maitland, 1986). It is not intended that this routine should be strictly adhered to, but it serves as a guide for beginning students, and even for experienced clinicians faced with solving new and challenging problems.

The order in which information is collected may affect its interpretation. It is suggested that our original hypotheses are made from the first information gained. With further information we then change or refine our early hypotheses. Often the order in which we collect information relates to the relative importance assigned to it, e.g. when a person presents with a knee problem, the mechanism of injury may be determined early in the history because this information is important diagnostically, whereas with low back pain this information may have less diagnostic value.

All pertinent information must be recorded. This includes noting questions that were asked but were negative, e.g. the patient had no arm pain on the first visit. There are many occasions when records need to be consulted, such as on subsequent treatment occasions, or if the problem relapses in the future, as well as for research, audit or legal

Table 5.1 The history: categories of questions asked, the information gathered and how this information is used by physiotherapists

Category (method of gaining information)	Information	Use of information
Area and type of symptoms (interview and questionnaires, e.g. McGill pain questionnaire)	Spatial distribution, referral patterns	Diagnosis, prognosis, monitor progress
	Type of symptoms: ● Pain ● Paraesthesia ● Anaesthesia	Diagnosis, monitor progress
	Constant or intermittent	Diagnosis, prognosis
	Quality, e.g. ● Dull ache ● Burning, sharp	Monitor progress (? diagnosis)
	Intensity	Monitor progress
	Depth	Diagnosis
	Relationship of symptoms	Diagnosis, treatment
Current history (interview)	When injury occurred	Treatment, prognosis
	Mechanism of injury	Diagnosis, treatment
	Progress of symptoms	Treatment, prognosis
	Previous treatment and effect	Diagnosis, treatment and prognosis
Behaviour of symptoms i.e. 24 h behaviour (interview and questionnaries, e.g. Roland–Morris)	Night pain ● Prevents getting to sleep? ● Wakens? ● Best/worst positions	Diagnosis, treatment
	Morning ● Pain ● Stiffness	Diagnosis
	Activities or positions aggravating symptoms	Diagnosis, treatment
	Activities or positions easing symptoms	Diagnosis, treatment
	Symptom behaviour during the day	Diagnosis, treatment
Irritability of symptoms (interview and questionnaire, e.g. Roland–Morris)	What activity (and how much) aggravates symptoms?	Physical examination: ● Which tests? ● Vigour ● Treatment ● Strategy ● Dose
	Intensity of symptoms	
	Continuation of symptoms after cessation of activity	

continued

Table 5.1   *continued*

Category (method of gaining information)	Information	Use of information
Past history (interview)	First episode: ● When did it occur? ● How did it occur? ● Previous treatment and effect?	Diagnosis, treatment and prognosis
	Subsequent episodes: are they changing in ● Frequency? ● Intensity? ● Duration?	Treatment, prognosis
Questions to determine precautions and contraindications to examination and treatment (interview and modified core questionnaire)	General health Presence of inflammatory disorders, cancer, osteoporosis X-rays and other investigations Medications, steroids Depression, abnormal illness behaviour	These questions are aimed at identifying pathology Certain pathologies may contraindicate all or selected treatment strategies and may require further medical investigation
For spinal conditions	Cord signs	
For lumbar spine	Cauda equina syndrome	
For cervical spine	Dizziness	
Cognitive factors (interview and questionnaire, e.g. acute low back pain screening questionnaire, Tampa scale)	Beliefs about the condition: ● Cause ● Responsibility and control ● Fear of hurting/harming Coping strategies Mood: ● Stress ● Anxiety ● Depression	Diagnosis, treatment prognosis
Social history (interview)	Age and gender	Diagnosis, treatment, prognosis
	Employment ● Status ● Type	Treatment
	Domestic role	Treatment
	Self-care	Other interventions
	Dependants	Treatment
	Leisure activities	Treatment
	Goals of treatment	Treatment

purposes. Records should therefore be complete, accurate and meet legal requirements.

Sometimes patients are not seeking treatment for symptoms that they currently suffer but are seeking advice regarding prevention of injury or strategies that could be used to maximize their function. For example, women may present following childbirth, requesting advice about suitable strategies for minimizing stress to the spine with childcare tasks. Another patient may attend with a teenage son who has scoliosis and wants advice about what to do. In these instances all aspects of the history provided in Table 5.1 may not be relevant and physiotherapists will need to customize their own history plan.

HOW DO WE TAKE A HISTORY?

In Table 5.1 you will have noticed that, following the category of information, the suggested method for obtaining information appears in brackets, i.e. either interview or questionnaire. In general the best way to obtain relevant, measurable information from the patient entails the use of both an interview and a standardized questionnaire. During an interview a large amount of data may be collected from the patient, some of which may have originally fallen outside the physiotherapist's frame of reference. However an interview is preferred by many patients to the simple completion of a questionnaire because of the necessary patient–therapist interaction.

During the interview a variety of different questioning styles may be used to obtain information, including dichotomous questions requiring a simple yes/no answer, forced-choice questions requiring the patient to choose one of the answers offered, e.g. is your pain better, worse or the same? or open-ended questions, e.g. could you describe the quality of your pain? Dichotomous questions will provide reliable information, but the information gained is severely limited and may provide little insight into the patient's problem (Waddell et al., 1982). Forced-choice questions should be used judiciously, for example, when a patient is unable to answer a specific question. In this instance providing the patient with several options may help. For example, if a patient, when asked to describe the pain, appears at a loss, the therapist may ask 'Is the pain sharp or dull?' Once supplied with possible options, patients may find it easier to choose between these or may spontaneously supply their own choice. Open-ended questions provide reliable and valid information (Waddell et al., 1982) and are often used when asking patients about the distribution of their symptoms and the onset and duration of their condition. Sometimes the reply may be complex, rambling and difficult to categorize, thus making it difficult to compare the patient's responses at subsequent treatments (French, 1988). In patients who appear reluctant to talk about their condition, open-ended questions may be used to encourage them to talk further, as well as reassuring them that talking will provide information and not be interpreted as complaining.

Disadvantages to using interviews include the difficulty in categorizing the patient's responses for subsequent comparison, and the difficulty in accurately establishing the reliability of this information. Use of a standardized questionnaire in addition to the interview will substantially overcome these difficulties. Questionnaires are less labour-intensive and are standardized to enable comparison of results. Many of the questionnaires used to assess patients with low back pain have demonstrated high reliability and validity (Melzack, 1975; Fairbank et al., 1980; Waddell et al., 1982; Gibson et al., 1985) and appear sensitive to change, i.e. a patient's score on the questionnaire improves as his or her condition improves (Melzack, 1975; Fox and Melzack, 1976; Linton and Gotestam, 1983). The main disadvantages of a questionnaire are that they may limit the response of the patient by using closed or forced-choice questions, they may not be useful in patients with poor English (although several questionnaires have been translated into other languages) and some are complex to score. However, despite this, the combination of both interview and questionnaire is likely be the most successful for obtaining high-quality data from the patient.

In the next section we will:

- review some of the questionnaires available for a patient with a musculoskeletal disorder. Most questionnaires relate to spinal pain but some can be used for any disorder, e.g. the patient-specific functional scale (Westaway et al., 1998)

- review important aspects of the interview process
- describe the procedure of taking a history from a patient with a musculoskeletal disorder, considering the categories of questions that need to be asked and how best to obtain this information.

THE HISTORY: QUESTIONNAIRES FOR DISABILITY AND PAIN

Disability measures

After initially greeting the patient, many physiotherapists ask a general question regarding the patient's main reason for attending physiotherapy. The response provided indicates the measurement that the therapist needs to perform and the outcome of interest. For example, if a patient with chronic low back pain tells you that the main reason for attending physiotherapy is to return to work or sport, we must measure the disability, as well as monitor the return to work or sport. Commonly used disability questionnaires include:

- Patient-specific functional scale (Westaway et al., 1998) for any musculoskeletal disorder
- Roland–Morris Scale (RM 24; Roland and Morris, 1983) for low back dysfunction
- Oswestry Disability Index (Roland and Fairbank, 2000) for low back dysfunction
- Vernon–Mior Neck Disability Scale (Vernon and Mior, 1991) for neck dysfunction
- Neck pain and disability scale (Wheeler et al., 1999) for neck dysfunction.

These questionnaires are reproduced below with an overview of the questionnaire and evaluation of reliability and validity. One of these questionnaires may be given to the patient either before the physical examination, or after the initial assessment and treatment. The results will provide a reliable and valid measure of the patient's presenting level of disability and can be used to reflect changes in disability after treatment and over time.

Disability questionnaires are most likely to be useful for patients with subacute and chronic musculoskeletal conditions who may require several weeks to months of treatment. It is unlikely that disability needs to be measured in patients presenting with acute musculoskeletal conditions such as an acute wry neck where rapid recovery is predicted and disability is usually temporary.

Patient–specific functional scale

Overview and scoring of test   Generic and condition-specific disability scales include a standard set of items that are used for all patients. The limitation of a standard list of items is that they may include items that are not relevant to a particular patient, e.g. the Quebec Back Pain Disability Scale item 'throw a ball' may not be useful because many patients would not routinely throw a ball. Patient-generated or patient-specific disability scales solve this problem by asking the patient to specify activities that are of concern to them.

The patient-specific functional scale is a self-report disability measure that is specific to individual patients. The original version described by Stratford and colleagues in 1995 (Stratford et al., 1995) required subjects to specify five important activities that they were unable to do or had difficulty with as a result of their condition and to rate their ability to perform each activity on a 0–10 scale. A revised version was later published in 1998 that only required the subject to specify three activities (Westaway et al., 1998; Fig. 5.1). This change was made because the authors found that subjects had difficulty specifying five activities. In addition, the scoring system has been reversed: in the original version inability to perform a task was allocated a score of 10/10, whereas in the later version, reproduced here, normal performance of a task is allocated a score of 10/10.

Reliability   The questionnaire has been shown to have acceptable reliability when used to assess patients with low back pain, neck pain and knee dysfunction. In 63 outpatients with mechanical low back pain test–retest reliability was excellent ($ICC_{1,1} = 0.97$; standard error of measurement = 0.41, Stratford et al., 1995). Similarly, high reliability was reported when the scale was used with patients with neck dysfunction (ICC = 0.92, Westaway et al., 1998). The test–retest reliability was excellent for patients with knee dysfunction ($ICC_{2,1} = 0.84$) with a 2–3-day interval between testing (Chatman et al., 1997).

Validity   There is little information to date regarding the validity of the patient-specific functional scale.

Instructions:
Clinician to read and fill in at the end of the history and prior to physical examination.

Read at initial assessment
I'm going to ask you to identify *up to 3 important activities* that you are unable to do or have difficulty performing as a result of your problem.

Today, are there any activities that you are unable to do or have difficulty with because of your problem? (show scale)

Read at follow-up visits
When I assessed you on (state previous assessment date), you told me that you had difficulty with (read 1, 2, 3 from list).

Today do you still have difficulty with activity 1 (have patient score this activity); 2 (have patient score this activity); 3 (have patient score this activity)?

Scoring scheme (show patient scale):

0	1	2	3	4	5	6	7	8	9	10

Unable to perform activity

Able to perform activity at pre-injury level

Date/score

Activity											
1.											
2.											
3.											
Additional											
Additional											

Figure 5.1   Patient-specific functional scale. (Reproduced from Westaway MD, Stratford PW, Binkley JM. The patient-specific functional scale: validation of its use in persons with neck dysfunction. *J. Orthop. Sports Phys. Ther.* 1998; **27**(5): 331–338, with permission of the Orthopaedic and Sports Physical Therapy Sections of the American Physical Therapy Association.)

Roland–Morris Disability Questionnaire (RM-24)

Overview and scoring of test   The Roland–Morris low back questionnaire (Roland and Morris, 1983) is a self-report measure of perceived disability due to back pain (Fig. 5.2). The questionnaire was constructed by selecting 24 yes/no items from the Sickness Impact Profile (SIP), which covers a range of aspects of daily living that may be affected by low back pain. The questionnaire is completed by the patient who is required to place a tick beside statements which currently describe the patient's functional status. The questionnaire takes 5 min to complete and score. Each statement that is ticked is worth one point, with the maximum score possible being '24' representing severe disability and the lowest score possible '0' representing no perceived disability.

Reliability   The questionnaire has been shown to have acceptable reliability in a number of studies. Roland and Morris (1983) evaluated the test–retest reliability within the same day for 20 low back

Roland–Morris Disability Questionnaire (RM-24)

Name: _____ Date: _____

When your back hurts, you may find it difficult to do some of the things you normally do.

This list contains some sentences that people have used to describe themselves when they have back pain. When you read them, you may find that some stand out because they describe you **today**. As you read the list, think of yourself **today**. When you read a sentence that describes you today, fill the box to the left of the sentence. If the sentence does not describe you, then leave the box blank and go on to the next one. Remember, only mark the sentence if you are sure that it describes you **today**.

☐ 1. I stay at home most of the time because of my back.
☐ 2. I change positions frequently to try and get my back comfortable.
☐ 3. I walk more slowly than usual because of my back.
☐ 4. Because of my back, I am not doing any of the jobs that I usually do around the house.
☐ 5. Because of my back, I use a handrail to get upstairs.
☐ 6. Because of my back, I lie down to rest more often.
☐ 7. Because of my back, I have to hold on to something to get out of an easy chair.
☐ 8. Because of my back, I try to get other people to do things for me.
☐ 9. I get dressed more slowly than usual because of my back.
☐ 10. I only stand up for short periods of time because of my back.
☐ 11. Because of my back, I try not to bend or kneel down.
☐ 12. I find it difficult to get out of a chair because of my back.
☐ 13. My back is painful almost all the time.
☐ 14. I find it difficult to turn over in bed because of my back.
☐ 15. My appetite is not very good because of my back pain.
☐ 16. I have trouble putting on my socks (or stockings) because of the pain in my back.
☐ 17. I only walk short distances because of my back pain.
☐ 18. I sleep less well because of my back.
☐ 19. Because of my back pain, I get dressed with help from someone else.
☐ 20. I sit down for most of the day because of my back.
☐ 21. I avoid heavy jobs around the house because of my back.
☐ 22. Because of my back pain, I am more irritable and bad-tempered with people than usual.
☐ 23. Because of my back, I go upstairs more slowly than usual.
☐ 24. I stay in bed most of the time because of my back.

Figure 5.2 Roland–Morris Scale (RM-24). (Reproduced from Roland and Fairbank, 2000.)

pain patients and noted a correlation coefficient of 0.91 between the two sets of scores and agreement within one point for 13 of the patients. Brodie et al. (1990) evaluated reliability over a 2-day period and found 89% exact agreement for the scale when delivered to 20 patients with non-specific low back pain. Similar results were found by Jensen et al. (1992) and Kopec et al. (1995). The largest reliability study was performed by Kopec et al. (1995) using 98 low back pain patients with a test–retest interval of 1–14 days. This study is of interest because it compared the reliability of the Quebec, Roland–Morris and Oswestry scales and noted that all had excellent reliability (ICC 0.91–0.92).

Stratford and colleagues conducted two studies (Stratford et al., 1996) designed to assist the therapist to interpret changes in RM scores. The studies provide information on how large a change score needs to be for the therapist to be confident that the change represents true change and not error. They expressed the results as the minimal detectable change (the minimum amount of change required between two points in time to be confident that a patient has truly changed). Stratford et al. (1996) reported that the minimum level of detectable change at the 90% confidence interval was 4–5 points on the scale. This result means that a therapist cannot be confident that true change has occurred until the difference in scores is 4–5 points on the scale. The implication of this result is that when a patient scores <4 it is not possible to document recovery and in such patients it would be wise to judge recovery in some other way. For patients who obtain a score of 20 or more the instrument is useful to document improvement but deterioration cannot be confidently ascertained.

Validity   There is good evidence for the construct validity of the RM-24 scale. Patients' scores on the Roland–Morris scale correlate highly with their scores on other low back pain disability scales such as the Quebec Scale (Kopec et al., 1995) and the Oswestry Disability Index (Co et al., 1993) and with the longer SIP (Deyo and Centor, 1986; Jensen et al., 1992). Correlations with pain were moderate and with physical impairments only fair.

The ability of the RM-24 to detect change over time has been shown in two studies using receiver operating characteristic curves (Deyo and Centor, 1986; Stratford et al., 1994) and another using the *t*-statistic (Jensen et al., 1992). Deyo and Centor (1986) found that the SIP and the RM-24 scale were equally sensitive to change over time in a study of patients with low back pain. A study by Kopec et al. (1995) found that the sensitivity to true change was, on average, similar for the Quebec and RM-24 but both were always superior to the Oswestry and the Short Form-36 (a measure of health-related quality of life). Beurskens et al. (1996) also found that the RM-24 was more sensitive than the Oswestry, although recent preliminary data show that the Patient Specific Functional Scale is more responsive to change than the RM-24 (Pengel et al., 2004).

The Oswestry disability index

Overview and scoring of test   The Oswestry is a self-report measure of perceived low back pain-related disability (Fig. 5.3) and was developed at the Robert Jones and Agnes Hunt Orthopaedic Hospital in Oswestry in the UK, hence the name.

The questionnaire consists of 10 sections which each contain six statements representing increasing levels of disability on that dimension or, in the case of section 1, pain intensity. The questionnaire can be filled in by the patient and then scored by the therapist in approximately 5 min. For each section the maximum score is five, with the first statement marked with 0 and the last statement with a 5. If all 10 sections are completed the maximum

score is 50 which is then converted to a percentage. High percentages represent high disability.

If a section is missed or not applicable the percentage is adjusted accordingly. Frequently the section on sex life is ignored by patients and so it is common for the maximum score to be only 45, which is then converted to a percentage. The Hudson Cook version of the Oswestry omits the sex life section and replaces it with a second pain section.

There are four English-language and nine non-English-language versions of the Oswestry. In the authors' recent review of the Oswestry disability index they advocate use of version 2.0 (Roland and Fairbank, 2000).

Reliability   The scale has been shown to have high test–retest reliability (Fairbank et al., 1980; Gronblad et al., 1993). The best result was a correlation of 0.99 for a 1-day test–retest interval and the worst an ICC value of 0.83 for a 1-week test–retest interval.

Validity   There is good evidence for the construct validity of the scale. As expected, patients' scores on the Oswestry scale correlate highly with their scores on other low back pain disability scales such as the Quebec (Kopec et al., 1995) and the Roland–Morris Disability questionnaires (Co et al., 1993) and also generic disability scales such as the Pain Disability Index (Gronblad et al., 1993). Oswestry scores correlate moderately with pain measures (Gronblad et al., 1993) but have only fair correlations with impairment measures such as muscle strength (Gronblad et al., 1997).

The scale has been used as an outcome measure in a variety of studies that have demonstrated an effect for treatment and, together with the Roland–Morris scale, is probably the most widely used disability outcome measure in back pain research. Stratford et al. (1994) have shown that the Roland–Morris and Oswestry scales have equally good ability to detect change over time in low back pain patients. However, a study by Kopec et al. (1995) found that the responsiveness to change of the Oswestry was lower than the Roland–Morris and Quebec scales. Beurskens et al. (1996) also found that the Roland–Morris was more sensitive than the Oswestry.

Oswestry Disability Index version .2.0

Name: _____   Date: _____

Please read:

This questionnaire has been designed to give information as to how your back pain has affected your ability to manage in everyday life. Please answer every section, and mark in each section only the *one box* which applies to you. We realize you may consider that two of the statements in any one section relate to you, but please just *mark the box which most closely describes your problem.*

Section 1 – Pain intensity
- ☐ I have no pain at the moment.
- ☐ The pain is very mild at the moment.
- ☐ The pain is moderate at the moment.
- ☐ The pain is fairly severe at the moment.
- ☐ The pain is very severe at the moment.
- ☐ The pain is the worst imaginable at the moment.

Section 2 – Personal care (washing, dressing, etc.)
- ☐ I can look after myself normally without causing extra pain.
- ☐ I can look after myself normally but it causes extra pain.
- ☐ It is painful to look after myself and I am slow and careful.
- ☐ I need some help but manage most of my personal care.
- ☐ I need help every day in most aspects of self-care.
- ☐ I do not get dressed, wash with difficulty and stay in bed.

Section 3 – Lifting
- ☐ I can lift heavy weights without extra pain.
- ☐ I can lift heavy weights but it gives extra pain.
- ☐ Pain prevents me from lifting heavy weights off the floor, but I can manage if they are conveniently positioned, e.g. on a table.
- ☐ Pain prevents me from lifting heavy weights but I can manage light to medium weights if they are conveniently positioned.
- ☐ I can lift only very light weights.
- ☐ I cannot lift or carry anything at all.

Section 4 – Walking
- ☐ Pain does not prevent me walking any distance.
- ☐ Pain prevents me walking more than 1 mile.
- ☐ Pain prevents me walking more than ½ mile.
- ☐ Pain prevents me walking more than 100 yards.
- ☐ I can only walk using a stick or crutches.
- ☐ I am in bed most of the time and have to crawl to the toilet.

Section 5 – Sitting
- ☐ I can sit in any chair as long as I like.
- ☐ I can only sit in my favourite chair as long as I like.
- ☐ Pain prevents me sitting more than 1 hour.
- ☐ Pain prevents me from sitting more than 1/2 hour.
- ☐ Pain prevents me from sitting more than 10 min.
- ☐ Pain prevents me from sitting at all.

Section 6 – Standing
- ☐ I can stand as long as I want without extra pain.
- ☐ I can stand as long as I want but it gives me extra pain.
- ☐ Pain prevents me from standing for more than 1 hour.
- ☐ Pain prevents me from standing for more than 30 min.
- ☐ Pain prevents me from standing for more than 10 min.
- ☐ Pain prevents me from standing at all.

Section 7 – Sleeping
- ☐ Pain does not prevent me from sleeping well.
- ☐ I can sleep well only by using tablets.
- ☐ Even when I take tablets I have less than 6 hours' sleep.
- ☐ Even when I take tablets I have less than 4 hours' sleep.
- ☐ Even when I take tablets I have less than 2 hours' sleep.
- ☐ Pain prevents me from sleeping at all.

Section 8 – Sex life
- ☐ My sex life is normal and causes no extra pain.
- ☐ My sex life is normal but causes some extra pain.
- ☐ My sex life is nearly normal but is very painful.
- ☐ My sex life is severely restricted by pain.
- ☐ My sex life is nearly absent because of pain.
- ☐ Pain prevents any sex life at all.

Section 9 – Social life
- ☐ My social life is normal and gives me no extra pain.
- ☐ My social life is normal but increases the degree of pain.
- ☐ Pain has no significant effect on my social life apart from limiting my more energetic interests, e.g. sport etc.
- ☐ Pain has restricted my social life and I do not go out as often.
- ☐ Pain has restricted my social life to my home.
- ☐ I have no social life because of pain.

Section 10 – Travelling
- ☐ I can travel anywhere without extra pain.
- ☐ I can travel anywhere but it gives me extra pain.
- ☐ Pain is bad but I manage journeys over 2 hours.
- ☐ Pain restricts me to journeys of less than 1 hour.
- ☐ Pain restricts me to short necessary journeys under 30 min.
- ☐ Pain prevents me from travelling except to receive treatment.

Figure 5.3   The Oswestry Disability Index (version 2.0). (Reproduced from Roland and Fairbank, 2000.)

Vernon–Mior Neck Disability Index

Overview and scoring of test   The Vernon–Mior Neck Disability Index is a modification of the Oswestry Low Back Pain Disability Questionnaire (Fig. 5.4). The questionnaire consists of 10 sections, each section containing six statements that represent problems of increasing severity on that dimension. The questionnaire can be filled in by the patient and then scored by the therapist in approximately 5 min. For each section the maximum score is five, with the first statement marked with 0 and the last statement with a 5. If all 10 sections are completed the maximum score is 50 points which is sometimes converted to a percentage. High scores or percentages represent high disability.

Reliability   The instrument has been repeatedly shown to have excellent test–retest reliability (Vernon and Mior, 1991) and internal consistency (Vernon and Mior, 1991; Hains et al., 1998). Stratford and colleagues (1999) reported that the minimal level of detectable or true change was 4.7 points (or 9.4% if expressed as a percentage), i.e. a patient needs to improve by more than 4.7 points to be confident that true change has occurred.

Validity   Riddle and Stratford (1998) administered the Short-Form 36 (SF-36) and the neck disability index (NDI) to 146 patients with neck pain. The NDI correlated moderately well with the mental component summary scale ($r = 0.47$) and with the physical component summary scale of the SF-36 ($r = 0.53$).

Vernon–Mior Neck Disability Index

Name: _____   Date: _____

This questionnaire has been designed to give the physiotherapist information as to how your neck pain has affected your ability to manage in everyday life. Please answer every section and mark in each section only the *one* box which applies to you. We realize you may consider that two of the statements in any one section relate to you, but please just mark the box which most closely describes your problem.

Section 1 – Pain intensity
- ☐ I have no pain at the moment.
- ☐ The pain is very mild at the moment.
- ☐ The pain is moderate at the moment.
- ☐ The pain is fairly severe at the moment.
- ☐ The pain is very severe at the moment.
- ☐ The pain is the worst imaginable at the moment.

Section 2 – Personal care (washing, dressing, etc.)
- ☐ I can look after myself normally without causing extra pain.
- ☐ I can look after myself normally but it causes extra pain.
- ☐ It is painful to look after myself and I am slow and careful.
- ☐ I need some help but manage most of my personal care.
- ☐ I need help every day in most aspects of self-care.
- ☐ I do not get dressed, I wash with difficulty and stay in bed.

Section 3 – Lifting
- ☐ I can lift heavy weights without extra pain.
- ☐ I can lift heavy weights but it gives extra pain.
- ☐ Pain prevents me from lifting heavy weights off the floor, but I can manage if they are conveniently positioned, for example on a table.
- ☐ Pain prevents me from lifting heavy weights, but I can manage light to medium weights if they are conveniently positioned.
- ☐ I can lift very light weights.
- ☐ I cannot lift or carry anything at all.

Section 4 – Reading
- ☐ I can read as much as I want to with no pain in my neck.
- ☐ I can read as much as I want to with slight pain in my neck.
- ☐ I can read as much as I want with moderate pain in my neck.
- ☐ I can't read as much as I want because of moderate pain in my neck.
- ☐ I can hardly read at all because of severe pain in my neck.
- ☐ I cannot read at all.

Section 5 – Headaches
- ☐ I have no headaches at all.
- ☐ I have slight headaches which come infrequently.
- ☐ I have moderate headaches which come infrequently.
- ☐ I have moderate headaches which come frequently.
- ☐ I have severe headaches which come frequently
- ☐ I have headaches almost all the time.

Section 6 – Concentration
- ☐ I can concentrate fully when I want to with no difficulty.
- ☐ I can concentrate fully when I want to with slight difficulty.
- ☐ I have a fair degree of difficulty in concentrating when I want to.
- ☐ I have a lot of difficulty in concentrating when I want to.
- ☐ I have a great deal of difficulty in concentrating when I want to.
- ☐ I cannot concentrate at all.

Section 7 – Work
- ☐ I can do as much work as I want to.
- ☐ I can only do my usual work, but no more.
- ☐ I can do most of my usual work, but no more.
- ☐ I cannot do my usual work.
- ☐ I can hardly do any work at all.
- ☐ I can't do any work at all.

Section 8 – Driving
- ☐ I can drive my car without any neck pain.
- ☐ I can drive my car as long as I want with slight pain in my neck.
- ☐ I can drive my car as long as I want with moderate pain in my neck.
- ☐ I can't drive my car as long as I want because of moderate pain in my neck.
- ☐ I can hardly drive at all because of severe pain in my neck.
- ☐ I can't drive my car at all.

Section 9 – Sleeping
- ☐ I have no trouble sleeping.
- ☐ My sleep is slightly disturbed (less than 1 h sleepless).
- ☐ My sleep is mildly disturbed (1–2 h sleepless).
- ☐ My sleep is moderately disturbed (2–3 h sleepless).
- ☐ My sleep is greatly disturbed (3–5 h sleepless).
- ☐ My sleep is completely disturbed (5–7 h sleepless).

Section 10 – Recreation
- ☐ I am able to engage in all my recreation activities with no neck pain at all.
- ☐ I am able to engage in all my recreation activities, with some pain in my neck.
- ☐ I am able to engage in most but not all of my usual recreation activities because of pain in my neck.
- ☐ I am able to engage in a few of my usual recreation activities because of pain in my neck.
- ☐ I can hardly do any recreation activities because of pain in my neck.
- ☐ I can't do any recreation activities at all.

Figure 5.4   Vernon–Mior Neck Disability Index. (Reprinted from *Journal of Manipulative and Physiological Therapeutics*, 14, Vernon H and Mior S, The Neck Disability Index: a study of reliability and validity, pp. 409–415, Copyright (1991), with permission from *International Association for the Study of Pain*.)

The Neck Pain and Disability Scale (Wheeler et al., 1999)

Overview and scoring of test   The Neck Pain and Disability Scale consists of 20 items that assess neck pain and neck pain-related disability (Fig. 5.5; Wheeler et al., 1999). The items measure the intensity of pain, its interference with self-care, work, social and recreational activities and associated emotional factors. Each item is scored on a 0–5 scale with the total score ranging from 0 to 100.

Reliability   The internal consistency was established in a sample of 100 patients seeking care for neck pain ($r = 0.93$). Factor analysis revealed four factors that accounted for 76% of the variance. The authors labelled the factors 'neck problems', 'pain intensity', 'effect of neck pain on emotion and cognition' and 'interference with life activities' (Wheeler et al., 1999).

Validity Evidence for face validity was demonstrated by higher scores in a group of patients with neck pain (mean = 60.5; range 8–89) compared to those with back pain (mean = 44; range 0–70) and a score close to zero for painfree subjects (mean = 0.78; range 0–7). Evidence for convergent validity was provided by correlations with the Oswestry Disability Questionnaire (0.78) and the Pain Disability Index (0.80).

Neck Pain and Disability Scale

Please circle a number to show how far from normal (0), toward the worst possible situation (5), your pain problem has taken you.

1. How bad is your pain today?

| 0 | 1 | 2 | 3 | 4 | 5 |
No pain   Most severe pain

2. How bad is your pain on average?

| 0 | 1 | 2 | 3 | 4 | 5 |
No pain   Most severe pain

3. How bad is your pain at its worst?

| 0 | 1 | 2 | 3 | 4 | 5 |
No pain   Cannot tolerate

4. Does your pain interfere with your sleep?

| 0 | 1 | 2 | 3 | 4 | 5 |
Not at all   Can't sleep

5. How bad is your pain with standing?

| 0 | 1 | 2 | 3 | 4 | 5 |
No pain   Most severe pain

6. How bad is your pain with walking?

| 0 | 1 | 2 | 3 | 4 | 5 |
No pain   Most severe pain

7. Does your pain interfere with driving or riding in a car?

| 0 | 1 | 2 | 3 | 4 | 5 |
Not at all   Can't drive or ride

8. Does your pain interfere with social activities?

| 0 | 1 | 2 | 3 | 4 | 5 |
Not at all   Always

9. Does your pain interfere with recreational activities?

| 0 | 1 | 2 | 3 | 4 | 5 |
Not at all   Always

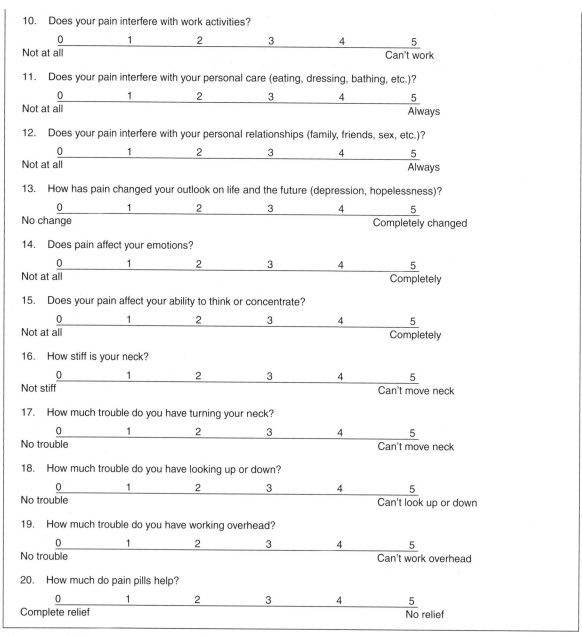

10. Does your pain interfere with work activities?

| 0 | 1 | 2 | 3 | 4 | 5 |

Not at all   Can't work

11. Does your pain interfere with your personal care (eating, dressing, bathing, etc.)?

| 0 | 1 | 2 | 3 | 4 | 5 |

Not at all   Always

12. Does your pain interfere with your personal relationships (family, friends, sex, etc.)?

| 0 | 1 | 2 | 3 | 4 | 5 |

Not at all   Always

13. How has pain changed your outlook on life and the future (depression, hopelessness)?

| 0 | 1 | 2 | 3 | 4 | 5 |

No change   Completely changed

14. Does pain affect your emotions?

| 0 | 1 | 2 | 3 | 4 | 5 |

Not at all   Completely

15. Does your pain affect your ability to think or concentrate?

| 0 | 1 | 2 | 3 | 4 | 5 |

Not at all   Completely

16. How stiff is your neck?

| 0 | 1 | 2 | 3 | 4 | 5 |

Not stiff   Can't move neck

17. How much trouble do you have turning your neck?

| 0 | 1 | 2 | 3 | 4 | 5 |

No trouble   Can't move neck

18. How much trouble do you have looking up or down?

| 0 | 1 | 2 | 3 | 4 | 5 |

No trouble   Can't look up or down

19. How much trouble do you have working overhead?

| 0 | 1 | 2 | 3 | 4 | 5 |

No trouble   Can't work overhead

20. How much do pain pills help?

| 0 | 1 | 2 | 3 | 4 | 5 |

Complete relief   No relief

Figure 5.5   Neck Pain and Disability Scale. (Reproduced with permission from Wheeler et al., 1999. Development of the Neck Pain and Disability Scale. Item analysis, face, and criterion-related disability. *Spine*, **24**, 1290–1294.)

MEASUREMENT OF PAIN

Pain measures

If, like the majority of patients with musculoskeletal conditions, the patient is seeking treatment for the relief of pain, then adequate measurement of pain must be performed. Several studies have demonstrated that there is little correlation between measures of disability and direct measures of pain, although disability may be related to attitudes and beliefs about pain (Meade et al., 1990; Strong et al., 1990). Therefore a disability measure cannot be used to infer information about pain or vice versa. Pain may be measured both directly and indirectly. Indirect measures include measures of analgesic intake or demand, and measures of the number of times a patient engages in pain behaviours such as moaning, contortion and facial expressions. Direct pain measures commonly used by physiotherapists include scales that measure either the sensory dimension or intensity of the pain, and scales that measure the affective dimension or unpleasantness of the pain. These scales are called unidimensional measures while scales that measure both the sensory and affective dimensions of pain are called multidimensional measures. The scales commonly used by physiotherapists are listed below.

Unidimensional measures

1. Pain drawings
2. Pain scales:
    (a) Visual analogue scale (VAS)
       - Sensory VAS
       - Affective VAS
    (b) Verbal rating scale
    (c) Numerical rating scale.

Multidimensional measures

1. Short-form McGill Pain Questionnaire (SFMPQ).

These measures are described below with an overview of the measure and information regarding their reliability and validity.

Unidimensional measures

Pain drawings Many authors have demonstrated the poor correlations between pain, disability and physical impairment. Therefore the decision to measure pain should be based upon an understanding that pain is the patient's main concern and that pain should change following an intervention. Physiotherapists commonly use body charts to map the areas of paraesthesia and anaesthesia. With pain drawings, patients are asked to shade in areas within an outline of a human figure which correspond to areas of their body which are in pain.

Reliability For the pain drawing to be used as a measure of treatment progress and outcome, the stability of painful areas depicted in the drawing needs to be high. Margolis and colleagues (1988) examined

the test–retest reliability of pain drawings in a group of 51 patients with chronic pain. They reported a test–retest reliability of $r = 0.85$ for patients evaluated over an average of 71 days, when raters estimated the number of body areas shaded.

Validity Pain drawings have been used to discriminate between pain of organic and non-organic origin (Margolis et al., 1986). Also Ransford et al. (1976) suggest that pain drawings may aid in the psychological evaluation of patients with back pain.

Pain scales
Visual analogue scales
Pain intensity The absolute visual analogue scale (AVAS) is widely used by physiotherapists to measure pain intensity. The AVAS consists of a 100-mm line bounded with verbal descriptors such as 'No pain' at one end and 'Pain as bad as it could possibly be' at the other end (Fig. 5.6; Scott and Huskisson, 1976).

Sensory and affective dimensions of pain The AVAS can also be used to separate the sensory and affective dimensions of pain by changing the descriptors. To help the patient understand the two dimensions of pain, the sensation of pain can be compared to the sensation of sound with the following analogy:

> There are two aspects of pain which we are interested in measuring: the intensity, how strong the pain feels, and the unpleasantness, how unpleasant or disturbing the pain is for you. The distinction between these two aspects of pain might be made clearer if you think of listening to a sound, such as a radio. As the volume of the sound increases, I can ask you how loud it sounds or how unpleasant it is to hear it. The intensity of pain is like loudness; the unpleasantness of pain depends not only on intensity but also on other factors which may affect you (Price et al., 1983).

To further assist the differentiation, the two VAS should preferably not be placed directly under each other but rather one aligned horizontally and the other vertically (Figs 5.7 and 5.8).

The anchors used in this scale are 'The most unpleasant feeling possible for me' and 'Not bad at all'. The distance from 'Not bad at all' to the mark made by the patient in millimetres represents the pain score.

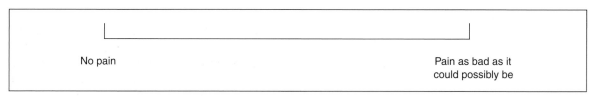

Figure 5.6 Simple visual analogue scale. A line 100 mm long is anchored with the descriptors 'No pain' and 'Pain as bad as it could possibly be'. The patient marks the line to indicate the magnitude of the pain.

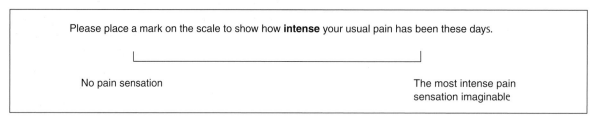

Figure 5.7 Visual analogue scale (VAS). The VAS is used to measure the sensory dimension of pain, ranging from 'No pain sensation' to 'The most intense pain sensation imaginable'.

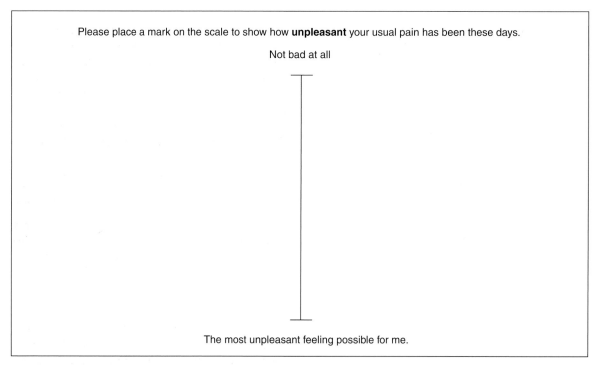

Figure 5.8 Visual analogue scale used to measure the affective dimension of pain. The anchors used reflect the domain ranging from 'Not bad at all' to 'The most unpleasant feeling possible for me'.

Reliability of AVAS   Although pain rating scales are reported to have high reliability (Zusman, 1986), few studies have clearly recorded the reliability coefficients of any of the pain rating scales.

Validity of AVAS   Validity is discussed for all pain rating scales together at the end of the section, after verbal and numerical rating scales.

Table 5.2   Intensity scales

5-point scale	15-point scale
None	Extremely weak
Mild	Very weak
Moderate	Weak
Severe	Very mild
Very severe	Mild
	Very moderate
	Slightly moderate
	Moderate
	Barely strong
	Slightly intense
	Strong
	Intense
	Very strong
	Very intense
	Extremely intense

Verbal rating scale for pain intensity   Verbal rating scales (VRS) contain a list of adjectives that are frequently used to describe different levels of pain intensity. Examples of a 5-point and a 15-point scale appear in Table 5.2 (Gracely et al., 1978a,b).

A pain score is obtained by assigning a number to each word according to its rank on the order of pain intensity. For example, on the 5-point scale, 'none' would be given a score of 0, 'mild' a score of 1.

Affective scale (Gracely et al., 1978a)   Verbal rating scales can also be constructed to measure the affective dimension of pain.

15-point scale:

- Bearable
- Distracting
- Unpleasant
- Uncomfortable
- Distressing
- Oppressive
- Miserable
- Awful
- Frightful
- Dreadful
- Horrible
- Agonizing
- Unbearable
- Intolerable
- Excruciating

Numerical rating scale (Ross and LaStayo, 1997)   Numerical rating scales require patients to rate their perceived level of pain intensity on a numerical rating scale from 0 to 10, i.e. an 11-point scale, or 0–100, a 101-point scale. The 0 represents no pain, and the 10 or 100 represents pain as bad as it could be.

101-point numerical rating scale   Patients are asked to identify the intensity of the pain experienced by choosing a number that reflects the intensity. The number should lie in the range 0–10 for the 11-point scale and 0–100 for the 101-point scale. For example:

Please indicate on the line below the number between 0 and 100 that best describes your pain. A zero (0) would mean 'no pain' and a one hundred (100) would mean 'pain as bad as it could be'. Please write only one response.

e.g.   _____59_____

11-point box scale   Another form of numerical rating scale is the box scale. Numbers between 0 and 10 appear in adjacent boxes of a table. Patients are asked to mark the box that reflects the pain intensity where zero (0) means no pain, and 10 means the worst pain ever.

e.g.: On the zero to 10 scale below, put an X through the number that best pinpoints your level of pain.

0	1	2	3	4	5	6	7	8	9	10

Reliability of pain scales   Although pain rating scales are reported to have high reliability (Zusman, 1986), few studies have clearly recorded the reliability coefficients of any of the pain rating scales.

Responsiveness of pain scales   A recent study has shown that the VAS is more responsive when used to rate average pain over the last 24 h rather than current pain (Scrimshaw and Maher, 2001). This result has also been shown for pain judged over 1 week (Bolton and Wilkinson, 1998) and a fortnight (Jensen et al., 1999). These results make sense because patients would typically be made comfortable during the interview so that their current pain may be quite unlike their typical pain.

Validity of pain scales The AVAS is highly correlated with verbal ($r = 0.81$) and numerical rating scales (Ohnaus and Adler, 1975; Kremer et al., 1981). When used to measure intensity, verbal and numerical scales are sensitive to change in pain (Jensen et al., 1986, 1989), and have high validity in terms of outcome measures (Jensen et al., 1986, 1989). Higher initial VAS scores were highly correlated with delayed recovery from low back pain (Gatchel et al., 1995).

VRS are highly correlated with intensity measures of pain using the AVAS.

Multidimensional pain measures

Short-form McGill Pain Questionnaire

Overview The SFMPQ (Fig. 5.9; Melzack, 1987) is designed to measure the sensory, affective and overall intensity of pain. The scale was developed from the standard McGill Pain Questionnaire to provide a measure of pain that provides more information than a simple VAS yet does not take the 5–10 min required for the standard McGill. The McGill has become the most widely used measure of pain in pain research and has had substantial investigation of its reliability and validity for a number of pain conditions. The SFMPQ and standard McGill are available in a number of languages, including French, Italian, Spanish and Norwegian.

The short-form uses the first 11 descriptors to represent the sensory dimension of the pain experience and descriptors 12–15 to represent the affective dimension. Each descriptor is ranked on an intensity scale from 0 = none to 3 = severe. A score is then obtained for the sensory descriptors, the affective descriptors and the total score. The SFMPQ also includes the present pain intensity of the standard scale and the VAS to provide overall pain intensity scores. The short form takes 2–5 min to administer and score.

Reliability The English version of the questionnaire has not been examined for reliability; however, the long form has repeatedly been shown to have good reliability. A Swedish version has been shown to have acceptably high internal consistency and test–retest reliability (Burckhardt and Bjelle, 1994).

Validity High correlations have been found between the standard McGill and the SFMPQ when used to measure pain in obstetric and post-surgical wards and to measure spinal pain in physiotherapy departments (Melzack, 1987). In the same study the scale was shown to be sufficiently sensitive to demonstrate differences due to treatment.

Evidence for the ability of the scale to measure the affective and sensory dimensions separately is provided by two studies (Melzack, 1987; Dudgeon et al., 1993) that showed high correlations between the long- and short-form scores for sensory pain and affective pain. Gronblad et al. (1990) further showed that SFMPQ affective and sensory scores were not correlated in a group of chronic low back pain patients. However the results may have been biased because on both instruments the sensory and affective descriptors are grouped together.

The results of a number of studies (Kremer et al., 1981, 1983; McCreary et al., 1981; Geisser et al., 1994) provide support for the opinion that the affective scale of the standard McGill can provide information about psychological impairments. For example, Kremer et al. (1983) found that patients who reported high affective scores on the standard McGill were more depressed and anxious than patients who reported low affective scores.

THE PROCESS OF TAKING A HISTORY FOR MUSCULOSKELETAL DISORDERS

The interview

The combination of an interview and completion of relevant, reliable and accurate questionnaires is the best way to obtain good-quality data from the patient regarding their presenting disorder (Table 5.1). Some categories of information are best gained by questionnaire, and other categories by interview (Table 5.1). Taking a good history, therefore, requires good interpersonal skills as well as a good knowledge base to interpret the information gained.

After charting the area of pain and rating its intensity and unpleasantness, physiotherapists generally proceed to interview patients regarding many other aspects of the pain and resultant disability such as the onset and progression of the disorder

Short-Form McGill Pain Questionnaire

Name: _____   Date: _____

Please read each word below, and decide whether it describes what your pain feels like. If a word *does not* describe your pain tick none, and go on to the next item. If a word does describe your pain, then rate how strongly you have felt that sensation by ticking the mild, moderate or severe box.

My pain felt like it was:

	None	Mild	Moderate	Severe
1. Throbbing	0	1	2	3
2. Shooting	0	1	2	3
3. Stabbing	0	1	2	3
4. Sharp	0	1	2	3
5. Cramping	0	1	2	3
6. Gnawing	0	1	2	3
7. Hot/burning	0	1	2	3
8. Aching	0	1	2	3
9. Heavy	0	1	2	3
10. Tender	0	1	2	3
11. Splitting	0	1	2	3
12. Tiring/exhausting	0	1	2	3
13. Sickening	0	1	2	3
14. Fearful	0	1	2	3
15. Punishing/cruel	0	1	2	3

Please put a mark on the scale to show how bad your *usual* pain has been *these* days.

No pain | _____ | Worst possible pain

How bad is your pain *now*?

0	No pain	_____
1	Mild	_____
2	Discomforting	_____
3	Distressing	_____
4	Horrible	_____
5	Excruciating	_____

Figure 5.9 Short-form McGill Pain Questionnaire. This questionnaire is used to measure sensory, affective and overall intensity of pain. (Reprinted from *Pain*, 30, Melzack R, The Short-form McGill Pain Questionnaire, pp. 191–197, Copyright (1987), with permission from *National University of Health Services*.)

and the presence of contraindications or precautions to treatment. Hypotheses regarding injured structures, useful treatments and expected outcome are generated based on the information obtained from the interview. It is essential therefore that this information is as accurate and reliable as possible.

There are many factors that may affect the reliability of information obtained during the interview. These include misinterpretation of information from the patient to the therapist and vice versa, poor patient memory or recall, lack of patient concentration due to severe pain or fatigue and patient motivation, including factors such as desire to please, or desire to appear stoic. Patient reporting may also be influenced by the non-verbal cues they receive from the physiotherapist. If the physiotherapist appears tired and uninterested, or judgemental, then this may affect how the patient responds. The therapist needs to be positioned at the same level and facing the patient so that he or she can best convey interest in the patient's problems. The therapist should shake hands or smile to welcome the patient. During the interview, maintaining appropriate eye contact with the patient and nodding in affirmation of what the patient says helps to reassure the patient that the therapist is interested in the problem and helps to promote a relationship of trust.

In summary, when taking a history from a patient with spinal pain you may prefer to interview the patient, use a series of relevant questionnaires, or use a combination of both. Reliable questionnaires provide the physiotherapist with a score that may be compared with the results of testing following treatment and over time. This will be more useful in determining outcome than relying solely on the therapist's impression of whether a patient's aggravating activities are resolving or not. Questionnaires may also be used to alert the therapist to historical features that the patient may have that suggest that manual therapy is contraindicated for that patient. The next section will discuss this in detail.

INTERPRETATION OF SPECIFIC INFORMATION

Area and type of symptoms (body chart)

The body chart is really a map of the patient's symptoms outlined on a chart of the body, as shown in

Figure 5.10, and discussed earlier in the section on measurement of pain. This chart may be completed by the patient or the area of pain reported to the physiotherapist who then completes the body chart for the patient. The purpose of completing such a map is to identify possible sources of symptoms by:

1. identifying clearly all areas and types of symptoms
2. initial determination of the relationship of symptomatic areas.

Hypotheses raised from the body chart will be pursued throughout the remainder of the examination.

Information mapped on the body chart includes the area, constancy, quality and severity of symptoms, and the relationship of symptoms if there is more than one area. The depth of pain is sometimes also determined.

Area

The area of symptoms gives much information about the source of the problem, and perhaps about prognosis. Knowledge of referral patterns (and receptive fields; see Schaible and Grubb, 1993) and of common patterns of presentation of particular pathologies is required to interpret the symptoms effectively. Dermatomes and myotomes are illustrated in Williams and Warwick (1980). Pain radiating down the lateral aspect of the calf and foot, for example, may indicate involvement of the fifth lumbar segment or spinal nerve (Williams and Warwick, 1980). Recently the pain referral patterns of the thoracic zygapophyseal joints have also been clearly documented (Dreyfuss et al., 1994), as have referral patterns for various lumbar spine somatic structures. Several studies have found that pain from the lumbar spine radiating below the knee is likely to be radicular in origin (McCulloch and Waddell, 1980; Austen, 1991).

The area and type of symptoms can also be used as a baseline measure to monitor treatment effects. For example, a decrease in area of pain or centralizing of pain towards the spine may indicate improvement in the condition (McKenzie, 1981), whereas a change from paraesthesia to anaesthesia would signify a worsening of the condition. For these reasons it is important to determine as accurately as possible all sites of symptoms. This

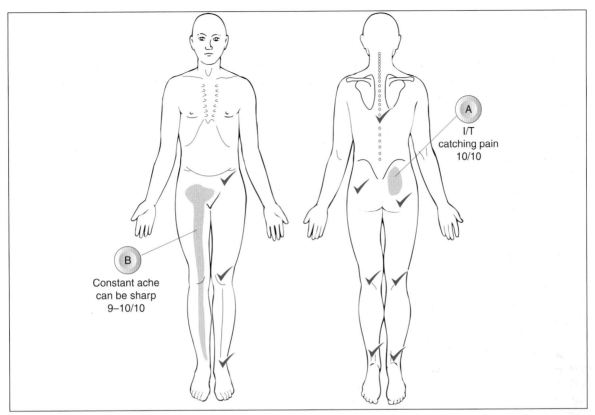

Figure 5.10   Body chart used to map spatial distribution and describe quality of patient's symptoms. I/T, intermittent.

often means asking specifically about the presence or absence of symptoms in the leg (in lumbar spine conditions) or arm (in disorders of the cervical spine). All possible sources of symptoms must be followed up throughout the examination.

Absence of symptoms should also be recorded. This indicates that the patient was asked about symptoms in these areas and they were not present.

The area of symptoms is also used to assist in determining the prognosis. It is generally considered that a large area of pain with many associated symptoms, such as pins and needles, would take longer to recover fully than would a small localized area of pain with no other symptoms. For a thorough review of spinal pain, see Schaible and Grubb (1993).

Anaesthesia or paraesthesia

Patients presenting with spinal musculoskeletal conditions are routinely asked whether they have any areas of paraesthesia (altered sensation such as pins and needles) or anaesthesia (absence of sensation or numbness). The presence of any altered sensation is strongly suggestive of nerve compromise, particularly when the distribution of symptoms is dermatomal (Helfet and Gruebel, 1978; Sunderland, 1978; see Ch. 6). Other conditions, including vascular compromise or perhaps altered afferent input from somatic structures, may also cause paraesthesia. However, the most common cause of altered sensation accompanying spinal disorders is compromise of the spinal nerve/nerve root (Bodguk, 1991).

Constancy

Constancy refers to whether the symptoms are continuously present and, more importantly, whether the intensity of the symptoms varies, particularly with movement or positioning. Generally, pain or paraesthesia that is made worse or better by certain movements or positions is likely to be musculoskeletal in origin or, as it is often described, has a mechanical component. This is because when the tissues involved are stressed they will transmit painful stimuli. Many pathologies will present with this pattern of signs and symptoms responding to movement, such as some skeletal metastases, notably osteoid osteoma (Martire, 1987; O'Connor and Currier, 1992), but other information from the history and physical examination should alert the physiotherapist that the condition may be due to serious or identifiable pathology. Patients may have pain at rest, that is, even when they are not moving, but if their pain does not vary (i.e. increase or decrease) with movement, the problem may not be a mechanical disorder of the musculoskeletal system. Rather, it may be systemic or organic, caused by pathologies like arthritis or cancer or diseases of the viscera. A patient may have constant pain (resting pain) because of accompanying inflammation or sensitization of receptors (Schaible and Grubb, 1993) but the pain will still vary with activity. Therefore, if symptoms are constant and unvarying, the physiotherapist should be suspicious about the nature of the problem. Such suspicions should be clarified throughout the remainder of the history, and followed up with further investigations if appropriate.

Constancy of symptoms may also give some idea of prognosis. It is generally considered that the presence of resting pain indicates that the problem may take longer to improve than intermittent pain. Also, resting pain that becomes intermittent in nature suggests that the patient's condition is improving.

Quality

The quality or description of pain (burning, throbbing, knife-like, dull ache, etc.) has often been interpreted in terms of pathology and structures producing pain. For example, throbbing pain is thought to characterize inflammation, whereas burning or knife-like pain is thought to characterize neural involvement, and a dull ache to indicate joint involvement. Quality of pain, however, is thought to have poor reliability and poor validity in detecting the structure or pathology involved, when investigating spinal problems with and without neural involvement (Dalton and Jull, 1989; Austen, 1991).

Quality of pain does have some uses, however. The quality of pain may be used to monitor a patient's progress with treatment. It is usually satisfying for the patient if the quality of the pain experience becomes less unpleasant. In addition, the quality of pain is used in disability questionnaires (e.g. the McGill Pain Questionnaire; Melzack, 1975). Combined with other information, then, the quality of the pain indicates the severity of the pain experience. In isolation, this information is probably of limited value.

Intensity

The usual way that physiotherapists determine the intensity of pain is to ask patients to rate the pain on a 0–10 rating scale, as described in detail earlier. Intensity of pain is used to indicate the severity of the symptoms as experienced by the patient and can be used as a reliable indicator of progress of the condition and effect of treatment. The intensity of symptoms possibly assists in determining prognosis; for example, more severe pain may take longer to full recovery than mild pain.

It is worthwhile remembering that intensity is not an objective measure of the pain experience. Different patients may nominate the same level on the scale for different pain experiences. However, it is a good indicator of change in pain. For example, if pain were originally rated as 8/10 on a numerical rating scale and this changed to 4/10 following intervention, the patient's pain has substantially reduced.

Depth

In the past it was thought that the depth of pain indicated the depth of the structure involved. However, this is not always a valid assumption (consider the superficial dermatomal symptoms caused by spinal nerve/nerve root compromise, the nerve root/spinal nerve being a deep anatomical complex). Pain from musculoskeletal conditions is often described as a deep dull ache (Austen, 1991), although pain in superficial muscles may feel local. To make most sense of this information, knowledge of referral patterns for anatomical structures is essential. Muscles, for example, do not refer superficially (Mense, 1993), whereas viscera generally do have a cutaneous referral pattern, remembering that not all viscera are sensitive to noxious stimuli (Gebhart and Ness, 1991), and skin rarely (if ever) refers pain (Lewis, 1942). Joints, such as the zygapophyseal joints, appear to refer symptoms superficially (Mooney and Robertson, 1976). Autonomic symptoms, such as drop in blood pressure, sweating and nausea, may also be associated with visceral, and sometimes muscle, pain (Feinstein et al., 1954). Since the source of spinal pain is not understood in most cases, but rarely seems to be originally from lesions in the muscles or skin, this information is probably less useful for diagnosis and treatment selection in disorders of the vertebral column than of the periphery.

Relationship of symptoms

A patient may have several symptomatic areas or several types of symptoms. The physiotherapist must establish whether the various symptoms appear to originate from one source, or whether several sources are involved. This can be done by determining whether symptoms are provoked independently (unrelated symptoms) or they all worsen together (related symptoms). If symptoms are related, the physiotherapist will potentially treat one area and expect all symptoms to improve. On the other hand, if there are two or more separate sources of symptoms, several areas may require treatment. For example, it may be necessary to treat both the hip and lumbar spine to resolve a patient's leg pain completely. It is not always easy to establish a relationship at this stage. If it is not possible, the relationship needs be clarified throughout the examination.

Current history

After clearly delineating the symptoms, physiotherapists often gain information about the current history. The current history (history of the presenting condition) includes all relevant information about the onset of the disorder, including when the injury happened, how it happened (the mechanism of injury), the progress of symptoms, and what treatment has been used (if any) and its effect. This information assists in decisions about diagnosis, treatment and prognosis.

When the injury occurred readily indicates whether the injury is acute, subacute or chronic. Acute injuries are defined as 0–7 days postinjury, subacute as 7 days to 7 weeks postinjury, and

chronic as more than 7 weeks postinjury, although definitions vary (le Blanc et al., 1987). This gives an idea of the stage of the pathology and the likelihood of the presence of inflammation, and thus indicates appropriate types of intervention. For example, a severe ligament injury that occurred within 24 h would most likely require rest, whereas an ankle sprain sustained 3 weeks ago would probably require exercise and mobilizing. The length of time since injury may also give some idea of prognosis – the longer the patient has had the problem, the longer it may take to resolve completely. However, for spinal pain, it is more common for the acute phase to be defined as up to 6 weeks after symptom onset, subacute as pain of 6 weeks to 3 months' duration, and chronic to refer to pain of more than 3 months' duration.

Mechanism of injury

Mechanism of injury is used in formulating a diagnosis, especially in the periphery. The tissue damaged may be indicated by the direction and position of applied forces. It is also valuable to compare the magnitude of the force with the severity of the injury sustained: a minor force causing a very severe injury may indicate abnormal tissue status, such as osteoporosis, prior to injury.

Progress of symptoms (whether the condition is better, worse or the same, and in what way)

Many musculoskeletal disorders improve with the normal process of healing and repair, usually within 6 weeks (Evans, 1980; Sheldon, 1984). However, other disorders may worsen or require intervention. It is not uncommon, for example, for pain to start in a small area and radiate over time (e.g. 48 h) or increase in severity. The condition would also be considered to be worsening if paraesthesia commenced after the initial pain. Such progression of symptoms may indicate specific pathologies. For example, symptoms from fragments of intervertebral disc tissue impinging on a nerve root and aggravated by a lifting injury may radiate down the limb some hours or days after the insult; the symptoms of intermittent claudication from spinal canal stenosis may increase with time, but symptoms from a muscle strain with no complications should be improving within 1–2 weeks. Thus, knowledge of progress of symptoms assists in diagnosis. It also probably assists in selecting the dose of treatment: a smaller dose may be applied if the problem is worsening, or a more vigorous dose may be selected if the problem is unchanged. Furthermore, progress of symptoms may indicate prognosis. Generally, the prognosis is better if the condition is currently improving rather than worsening.

Previous treatment and effect

It is efficient to use all possible information to select a treatment, therefore, if the patient has previously been treated for a similar disorder it is important to establish the treatment used and its effect. A treatment that has already been used successfully may again be an appropriate choice. On the other hand, if the condition worsened, or did not respond as quickly as predicted with treatment, this is an indication to alter the dose of the treatment or change the intervention strategy altogether. In addition, if the patient has already been treated well and responded poorly, the prognosis is poorer than if the condition had responded well. Knowing about previous treatments and their effects thus gives us ideas about treatment selection, dose and prognosis.

Behaviour of symptoms during the day and night (24–h behaviour)

Appreciation of the 24-h behaviour of symptoms includes knowing the status of symptoms at night and when the patient first wakes in the morning, how symptoms alter during the day and specific activities that aggravate or alleviate symptoms. Understanding how symptoms behave during the day and at night assists in formulating a diagnosis, a treatment plan and, to a lesser extent, assists in determining prognosis. Information about response of symptoms to various activities, often obtained from the completed disability questionnaire, is used to monitor progress of the condition.

Specific syndromes or diseases, such as spinal canal stenosis, vertebrobasilar insufficiency, the arthritides or other inflammatory diseases, can frequently be recognized based on the response of symptoms to various activities, since such conditions often have a characteristic presentation. Symptoms of spinal canal stenosis, for example, typically worsen when the patient walks, and are relieved on squatting or spinal flexion (Grieve, 1986). Commonly, however, most spinal conditions seen by physiotherapists have no specific pathology: current knowledge is insufficient to identify the anatomical structure or pathology involved. Having determined that the condition originates in the musculoskeletal system, that there is apparently no specifically identifiable pathology, and that the condition is 'mechanical', further information about response of symptoms to various activities and positions becomes increasingly important because this may be used to formulate the clinical diagnosis and to form the basis of the treatment plan.

Specific information gained

Night pain: does the patient get to sleep normally, and once asleep, does the patient stay asleep? Establish whether the patient has more difficulty than usual getting to sleep, remembering that many people normally have trouble sleeping. Difficulty in getting to sleep may be caused by an inappropriate pillow or bed, or by particular sleeping positions. Before giving advice about pillows or beds, determine the status of the symptoms when the patient wakes in the morning (see below). If the bed or pillow is inappropriate (for example, some thoracic spine conditions are more comfortable in a soft bed and some cervical spine conditions may prefer a slim feather pillow), advise your patient about changing them. Choice of bed and pillow, however, is related to individual comfort: there is no variable that will satisfy all painful conditions.

Sleeping positions or postures also often cause discomfort. Patients frequently report, for example, that lying on the symptomatic side is painful. Determine the worst and best sleeping positions. Information about sleeping positions is mainly used in determining a management plan. Intervention to enhance the patient's comfort and ability to sleep may be required, for example by using a pillow to avoid rolling on to the painful side. In addition, the provocative position may be used in treatment. If, for example, a patient cannot lie on the left side because it brings on left-leg pain, this position may be used as a treatment. On the other hand, if the condition is severe, this position may be avoided initially, and the most comfortable position used.

Does the pain wake the patient during the night? The answer to this question is extremely important because intractable night pain is generally indicative of serious pathology (O'Connor and Currier, 1992). This type of pain not only wakes the patient, but may force him or her to get out of bed, because nothing eases the pain. Unremitting pain may be caused by pathology such as the inflammation of rheumatoid arthritis or ankylosing spondylitis during exacerbation, or severe infections such as osteomyelitis, or advanced carcinomas. The reasons for the severity of the pain and its worsening during the night are largely unknown at this stage. Therefore, if patients tell you about pain at night that is very severe and unremitting, it is extremely important to follow up the possibilities of other, more serious pathologies with further questioning and tests throughout the examination. In such cases referral to a medical practitioner would be the appropriate course of action. Patients with musculoskeletal disorders often have night pain, but this can usually be relieved by changing position. This pain needs to be differentiated from the unremitting night pain indicative of severe inflammation or other serious pathologies.

Morning pain and stiffness   The status of symptoms when the patient first wakes establishes whether the symptoms are better with rest. Generally, 'mechanical' musculoskeletal conditions respond well to rest. Although there may be some stiffness in the morning it usually resolves quickly, often with a warm shower. Pain is also usually reduced in the morning. In contrast some arthritides, such as rheumatoid arthritis, respond poorly to rest. For example, when patients with rheumatoid arthritis wake in the morning, they often have marked stiffness lasting for more than 30 min (Kannangara and Shenstone, 1988; Schumacher, 1988). Therefore, the possibility of an inflammatory arthritis should be considered in patients who complain of morning stiffness lasting for more than 30 min. If patients with a musculoskeletal disorder wake with increased pain in the morning, it is possible that the bed or pillow is inappropriate, or

that the patient has slept in a provocative position. It seems wise not to recommend a change in bed or pillow unless you have determined that these factors are aggravating the condition.

Aggravating and easing activities   The activities that make the condition better or worse should be identified. Much of this information can be obtained from the completed disability questionnaires, but can also be obtained or expanded in the interview. This information is particularly important, because the decision about whether or not the condition is 'mechanical' largely rests on this information. Therefore, the treatment approach to some extent also relies on this information. Pain from 'mechanical' musculoskeletal conditions generally decreases with rest in a position of comfort, and there is generally a particular movement or movements that will consistently cause pain or difficulty when attempted. For example, the pain from a sprained ankle often feels better after elevation for some time, and feels worse after walking for some distance. The ankle pain will respond in this same way consistently, until it has recovered. Systemic inflammation or arthritides such as ankylosing spondylitis or osteoarthritis will behave quite differently once the disease process is established. Such pathologies cause the patient to become stiffer and perhaps more painful after rest, and to become more mobile and less painful after appropriate exercise and movement (Kannangara and Shenstone, 1988; Schumacher, 1988). Too much exercise may exacerbate such conditions, all movements and positions probably becoming painful. Thus, the behaviour of the symptoms assists in diagnosis. When the condition is mechanical with non-specific pathology the movements aggravating the symptoms may also suggest the type of treatment that is appropriate. If activities involving spinal rotation aggravate the symptoms and the condition is not severe, then rotation may be a useful treatment option. If symptoms are severe, rotation may initially be avoided.

During the day symptoms may also behave in a manner typical of certain pathologies. Musculoskeletal mechanical conditions are generally better in the morning than in the evening, whereas inflammatory disorders and other pathologies may be worse in the morning, improve as the day progresses and become worse again in the evening. This behaviour depends to some extent on the balance between exercise and rest.

It is often difficult to distinguish definitively between non-specific mechanical disorders and inflammatory joint pathology, since many musculoskeletal conditions may have an inflammatory component: lesions in the tissues of the musculoskeletal system heal with inflammation, and therefore musculoskeletal disorders would usually be accompanied by some symptoms of inflammation (Evans, 1980; Kannangara and Shenstone, 1988). Therefore, in many pathologies, features of inflammation may coexist with features of a non-specific mechanical musculoskeletal disorder. An important feature of systemic inflammatory disease, however, is stiffness on first waking in the morning that lasts for more than 30 min (Kannangara and Shenstone, 1988; Schumacher, 1988).

Any functional activity that aggravates symptoms should be further examined in the physical examination. The patient may tell you, for example, that sitting causes immediate pain in the back, the buttock and the leg. Sitting and spinal flexion would therefore be examined in the physical examination, anticipating a painful response. In this patient, sitting can be used to monitor the patient's progress. After treatment, the patient may be able to sit for 10 min before any pain onset, and only pain in the back and the buttock is provoked. This represents a functional improvement, the most important improvement from the patient's point of view.

Irritability

Irritability is a theoretical concept proposed by Maitland (1986) to describe the ease with which a condition is exacerbated by movement. It provides a guide about how to approach the physical examination of a musculoskeletal condition. It is inappropriate to apply rigid rules to this concept since it is of undetermined reliability and validity.

There are three key questions which are asked to determine the irritability of a condition:

1. What activity (and how much) aggravates symptoms?
2. How severe is the pain?
3. After cessation of the activity, how long until the pain returns to resting level?

It is the combination of this information that determines irritability. Probably the most important information, however, is the level of difficulty of the activity that aggravates symptoms. A condition that is considered irritable will prevent the patient from doing most activities. So, if a patient suggests that running, sporting activities or sitting for long periods aggravates symptoms, it is most unlikely that the condition is irritable. On the other hand if pain in the neck and arm is provoked on the slightest movement, it is probable that the condition is very irritable. Severe pain alone does not indicate irritability of a condition. Severe pain may be provoked by a very stressful activity such as playing tennis, but the patient may be painfree most of the time. The time the pain takes to settle suggests the ease with which symptoms will settle if they are provoked during examination. The physiotherapist may be unwilling to provoke symptoms that will take a long time to settle.

The condition is then interpreted as irritable or non-irritable. Unfortunately most conditions are not so easily categorized and may be slightly irritable or moderately irritable. It may be easier to think of irritability as a continuum, with two extremes; irritable conditions and non-irritable conditions. Most disorders will fall between the two extremes.

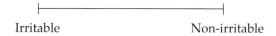

Irritable   Non-irritable

Irritable conditions require particular care when planning and executing the physical examination. For irritable conditions, only those examination procedures that give essential information, usually about diagnosis and treatment, will be performed. For non-irritable conditions, on the other hand, a vigorous examination exploring extremes of range of movement and various combinations of activities would generally be required. By predicting the response of symptoms to movement, the concept of irritability is useful for determining the appropriate vigour of the physical examination of musculoskeletal conditions, ensuring that the examination is neither too gentle nor too vigorous for individual patients. With increasing clinical experience physiotherapists reach many of their examination and management decisions without rigidly adhering to these concepts.

Physical examination decisions affected by irritability

How many active movements should be examined? The number of active movements examined is guided by the time taken for symptoms to settle to the usual level, but it is frequently possible to examine all movements. It is important to recognize when the condition is being exacerbated, because this is the signal to stop performing movement testing. If it is not possible to examine all active movements, the physiotherapist would normally first examine those movements predicted to give the most useful information. Such movements have been identified based on knowledge of the activities that aggravate the patient's symptoms.

How far through range to examine movements (active and passive)? When dealing with irritable conditions, physiotherapists would usually examine several movements stopping at the initial onset/increase in pain rather than one or two movements to end of range or until full reproduction of the symptoms.

Which examination procedures to perform? Physiotherapists usually prioritize examination procedures when assessing irritable conditions, ensuring that important procedures are performed early in the examination. Tests considered important for diagnosis or for treatment decisions, such as neurological testing, ligament tests or muscle tests, may be performed, even if symptoms may be exacerbated. Decisions to perform tests that will exacerbate an irritable condition are made based on the certainty with which the test results can be interpreted (reliability and validity) and the importance of the test results to management decisions. If the results of tests are essential, then they will be performed, despite the probability of increasing symptoms. If the tests will have little immediate impact on diagnostic or treatment decisions, they will probably not be performed until pain has settled at a subsequent visit. Consider the example of testing ligaments when your patient presents with an acute knee injury: ligament disruption may require surgical intervention, but the tests may be very painful for the patient. Some ligament tests are not reliable indicators of ligament disruption (such as the anterior draw test; Feagin and Curl,

1976) although instrumented measuring devices provide reliable indicators of anterior cruciate ligament disruption (Daniel et al., 1985). A physiotherapist experienced in treating knee injuries would probably choose to perform an instrumented ligament test, to decide the most appropriate method of management (which may require consultation with an orthopaedic surgeon), but may choose not to perform an anterior draw test.

In patients presenting with an irritable disorder of the vertebral column, it is usually best to examine first the patient's most symptomatic active movement, as identified from the aggravating activities. This will ensure that, should it be possible to examine only two or three active movements in these patients, information regarding the worst active movement, i.e. the active movement on which management and patient progress decisions are based, will have been examined.

The concept of irritability probably does not apply to all musculoskeletal conditions. In the presence of pathology such as rheumatoid arthritis, fractures, muscle rupture, joint replacements and other orthopaedic surgery, this concept is probably not very useful since treatment will be largely guided by the existing pathology, and the dose determined by the stage of healing and repair.

Past history

Patients may never have experienced the presenting condition before, or they may have had the same problem on one or several previous occasions. Previous episodes of the same problem may guide expectations for treatment and prognosis, and occasionally diagnosis. For example, a history of previous episodes of back pain is thought to worsen the prognosis for a current episode of back pain. Sometimes patients may have had a different condition that may have an impact on the prognosis of the presenting condition, e.g. a patient may have had a fusion of the lumbar spine and now be presenting with thoracolumbar pain. The key features of the history of other relevant conditions should be understood, such as how and when the disorder started, and the patient's normal health status. Some patients, for example, may 'normally' limp from a previous femoral fracture; the limp is not a feature of the presenting lumbar spine disorder and would not change with lumbar spine treatment, but may have implications for future recurrence of the presenting disorder and for prognosis.

For previous episodes of the same disorder, a detailed history of the first episode should be taken, including when and how the symptoms first started, and the type and effect of any previous treatment. In addition, information should be sought about subsequent episodes: are they increasing or decreasing in frequency, intensity or duration? This information provides guidelines for:

- prognosis: the duration of the current disorder will probably be similar to previous episodes if appropriate treatment had been administered, and other features are similar
- treatment: based on knowledge about effective and/or ineffective treatments used in the past
- diagnosis: there may be diagnostic information from previous episodes.

Recurrent problems may require further intervention to prevent future recurrence if factors contributing to onset can be identified.

Screening questions to determine precautions and contraindications (red flags)

All patients are routinely screened for serious pathology or for any health state that would constitute a precaution or contraindication to any examination or treatment strategy. The simplest form of these screening questions is:

1. state of general health
2. recent unexplained weight loss
3. results of recent X-rays or other investigations relevant to the presenting disorder
4. medications the patient is currently taking
5. use of oral steroids (presence of osteoporosis).

For all spinal conditions, additional questions are asked about:

6. Cord signs, i.e. bilateral non-dermatomal symptoms and ataxia.

For lumbar spine disorders:

7. Presence of cauda equina syndrome, i.e. disturbed bladder or bowel function, saddle anaesthesia.

For cervical spine disorders:

8. Dizziness (vertebrobasilar insufficiency).

In addition to the information gained from these questions, there are other sections of the history that have value in screening for pathology, such as behaviour of the symptoms at night and in the morning. A more extensive protocol for screening patients with low back pain is provided by the modified Core network low back pain medical screening questionnaire (see Fig. 5.13, later in this chapter).

A compilation of the red flags that indicate inflammatory disorders, spinal cord or cauda equina lesion or other serious pathology from three recent clinical practice guidelines is provided in Table 5.3.

Background to screening (red flags) questions

In this section we examine which clinical features should alert us to the presence of specific pathology in patients with musculoskeletal conditions. We also provide the reasons why we obtain information about patients' general health, medications and past investigations and what important additional information we require when examining patients with a disorder arising in the cervical, thoracic or lumbar spine.

General health   The general health of a person is an indicator of many systemic diseases. A general question about the patient's health is therefore asked. Many diseases have extra-articular features, usually late in the disease process. For example, patients with rheumatoid arthritis may have eye or gastrointestinal involvement and may feel unwell, nauseated or lethargic (Schumacher, 1988), patients with cancer may feel unwell or fatigued (O'Connor and Currier, 1992), and other diseases may manifest with fever or vomiting. Since patients may present to the physiotherapist as the first health practitioner, the physiotherapist must know when to refer patients to other specialized care, and therefore to recognize early symptoms of pathology. If the physiotherapist suspects a particular pathology, further questions will be asked about symptoms relevant to that disease, such as swelling in other joints for no reason, which may accompany rheumatoid arthritis. In addition, certain illnesses, such as viral illnesses, may cause joint pain, but do

Table 5.3   Red flags for inflammatory disorders, spinal cord and cauda equina lesions and other serious pathologies

Possible inflammatory disorders	Possible spinal cord or cauda equina lesion
<ul><li>Gradual onset before age 40</li><li>Marked morning stiffness</li><li>Iritis, skin rashes (psoriasis), colitis</li><li>Urethral discharge</li><li>Peripheral joint involvement</li><li>Persisting limitation of spinal movements in all directions</li><li>Family history</li></ul>	<ul><li>Recent onset of bladder dysfunction, such as urinary retention, increased frequency or overflow incontinence</li><li>Loss of anal sphincter tone or faecal incontinence</li><li>Saddle anaesthesia about the anus, perineum or genitals</li><li>Widespread (> one nerve root) or progressive motor weakness in the legs or gait disturbance</li><li>Sensory level</li></ul>

Possible serious spinal pathology (fracture, tumour, infection, etc.)	
<ul><li>Age over 50 (55) or under 20</li><li>History of cancer</li><li>Constitutional symptoms, such as recent fever or chills or unexplained weight loss</li><li>Risk factors for spinal infection: recent bacterial infection (e.g. urinary tract infection); intravenous drug abuse; or immune suppression (from steroids, transplant or HIV)</li><li>Major trauma, such as vehicle accident or fall from height</li></ul>	<ul><li>Minor trauma or even strenuous lifting in older and potentially osteoporotic patient</li><li>Constant, progressive non-mechanical pain</li><li>Thoracic pain</li><li>Systemic steroids</li><li>Systemically unwell</li><li>Persisting severe restriction of lumbar flexion</li><li>Pain that worsens when supine; severe nighttime pain</li><li>Structural deformity</li><li>Widespread neurology</li></ul>

HIV, human immunodeficiency virus.
Adapted from Bigos et al. (1994), Kendall et al. (1997) and Waddell et al. (1996)

not respond well to manual therapy. Other forms of physiotherapeutic intervention may be appropriate in many cases.

Weight loss   Weight loss occurring for no apparent reason can be a further indicator of systemic pathology. People may lose weight because they feel unwell or nauseated. However, loss of weight for no apparent reason generally suggests the presence of some pathology, e.g. late in the disease process of many cancers. Generally, by the time patients have started losing weight for no apparent reason, the disease is fairly advanced and has been diagnosed. Despite the fact that most people seem to want to lose weight, it is quite frightening when it happens for no apparent reason, and continues, perhaps because it signifies serious pathology. If patients say they have lost weight, check they

haven't been on a diet, or been particularly stressed. Weight loss should be investigated by the patient's medical practitioner.

X-rays and other medical investigations   X-rays and other imaging procedures will provide evidence of some diseases or abnormalities that may contraindicate certain procedures, or advise caution in others. The identification of spondylolisthesis or spondylolysis on X-ray, for example, may indicate a poor response to posterior–anterior mobilizations at the level of the abnormality. Other medical tests, such as blood tests or liver function tests, indicate the presence of pathology and the patient's general health status. If they have had such investigations, read the accompanying report, and view images (X-rays or computed tomography scans, for example) in light of the report. Any queries should be directed to the referring radiologist, remembering that physiotherapists are not professionally qualified to read such scans. Chapter 3 details common findings using various imaging techniques relevant to musculoskeletal physiotherapy.

Medications Determine what medications the patient is taking, the dose and the effect. Patients may be taking medication to control blood pressure or diabetes, but may have omitted to tell you that they have these conditions. This is therefore a further check on their health status. In addition, patients with musculoskeletal disorders are often prescribed analgesics or non-steroidal anti-inflammatories. For a discussion of these pharmaceutical agents, see Chapter 2. The physiotherapist needs to know the effect of these drugs on the presenting condition. A good response to anti-inflammatories suggests that there is an inflammatory component involved in the condition. If patients are taking analgesics, it may be wise in some cases to examine them before they take an effective medication so that signs and symptoms are not masked by the analgesic effect. In other cases, you may wish to treat after they have achieved some medication-induced analgesia, allowing a more vigorous intervention.

Steroid use (to identify the presence of osteoporosis) Oral and intra-articular steroids are fully discussed in Chapter 2. The main purpose of asking whether patients have taken oral steroids in the past is to determine the risk of osteoporosis. Vigorous manual treatments are contraindicated in osteoporosis because the diminished bone density places the patient at greater risk of fracture (Pocock et al., 1986), particularly if doses of >7.5 mg daily have been taken (Spector and Sambrook, 1993). There are other factors contributing to reduced bone density, including hormonal status (particularly postmenopausal women; Chow et al., 1986), lack of calcium in the diet, smoking, slim build in early life and lack of exercise (Bailey et al., 1986). In the presence of osteoporosis, manual treatments should be applied using small doses (with gentle forces).

Cord signs (questions to determine pathology in the central nervous system, particularly at spinal cord level) The central nervous system (CNS) is that part of the nervous system proximal to the anterior horn cell in the spinal cord (Williams and Warwick, 1980). Disorders of the CNS may therefore be the result of pathology anywhere in this part of the nervous system, including the brain and spinal cord. The location of the pathology must be established, because the cause of the CNS disorder may be pathology in the painful region of the spine. For example, cord compression secondary to rheumatoid arthritis in the upper cervical spine contraindicates management of upper cervical spine pain by manual therapy. CNS disorders will present with a variety of signs and symptoms, which include ataxia and diffuse (and, therefore, non-dermatomal) bilateral symptoms. When pathology affects the spinal cord at the level of the cervical spine, these symptoms will appear in both the arms and the legs, whereas disturbances at the level of the lumbar spine will only affect the legs. The patient should therefore be asked about ataxia or unsteady gait, and bilateral, non-dermatomal distribution of symptoms in the lower extremities for lumbar spine conditions, and in the upper and lower extremities for cervical spine conditions.

Further discussion of the CNS, testing and implications for treatment appears in Chapter 6.

Cauda equina syndrome The spinal cord terminates at approximately the first lumbar segment in the adult. The long nerve roots continue to exit at their appropriate intervertebral foramina and are collectively termed the cauda equina (Williams and Warwick, 1980). Cauda equina syndrome results from compromise of these nerve roots (Coscia et al., 1994). Compromise of the cauda equina will therefore affect motor and sensory function in the whole lower extremity. Of particular importance is compromise of the S2 spinal segment, since S2 supplies the bladder and sphincters (Williams and Warwick, 1980; Coscia et al., 1994). Compression of S2 will therefore result in loss of bladder and sphincter control, with a sensory loss in the genital region, commonly termed a 'saddle' distribution. Rarely, patients may present with urological dysfunction as the only sign or symptom (Coscia et al., 1994). Since prolonged compromise of S2 may result in permanent dysfunction, acute cauda equina syndrome is considered a medical emergency. Return of optimal neurological functioning requires surgical intervention, usually decompression (Coscia et al., 1994). It is imperative that cauda equina syndrome is recognized immediately.

To determine the presence of acute cauda equina syndrome, questions are directed at ascertaining conduction in the S2 spinal segment. Patients are asked about alterations in voiding (frequency or absence of micturition, and perhaps bowel movements) and the presence of altered sensation (paraesthesia or anaesthesia) in the saddle area.

Cauda equina syndrome is further discussed in Chapter 6.

Dizziness (adequacy of cerebral blood flow) The presence of vertebrobasilar insufficiency causing inadequate blood supply to the brain is a contraindication or precaution to many physiotherapeutic procedures applied to the cervical spine. The most common presenting symptom is dizziness. Other disorders such as postural (orthostatic) hypotension, Ménière's disease, vestibular or labyrinthine disorders and cervical vertigo (also termed benign positional vertigo) may also cause dizziness. The vertebrobasilar system supplies many intracranial structures. Ischaemia will result in symptoms from each of the affected structures and could include paralysis of gaze to side of lesion, diplopia (double vision), dysphagia, dysarthria, impaired trigeminal sensation (snout paraesthesia or anaesthesia) or transient ischaemic attacks. Vertebrobasilar insufficiency is caused by reducing the volume of blood passing through the vertebrobasilar system. One cause of reduced blood flow may be a reduction in diameter of the vertebral arteries during cervical spine extension and/or rotation (Toole and Tucker, 1960; Refshauge, 1994). Therefore, if the cause of dizziness is vertebrobasilar insufficiency, patients will usually complain of dizziness, perhaps occurring with a slight delay, on assuming the provoking head position.

Postural hypotension (orthostatic hypotension), on the other hand, will occur with a sudden decrease in blood pressure resulting in a decrease in cerebral blood flow (Burton, 1965). The decreased blood pressure will usually result from changes in position from low to high, such as sitting up after lying down. Dizziness will not, therefore, be increased with cervical spine movements, but rather by positional changes. (For review see Rushmer, 1976; or Rowell, 1986.)

Ménière's disease is associated with other signs and symptoms such as fluctuating hearing loss, tinnitus and a feeling of pressure in the ears. Dizziness associated with Ménière's disease is unlikely to be associated with head movements, but will be associated with these other symptoms (Coman, 1986).

Vestibular disorders also cause dizziness. Usually dizziness will be reproduced on specific head movement(s); the affected head movement(s) will be those causing movement of fluid to displace hairs in the affected canal (Kelly, 1991). The dizziness usually occurs immediately on head movement (unlike the slight delay associated with decreased blood flow). In addition, dizziness will not usually result from body movement that does not involve head movement (unlike vertebrobasilar insufficiency). However, it is sometimes difficult to distinguish vestibular or labyrinth disorders from vertebrobasilar insufficiency. The presence of pathological nystagmus (occurring even when the head is kept still) may assist in differentiation, since pathological nystagmus is a cardinal sign of disease of the labyrinth and its central connections (Goldberg et al., 1991).

Cervical vertigo arises from abnormal afferent impulses from deep cervical spine structures such as muscles, zygapophyseal joints and the posterior longitudinal ligament (de Jong et al., 1977). The disturbed afferent input can result in dizziness on head movement. It is therefore virtually impossible to differentiate between dizziness caused by vertebrobasilar insufficiency and that caused by cervical vertigo on the first treatment session: differential diagnosis is usually confirmed after investigation or response to treatment is known.

Patients are questioned about the presence of dizziness. If they affirm that they experience periods of dizziness, further questioning will elicit the provocative manoeuvres. It is then important to follow up with questions about head movement, body movement and other signs and symptoms to determine the cause of the symptoms.

A full discussion of vertebrobasilar insufficiency appears in Chapter 6.

What is the diagnostic accuracy of these features (red flags) for serious diseases?

Cancer The diagnostic accuracy of various clinical features to screen for cancer has been evaluated by Deyo and Diehl (1988) and Fernbach et al.

(1976). Deyo and Diehl (1988) studied 1975 patients at a 'walk-in' clinic in a USA public hospital using a standardized format. Of these, 13/1975 were eventually found to have cancer. Fernbach et al. (1976) studied 518 low back pain patients presenting to an orthopaedic surgeon at a university teaching hospital. The test performance is shown in Table 5.4.

A later paper reporting on the same study noted that a combination of age > 50 years or history of cancer or unexplained weight loss, or failure of conservative therapy had a sensitivity of 1.00 and specificity of 0.60 (Deyo et al., 1992). These items in Table 5.4 appear in both the original and modified Core.

Using the likelihood ratios (LR: see Ch. 4) provided in Tables 5.4 and 5.5, you will note that, if a patient presenting with acute low back pain has a pretest probability of 1% that a spinal tumour is the source of their back pain, knowing that the patient complains of unexplained weight loss (positive LR = 2.5) will result in a posttest probability of only 2.4%, providing little assistance to you in determining the diagnosis. Similarly, the small positive LR for presence of thoracic pain, and the fact that the negative LR is close to 1, suggest that this clinical feature is not going to be useful in determining whether the patient's low back pain is due to a possible tumour. A previous history of cancer is likely

Table 5.4 Accuracy of selected clinical features for diagnosis of cancer

Clinical feature	Sensitivity	Specificity	+LR	−LR
Age > 50 years	0.77	0.71	2.7	0.3
Age ⩾ 50 years	0.85	0.49	1.7	0.3
Unexplained weight loss (of more than 10 lbs (4.5 kg) in 6/12)	0.15	0.94	2.5	0.9
Previous history of cancer	0.31	0.98	15.5	0.7
Sought medical care during past month, not improving	0.31	0.90	3.1	0.8
Tried bedrest, but no relief	1.00	0.46	1.9	0.0
Insidious onset	0.61	0.42	1.1	0.9
Duration of this episode > 1 month	0.50	0.81	2.6	0.6
Recent back injury (including lifting, fall, blow)	0.00	0.82	0.0	1.2
Thoracic pain versus lumbar	0.17	0.84	1.1	1.0

LR, Likelihood ratio.
Data from Deyo and Diehl (1988) and Fernbach et al. (1976).

Table 5.5 Accuracy of selected laboratory findings for diagnosis of cancer

Laboratory test finding	Sensitivity	Specificity	+LR	−LR
ESR ⩾ 20 mm/h	0.78	0.67	2.4	0.3
ESR ⩾ 50 mm/h	0.56	0.97	18.7	0.5
ESR ⩾ 100 mm/h	0.22	0.996	55.0	0.8
Anaemia	0.54	0.86	3.9	0.5
Haematocrit < 30%	0.09	0.994	15.0	0.9
WBC ⩾ 12 000/mm^3	0.22	0.94	3.7	0.8
X-ray: lytic or blastic lesion	0.60	0.995	120.0	0.4
X-ray: compression fracture	0.20	0.957	4.7	0.8
X-ray: either compression fracture or lytic/blastic lesion	0.70	0.953	14.9	0.3

LR, Likelihood ratio; ESR, erythrocyte sedimentation rate; WBC, White blood cell.
Data from Deyo and Diehl (1988).

to be the most useful clinical feature in determining the diagnosis. For example, a 1% pretest probability that the patient has a spinal tumour may be increased to approximately 13% if the patient has had a previous history of cancer. Also, the presence of an erythrocyte sedimentation rate $\geqslant 100$ mm/h is likely to be a useful laboratory finding indicating the presence of cancer: 1% pretest probability is increased to a posttest probability of having the disease of approximately 35%. The low pretest probability of spinal tumour means that many of the clinical features or red flags suggested for this condition provide little useful information when interpreted individually. For example, a positive LR of 55 produces posttest probabilities of only 35% in suggesting the presence of a spinal tumour, making it difficult to decide strongly whether the patient has or does not have the disease. This is in contrast to instability testing of the knee where, at the conclusion of the history, the patient may have a pretest probability of 50% of having a rupture of the anterior cruciate ligament. Even though the Lachman test has a positive LR of only 27, this results in a posttest probability of approximately 96% that the patient has an anterior cruciate ligament disruption and hence the results of this test will greatly influence the clinical decisions made.

Ankylosing spondylitis Four studies have examined the diagnostic accuracy of the clinical examination in diagnosing ankylosing spondylitis (AS). Gran's data (1985) are based upon an epidemiological survey in Norway, and examined how well a clinical examination discriminated subjects with AS from those with back pain but no AS. In Calin et al.'s study (1977) three groups of subjects were studied; those with AS (source of recruitment not stated), low back pain patients attending an orthopaedic clinic and low back pain-free controls. Because it is irrelevant to know how to discriminate patients with AS from healthy control subjects without low back pain, these results are not reported (although if diagnostic tests were positive in the healthy controls this would be cause for concern). Sadowska-Wroblewska and colleagues (1983) studied 102 subjects with low back pain and/or limitation of spinal mobility of greater than 3 months' duration, of whom 70 had AS and 32 'lumbar disc disease'. Van der Linden et al.'s

study (1984) is of unknown value because the cases were relatives of patients with AS (not patients with AS) and the controls were volunteers, not patients seeking care for low back pain. The inadequacy of the study is clear from the sensitivity and specificity values quoted for the question 'Do you have pain in your lumbar spine?' Only 62% of the cases said yes and 57% of the controls said yes.

'Do you have any pain or stiffness in the morning that lasts longer than half an hour' is contained in the modified Core but not the original. Deyo et al. (1992) reported the test performances shown in Table 5.6, taken from a study by Gran (1985), for the detection of ankylosing spondylitis using items that include morning stiffness.

Compression fracture Identification of compression fracture is important for ensuring appropriate management of the patient. After one compression fracture, intervention should be aimed at reducing bone loss (or increasing bone mineral density) and reducing the risk of falls. Furthermore, several physiotherapy treatments would be contraindicated in the presence of osteoporosis and particularly in the presence of compression fracture. The modified Core (see Fig. 5.13, later in this chapter), but not the original, contains the item 'Have you ever taken steroids?' This item has been evaluated for its ability to screen for compression fracture (Deyo et al., 1992). In unpublished data on 833 patients who attended a 'walk-in' clinic and who subsequently had plain lumbar radiographs taken, Deyo et al. report the test properties shown in Table 5.7.

Cognitive factors

Depression and other mood disorders

The presence of depression or other mood disorders in patients suffering from musculoskeletal disorders is thought to be predictive of high disability and poor outcome from physiotherapy treatment. However, physiotherapists are not well skilled in identifying those patients suffering a mood disorder such as depression (Haggman et al., 2004), nor in the appropriate treatment or referral of such patients, although depression is known to be highly prevalent in patients with some musculoskeletal conditions such as low back pain.

Table 5.6   Accuracy of selected clinical findings for possible ankylosing spondylitis

Clinical feature	Sensitivity	Specificity	+LR	−LR
Marked morning stiffness				
Morning stiffness, 0.5 h or more[a]	0.64	0.59	1.56	0.61
Has the back been stiff, especially in the morning?	0.95	0.19	1.17	0.26
Morning back stiffness[b]	0.93	0.43	1.63	0.16
Gradual onset before age 40 years				
Age at onset < 40 years[a]	0.98	0.07	1.06	0.28
Did the problem begin slowly	0.88	0.76	3.67	0.16
Peripheral joint involvement				
Knee joint stiffness[b]	0.41	0.94	6.83	0.62
Hip pain[b]	0.30	0.94	5.00	0.74
Family history				
Have any members of your family had persistent back pain (include only immediate family members)?	0.58	0.76	2.42	0.55
Ankylosing spondylitis in family[b]	0.07	0.98	3.50	0.95
Extra–articular features				
Heel pain[b]	0.16	0.90	1.60	0.93
Iritis[b]	0.15	0.98	7.50	0.87
Persistent limitation of spinal movement in all directions				
Limitation of spinal movement	0.74	0.06	0.78	4.3

Data from Gran (1985), Calin et al. (1977) and Sadowska-Wroblewska et al. (1983).
[a]Gran (1985) cites the sensitivity as 1. A sensitivity of 1, however, makes it impossible to calculate the −LR, therefore the convention of adding 0.5 to each cell in the original data was performed in order to determine a value for −LR.
[b]Sadowska-Wroblewska et al. (1983), cite the specificity as 1. A specificity of 1 however, makes it impossible to calculate the +LR, therefore the convention of adding 0.5 to each cell in the original data was performed in order to determine a value for +LR.

Table 5.7   Accuracy of selected clinical features for diagnosis of compression fracture associated with osteoporosis

Clinical feature	Sensitivity	Specificity	+LR	−LR
Age > 50 years	0.84	0.61	2.2	0.3
Age > 70 years	0.22	0.96	5.5	0.8
Trauma	0.30	0.85	2.0	0.8
Corticosteroid use	0.06	0.995	12.0	0.9

LR, Likelihood ratio.

The modified Core questionnaire at the end of this section contains questions specifically aimed at identifying those patients who may be depressed. Questions 12 (a) and (b) in the modified Core questionnaire are used to detect major depression, with a positive test result being a yes response to either of the two questions. Whooley and colleagues (1997) demonstrated that these two questions, when used as part of a self-report questionnaire, had a very good ability to detect depression in patients presenting to a USA Veterans' Affairs urgent care clinic. Using the National Institutes of Mental Health Quick Diagnostic Interview Schedule (QDIS-III-R) as the gold standard, the study noted a prevalence of major depression of 18%. The two screening questions had a sensitivity of 96% (negative LR

0.07) and specificity of 57% (positive LR 2.2). The first question alone had a sensitivity of 93% (negative LR 0.11) and specificity of 62% (positive LR 2.4); the second question alone had a sensitivity of 71% and specificity of 72%.

Yellow flags

In addition to screening for potentially serious spinal pathology (red flags) it is possible to screen for psychosocial and other risk factors that are likely to delay recovery. To distinguish predictors of delayed recovery from red flags, the New Zealand Guideline (Kendall et al., 1997) coined the term 'yellow flags'. That is, 'red flags' relate to factors associated with serious disease and 'yellow flags' refer to factors that increase the risk of developing or perpetuating long-term disability and work loss associated with pain. The benefit of screening for such factors is that, once recognized, it becomes possible to address these issues in physiotherapy treatment directly and/or refer the patient to a clinical psychologist. The real problem is that these factors can go unrecognized and treatment failure is then attributed to other causes such as poor physiotherapist skill in performing a treatment or patient malingering.

The significance of a particular factor needs to be interpreted. Immediate notice should be taken if an important red flag is present. The same is true for yellow flags. The presence of red flags should lead to appropriate medical intervention, whereas the presence of yellow flags is more likely to indicate active treatment with appropriate behavioural management.

Interest in yellow flags has increased recently because many of the predictors of poor outcome are factors in the cognitive domain, such as patients' beliefs and their cognitive appraisal of their pain. For example, it has been shown that fear of pain, negative attitudes towards pain and catastrophizing are associated with poor outcome (Turner and Clancy, 1986; Nicholas et al., 1992; Jensen et al., 1994).

Assessing the presence of yellow flags should produce two key outcomes:

1. a decision about whether more detailed assessment is needed or referral to an appropriate health professional

2. identification of any salient factors that can become the subject of specific intervention, thus saving time and appropriately concentrating the use of resources.

Red and yellow flags are not mutually exclusive: an individual patient may require intervention for both pathology and disturbed mood (Kendall et al., 1997).

What are the psychosocial yellow flags? Yellow flags include:

- unhelpful attitudes and beliefs about low back pain, e.g. belief that pain is harmful or disabling, resulting in fear-avoidance behaviour
- unhelpful behaviours, e.g. use of extended rest and disproportionate downtime
- compensation issues, e.g. history of extended time off work due to injury or other pain problem (more than 12 weeks)
- inappropriate diagnosis and treatment, e.g. diagnostic language leading to catastrophizing and fear, such as fear of ending up in a wheelchair
- unhelpful emotions, e.g. feeling under stress and unable to maintain sense of control
- inappropriate family response, e.g. overprotective or socially punitive responses from spouse
- work issues, e.g. belief that work is harmful or poor job satisfaction.

For further information, see *Guide to Assessing Psychosocial Yellow Flags in Acute Low Back Pain* (Kendall et al., 1997). A questionnaire that may be used to assess some of these risk factors is reproduced below (the Tampa scale).

Several questionnaires have been developed to help identify those patients with unhelpful attitudes and beliefs. These include the:

- Tampa scale for kinesiophobia
- Fear-avoidance beliefs questionnaire (FABQ)
- Waddell's signs

These questionnaires are described below.

Tampa scale for kinesiophobia
Overview and scoring of test   The Tampa scale for kinesiophobia was developed by Miller and colleagues in 1991 (unpublished) as a measure of fear of movement/reinjury and subsequently reported

by Vlaeyen et al. (1995a). The questionnaire consists of 17 statements about pain and patients are asked to signal the extent to which they agree with each statement using a four-point scale (Fig. 5.11). The scores for items 4, 8, 12 and 16 are reversed when scoring.

Reliability The questionnaire items have been found to have moderate internal consistency (Cronbach's alpha = 0.77: Vlaeyen et al., 1995a).

Validity Evidence for the construct validity of the questionnaire is provided by Vlaeyen and colleagues (1995a), in a study in which the Tampa questionnaire was administered to 103 patients with chronic low back pain (CLBP) along with other psychological measures. Tampa scores were significantly correlated with three items on the Fear Survey Schedule, the Beck Depression Inventory, the reinterpreting pain and positive self-talk items of the Coping Strategies Questionnaire, VAS pain intensity and the pain impact and catastrophizing scales of the Pain Cognitions list. In multivariate analysis, where compensation status, gender and pain intensity are taken into account, catastrophizing and depression are most predictive of Tampa scores.

A factor analysis study of 129 patients with CLBP by Vlaeyen and colleagues (1995b) suggested that the Tampa scale contains four factors (accounting for 36.2% of total variance) that the authors labelled harm, fear of (re)injury, importance of exercise and avoidance of activity. The internal consistency of the factors ranged from 0.53 to 0.71. The Tampa scores were significantly correlated with the pain impact and catastrophizing scales of the pain cognitions list, pain intensity and the fear of blood/injury scale of the Fear Survey Schedule.

In a cross-sectional study of 33 CLBP patients, Vlaeyen and colleagues (1995b) demonstrated significant correlations between RM-24 disability scores and Tampa scores ($r = 0.49$, $P < 0.001$) but not pain intensity, pain duration, age or a measure of impairment. Tampa scores were the best predictor of disability (as measured by the Roland–Morris scale), explaining 13% of variance compared to the 4% explained by pain duration and gender.

Fear–avoidance beliefs questionnaire
Overview of test The FABQ (Waddell et al., 1995) was developed to assess patients' beliefs about

pain and work/physical activity. The questionnaire evolved from Waddell's earlier work that demonstrated that the severity of pain and the extent of physical impairment only explained a small proportion of self-reported low back disability. A better explanation of the disability resulted when psychological distress and illness behaviour were also considered. Waddell developed the questionnaire from fear theory and fear-avoidance cognitions and the concepts of disease conviction, somatic focusing and increased somatic awareness.

The questionnaire consists of 16 statements about pain and patients are asked to signal the extent to which they agree with each statement, using a seven-point scale (Fig. 5.12). Waddell suggests that items 6, 7, 9, 10, 11, 12 and 15 should be scored separately as scale 1, FABQ1 (fear avoidance beliefs about work) while items 2, 3, 4 and 5 form scale 2, FABQ2 (fear avoidance beliefs about physical activity).

Reliability Reliability has been assessed on 26 outpatients referred to a hospital physiotherapy department with low back pain (Waddell et al., 1995). The test–retest interval was 48 h. All 16 items of the questionnaire were shown to have acceptable reliability. The average kappa value for all 16 items was 0.74, with 71% of individual answers identical on retest.

Validity Factor analysis by Waddell et al. (1995) suggested a two-factor solution with factor one representing beliefs about work (items 6, 7, 9, 10, 11, 12 and 15) and factor two representing fear-avoidance beliefs about physical activity (items 2, 3, 4 and 5) with some items being redundant (13, 14 and 16) and others not fitting either factor well (1 and 8).

In a cross-sectional study of 184 patients with CLBP referred to hospital outpatient departments, Waddell noted, at best, weak correlations between FABQ1 or FABQ2 and pain characteristics but, in contrast, much stronger correlations between these scales and disability and psychological distress. For example, scores on FABQ1 (work beliefs) produced a correlation of 0.55 with the extent of work loss in the past year. A hierarchical regression analysis showed that, while pain characteristics explained 14% of disability in activities of daily living, the FABQ1 and FABQ2 explained a further

Tampa scale for kinesiophobia

Here are some of the things which other patients have told us about their pain. For each statement please circle any number from 1 to 4 to signify whether you agree or disagree with the statement.

	Strongly disagree	Somewhat disagree	Somewhat agree	Strongly agree
1. I'm afraid that I might injure myself if I exercise	1	2	3	4
2. If I were to try to overcome it, my pain would increase	1	2	3	4
3. My body is telling me I have something dangerously wrong	1	2	3	4
4. My pain would probably be relieved if I were to exercise	1	2	3	4
5. People aren't taking my medical condition seriously	1	2	3	4
6. My accident has put my body at risk for the rest of my life	1	2	3	4
7. Pain always means I have injured my body	1	2	3	4
8. Just because something aggravates my pain does not mean it is dangerous	1	2	3	4
9. I am afraid that I might injure myself accidentally	1	2	3	4
10. Simply being careful that I do not make any unnecessary movements is the safest thing I can do to prevent my pain from worsening	1	2	3	4
11. I wouldn't have this much pain if there weren't something potentially dangerous going on in my body	1	2	3	4
12. Although my condition is painful, I would be better off if I were physically active	1	2	3	4
13. Pain lets me know when to stop exercising so that I do not injure myself	1	2	3	4
14. It's really not safe for a person with a condition like mine to be physically active	1	2	3	4
15. I can't do all the things normal people do because it's too easy for me to get injured	1	2	3	4
16. Even though something is causing me a lot of pain, I don't think it's actually dangerous	1	2	3	4
17. No one should have to exercise when he/she is in pain	1	2	3	4

Figure 5.11   Tampa scale for kinesiophobia, indicating fear of movement. (Reprinted from *Pain*, **62**, Vlaeyen J, Kole-Snijders A, Boersen R and van Eek H, Fear of movement/(re)injury in chronic low back pain and its relation to behavioural performance, pp. 363–372, Copyright (1995), with permission from *National University of Health Services.*)

32%, and depressive symptoms a further 5%. While pain characteristics explained only 5% of work loss in the past year the FABQ1 (work beliefs) explained a further 26% of the variance, with measures of depressive symptoms contributing only 2%. Interestingly, there was a gender effect, with the FABQ1 much more predictive in males than females of work loss in the past year (35% for males, 18% for females) and disability (27% for males, 17% for females; Simmonds et al., 1998).

While the results of this study are impressive, it needs to be noted that the correlational design prohibits inferences about causation. However, allowing for these limitations, the study suggests that fear of pain and what we do about pain may be more disabling than pain itself. The study provides

Fear-avoidance beliefs questionnaire

Here are some things which other patients have told us about their pain. For each statement please circle any number from 0 to 6 to say how much physical activities such as bending, lifting, walking or driving affect or would affect *your* back pain.

	Completely disagree		Unsure			Completely agree	
1. My pain was caused by physical activity	0	1	2	3	4	5	6
2. Physical activity makes my pain worse	0	1	2	3	4	5	6
3. Physical activity might harm my back	0	1	2	3	4	5	6
4. I should not do physical activities which (might) make my pain worse	0	1	2	3	4	5	6
5. I cannot do physical activities which (might) make my pain worse	0	1	2	3	4	5	6

The following statements are about how your normal work affects or would affect your back pain.

6. My pain was caused by my work or by an accident at work	0	1	2	3	4	5	6
7. My work aggravated my pain	0	1	2	3	4	5	6
8. I have a claim for compensation for my pain	0	1	2	3	4	5	6
9. My work is too heavy for me	0	1	2	3	4	5	6
10. My work makes or would make my pain worse	0	1	2	3	4	5	6
11. My work might harm my back	0	1	2	3	4	5	6
12. I should not do my normal work with my present pain	0	1	2	3	4	5	6
13. I cannot do my normal work with my present pain	0	1	2	3	4	5	6
14. I cannot do my normal work until my pain is treated	0	1	2	3	4	5	6
15. I do not think that I will be back to my normal work within 3 months	0	1	2	3	4	5	6
16. I do not think that I will ever be able to go back to that work	0	1	2	3	4	5	6

Figure 5.12   Fear-avoidance beliefs questionnaire. This questionnaire is designed to assess patients' beliefs about pain and physical activity, including work. (Reprinted from *Pain*, 52, Waddell G, Newton M, Somerville D and Main C, A fear-avoidance beliefs questionnaire (FABQ) and the role of fear-avoidance beliefs in chronic low back pain and disability, pp. 157–168, Copyright (1995), with permission from *National University of Health Services.*)

support for Waddell's view that factors such as unjustified restriction of activity, prescription of rest, advice to avoid pain and passive treatment may all cause or reinforce fear-avoidance beliefs and so lead to iatrogenic disability. Waddell suggests that inappropriate fear-avoidance beliefs need to be recognized from the acute stage, tackled directly and changed early before they become fixed.

Support for this advice is indirectly provided by the number of studies that have noted good results from encouraging activity or active treatment rather than rest or passive treatment in acute low back pain (Malmivaara et al., 1995), subacute low back pain (Lindstrom et al., 1992) and CLBP (Frost et al., 1995). Lindstrom et al.'s study (1992) is particularly supportive of Waddell's model because this study employed a gradually increased exercise programme with an operant conditioning behavioural approach that aimed to teach the patients that it was safe to move while regaining function. The study noted much better results in males, which is in accord with Waddell's finding that fear-avoidance beliefs about work and physical activity were much more predictive of disability and work loss in males. Malmivaara et al.'s study (1995) is of note because it produced good results simply by telling patients to avoid bedrest and to resume normal duties as soon as possible. Even more compelling are the findings of Indahl et al. (1995) that giving patients with sub-acute LBP simple advice about the benign nature of LBP, and telling them that they should not be afraid of their back or be overcautious, provided better results than conventional medical treatment.

Perhaps not surprisingly this approach has also been used successfully in the treatment of whiplash injuries (McKinney, 1989; McKinney et al., 1989; Borchgrevink et al., 1998). The FABQ is however unsuitable for administration to non-low back pain patients because some of the items are specific to low back pain. A useful alternative for such cases is the Tampa scale.

Waddell's signs

Overview   Waddell et al. (1989) developed a series of tests incorporating both signs and symptoms to screen for abnormal illness behaviour. However, to identify abnormal illness behaviour, it is essential to recognize normal illness behaviour. The authors defined normal illness behaviour as follows: 'In normal illness behaviour the type of sick role accepted or sought by the patient is proportionate to the doctor's assessment of objective pathology and congruent with the sick role offered'. In contrast, they defined abnormal illness behaviour as follows: 'If the patient's illness behaviour is disproportionate to the doctor's assessment of objective pathology and the patient persists in the sick role, rejecting the doctor's view of what is appropriate, then this constitutes "abnormal illness behaviour"'. However, if the patient's illness behaviour is

merely unusual but not maladaptive or inflexible, it should not be regarded as abnormal.'

Waddell et al. (1980) originally described five types of signs that could be used as a simple clinical screening tool to assist in the identification of patients with non-organic signs, and who may require further detail assessment. Waddell et al. (1980) regarded the presence of three or more of the five types of signs as clinically significant. An alternative approach that has been used by some authors is to allocate a score of 1 for each item that is positive, giving a score that ranges from 0 to 8. However, it is more usual to use Waddell et al.'s criterion of three or more types of signs to signify a positive result for Waddell's non-organic signs test. A good summary of Waddell's non-organic signs is provided by Scalzitti (1997) (Table 5.8).

In addition to the signs presented in Table 5.8, Waddell described a set of symptoms that indicate a non-organic condition. Both the modified and original Core questionnaire (see Fig. 5.13, below) contain eight items to identify Waddell's non-organic symptoms. While Waddell's signs have been widely evaluated, there is little work on Waddell's symptoms. Waddell et al.'s (1980) original study reported that a composite score for illness behaviour formed from both non-organic signs and symptoms, as well as from the body chart, was the best predictor of the amount of treatment a patient received. Illness behaviour accounted for 15.2% of the total 49.8% that was accounted for by a multivariate model. Unfortunately this study did not state the variance that was explained by Waddell's symptoms.

Reliability   Waddell et al. (1980) examined the interrater reliability of the above tests by asking two observers to examine 50 consecutive patients with order of examination randomized. They reported good interrater reliability for assessment of each item, with exact agreement ranging from 78 to 86%; they also reported 86% agreement for a positive test result based on the criterion of three out of five types of signs being positive. McCombe et al. (1989) found poorer reliability, with kappa ranging from −0.16 to 0.48 for individual items; however, reliability for determining the presence of three or more types of signs was not evaluated.

While there is contradictory information on reliability, it is likely that the test is highly reliable

Table 5.8   Signs of abnormal illness behaviour (Scalzitti, 1997)

Test	Signs
Tenderness	Superficial: the skin is tender to light pinch over a wide area of lumbar skin Non-anatomic: deep tenderness felt over a wide area is not localized to one structure
Simulation tests	These tests give the impression that a particular examination is being carried out when in fact it is not Axial loading: low back pain reported on vertical loading of the standing patient's skull Rotation: back pain is reported when shoulders and pelvis are passively rotated in the same plane when the patient stands relaxed with the feet together
Distraction tests	A positive physical finding is demonstrated in the routine manner. This finding is then checked while the patient's attention is distracted; a non-organic component may be present if the finding disappears when the patient is distracted Straight leg raising: marked improvement in straight leg raising with distraction, e.g. variations based on sitting
Regional disturbances	Regional disturbances involve a widespread region of neighbouring parts such as the leg below the knee, the entire leg or a quarter or half the body. The essential feature is divergence from accepted neuroanatomy Weakness: weakness is demonstrated on formal testing by a partial cogwheel 'giving way' of many muscle groups that cannot be explained on a localized neurologic basis Sensory: include diminished sensation to light touch, pinprick or other neurologic tests fitting a 'stocking' rather than a dermatomal pattern
Overreaction	Overreaction may take the form of disproportionate verbalization, facial expression, muscle tension and tremor, collapsing or sweating. Judgements should be made with caution, minimizing the examiner's own emotional reaction; there are considerable cultural variations, and it is very easy to introduce observer bias or to provoke this type of response unconsciously

because there is considerable evidence for the validity of the test (see below).

Validity
Construct validity   Waddell's original study investigated the incidence of a positive test result (three out of five positive) in five groups of subjects:

1. a group with poor results following repeat back surgery
2. a group with prolonged disability
3. a group whose treatment had failed
4. a group with a first episode of low back pain
5. a group of normal subjects.

The prevalence of positive test results was 0% in the normal group, 12% in the group with first-episode low back pain and from 33 to 50% in the three failed treatment groups (Waddell et al., 1980). Concurrent validity   Waddell's original study also found weak to good correlations (0.27–0.73) between a positive test result and five other clinical tests to identify non-organic presentations. Waddell et al. also noted weak correlations (0.19–0.29) between the presence of non-organic signs and scores on the hypochondriasis, depression and hysteria scales of the Minnesota Multiphasic Personality Inventory (Hathaway and McKinley, 1943). A later study (Waddell et al., 1989) found a correlation between the presence of non-organic signs and scores on the Illness Behaviour Questionnaire (29% common variance). Chan et al. (1993) noted that subjects with a higher Waddell score were much more likely to have a non-organic pain drawing.
Predictive validity   Karas et al. (1997) studied 126 patients receiving physiotherapy for low back pain and found that a positive test result at initial examination was associated with a lower return to work rate. Ohlund et al. (1994) and Lancourt and Kettelhut (1992) also found evidence for the predictive validity of the tests. Bradish et al. (1988) found a similar result for patients with

non-specific low back pain but not for subjects with radiographic signs of degeneration. Unfortunately, Bradish et al.'s study had a high drop-out rate (23/120) and this may have limited their ability to find an effect in the second group. In each of these studies the treatment was not well described but two (Bradish et al., 1988; Karas et al., 1997) appeared to be traditional and pain-focused while none of the four studies mentioned psychological interventions.

Werneke et al. (1993) calculated a composite item score for Waddell's signs (maximum score 8) at entry and discharge for a group of 170 patients undergoing a work-oriented rehabilitation programme and found that 82% of the subjects who returned to work within 3 months reduced their Waddell's score, whereas only 44% of those who did not return to work reduced their score. Additionally those who had no Waddell's signs at discharge from the programme were more likely to return to work (RTW) than those patients where one or more Waddell's signs remained (78% RTW versus 35% RTW). However, Werneke et al. (1993) did not report the predictive ability of subjects' initial Waddell's score. Polatin et al. (1997) found that for subjects undergoing a functional restoration programme, the initial Waddell's score was not predictive of recovery. Thus it appears that it is the failure to improve Waddell's score or the persistence of Waddell's signs rather than the initial presence of Waddell's signs that is predictive of treatment failure in functionally oriented programmes where psychological factors are specifically addressed.

The modified Core network low back pain medical screening questionnaire (Fig. 5.13)   The modified Core network low back pain medical screening questionnaire was developed from the original described by Delitto and colleagues (1995) and has been modified to include the red flags suggested in subsequent clinical practice guidelines. The questionnaire provides one option for screening for red flags and consists of questions designed to screen for specific disease processes such as cancer (questions 1–11), questions to screen for depression (questions 12a and 12b) and inappropriate illness behaviour (questions 13–20) (Waddell's symptoms).

Reliability   No studies have evaluated the reliability of the modified Core network low back pain medical screening questionnaire.

Validity   The validity of the modified Core network low back pain medical screening questionnaire has not been assessed but there is information available on the sensitivity and specificity of individual items in screening. To emphasize the fact that effective screening requires information additional to that obtained with the modified Core, we have provided information on a range of items.

Social history

The social history provides useful information about management of the presenting disorder, and occasionally cues regarding diagnosis or the presence of coexisting pathology. Pathology is sometimes exclusive to a particular age group or gender. For example, postmenopausal women are more likely to suffer symptoms of osteoporosis than men in the same age group, and Scheuerman's disease most commonly affects young people.

Understanding the patient's social circumstances will ensure that overall management of the patient is appropriate and relevant. This requires learning about the patient's employment status (whether he or she works, and the type of work engaged in), domestic role, requirements for assistance with self-care, existence of dependants and leisure pursuits. There may be other relevant aspects to the patient's life that need to be explored to ensure that home programmes and treatment goals are realistic, remembering that physiotherapists need to work within the constraints imposed upon their patients.

Details about employment status inform about the physical demands placed daily on the patient. This determines our treatment goals to some degree. A patient may be unemployed and depressed, but have few other constraints in carrying out a home programme of exercises or rest. The goals of treatment will probably not be to return this patient to a particular work situation. For a patient who is currently employed, aspects of the work routine or postures adopted during the work day may require changing to benefit the patient in terms of avoiding reinjury or providing the optimal environment for tissue healing and repair. The demands placed

Modified Core network low back pain medical screening questionnaire

Name:_____   Date:_____

1. Is your general health good?   ❐ Yes   ❐ No

    If no, what problems do you have?:   _____

    _____

    _____

    _____

2. Do you have any ongoing disease process such as arthritis, osteoporosis

    or cancer?   ❐ Yes   ❐ No

    If yes, please specify: _____

    _____

    _____

    _____

3. Have you ever been treated for cancer?   ❐ Yes   ❐ No

4. Have you had any recent medical tests, e.g. blood tests, X-rays, etc.?   ❐ Yes   ❐ No

5. Have you lost more than 4 kg (10 lb) in the last 6 months?   ❐ Yes   ❐ No

6. Do you have any:

    numbness or tingling in your buttock or genital region?   ❐ Yes   ❐ No

    bladder or bowel problems?   ❐ Yes   ❐ No

    pain, swelling or redness in other joints?   ❐ Yes   ❐ No

    skin rashes?   ❐ Yes   ❐ No

    eye discomfort, watery eyes, eye pain with light?   ❐ Yes   ❐ No

    weakness in your legs?   ❐ Yes   ❐ No

    balance problems?   ❐ Yes   ❐ No

7. Have you had a:

    recent fever or chill?   ❐ Yes   ❐ No

    recent infection?   ❐ Yes   ❐ No

8. Do you get pain in your legs that is caused by walking and that is relieved by resting?   ❐ Yes   ❐ No

9. Is your back stiff in the morning for longer than half an hour?   ❐ Yes   ❐ No

10. Have you ever taken steroids, e.g. prednisone, cortisone?   ❐ Yes   ❐ No

11. Are you currently taking any medication?   ❐ Yes   ❐ No

    If yes, please specify: _____

    _____

    _____

    _____

12. During the past month:

    (a) have you often been bothered by feeling down, depressed or hopeless?   ❒ Yes   ❒ No

    (b) have you often been bothered by little interest or pleasure in doing things?   ❒ Yes   ❒ No

13. Do you get pain at the tip of your tailbone?   ❒ Yes   ❒ No

14. Does your entire leg ever become painful (front, sides and back at the same time)?   ❒ Yes   ❒ No

15. Does your entire leg ever become numb (front, sides and back at the same time)?   ❒ Yes   ❒ No

16. Does your whole leg ever give way?   ❒ Yes   ❒ No

17. Have you had any periods of time in the past year or during this episode when you have had very little pain?   ❒ Yes   ❒ No

18. Have you ever had to report to a hospital emergency room because of back pain?   ❒ Yes   ❒ No

19. Have you had any treatment for your problem that has helped you?   ❒ Yes   ❒ No

20. Have all treatments for your back made you worse?   ❒ Yes   ❒ No

Figure 5.13 Modified Core network low back pain medical screening questionnaire. The questions can be asked during the interview or the questionnaire can be administered. (Reproduced with permission from Maher et al., 2001.)

on a patient at work may be identified during other sections of the history (e.g. aggravating activities in the behaviour of symptoms over a 24-h period). Other features of the patient's employment situation may need to be considered. For example, it is not always possible to make changes to a patient's work situation; employees might be frightened of losing their job, a busy executive may be leading a company through organizational change, or an athlete may face losing his or her position in the team. Although not ideal, physiotherapists often need to work with patients within these constraints.

Leisure activities provide further information about desirable treatment outcomes. Type and level of activity, including specific requirements such as endurance of particular muscle groups, should be clearly ascertained. Retraining for these specific activities may form a necessary part of the management regimen.

Determining the patient's goals of treatment will provide guidance in how treatment programmes and outcome measures should be considered, and may influence an education programme.

When advising patients about home programmes and appropriate rest, account must be taken of the patient's dependants. This may mean incorporating appropriate advice, e.g. mothers with small children may be unable to avoid specific activities when it would be most desirable. They may also need advice about, for example, lifting and bathing small children. Compliance with home programmes is impossible if consideration is not given to these factors.

Some patients may require domestic assistance. Sometimes this can be achieved by modifying the activity, but often means assistance from another person. If the patient lives alone, assistance may be required from other health personnel, e.g. from occupational therapists or nurses.

It is important to be professional when discussing personal details with patients because it is easy to appear curious rather than proficient. In addition, a patient must trust you to give you honest personal details. It should also be remembered that it is unethical, and in come cases unlawful, to discuss your patients publicly or disclose any information about a patient to unauthorized people.

A good knowledge of the patient's social history is particularly relevant when designing home programmes and setting treatment goals. Details about occupation and leisure activities are frequently a source of diagnostic information. Even when this is not the case physiotherapists should understand the pressures the patient is facing to enhance the possibility of successful treatment outcomes.

REFERENCES

Austen, R. (1991). The distribution and characteristics of lumbar–lower limb symptoms in subjects with and without a neurological deficit. In: *Proceedings of Manipulative Physiotherapists Association of Australia 7th Biennial Conference*, NSW, pp. 252–257.

Bailey, D.A., Martin, A.D., Houston, C.S. and Howie, L.J. (1986). Physical activity, nutrition, bone density and osteoporosis. *Aust. J. Sci. Med. Sports*, **18**, 3–7.

Beurskens, A., De Vet, H. and Koke, A. (1996). Responsiveness of functional status in low back pain: a comparison of different instruments. *Pain*, **65**, 71–76.

Bigos, S., Bowyer, O., Braen, G. et al. (1994). *Acute Low Back Problems in Adults*. Clinical practice guideline no. 14. Rockville, MD: Agency for Health Care Policy and Research.

Bogduk, N. (1991). Innervation, pain patterns and mechanisms of pain production. In: *Clinics in Physical Therapy. Physical Therapy of the Low Back*, ed. L.T. Twomey and J.R. Taylor. London: Churchill Livingstone.

Bolton, J. and Wilkinson, R. (1998). Responsiveness of pain scales: a comparison of three pain intensity measures in chiropractic patients. *J. Manip. Physiol. Ther.*, **21**, 1–7.

Borchgrevink, G., Kaasa, A., McDonagh, D., Stiles, T., Haraldseth, O. and Lereim, I. (1998). Acute treatment of whiplash neck sprain injuries. A randomised trial of treatment during the first 14 days after a car accident. *Spine*, **23**, 25–31.

Bradish, C., Lloyd, G., Aldam, C. et al. (1988). Do nonorganic signs help to predict the return to activity of patients with low back pain? *Spine*, **13**, 557–560.

Brodie, D., Burnett, J., Walker, J. and Lydes-Reid, D. (1990). Evaluation for low back pain by patient questionnaires and therapist assessment. *J. Orthop. Sports Phys. Ther.*, **11**, 519–529.

Burckhardt, C. and Bjelle, A. (1994). A Swedish version of the Short-Form McGill Pain Questionnaire. *Scand. J. Rheumatol.*, **23**, 77–81.

Burton, A.C. (1965). Total fluid energy, gravitational potential energy, effects of posture. In: *Physiology and Biophysics of the Circulation – An Introductory Text*, ed. A.C. Burton, pp. 95–101. Chicago, IL: Year Book Medical.

Calin, A., Porta, J., Fries, J. and Schurman, D. (1977). Clinical history as a screening test for ankylosing spondylitis. *J.A.M.A.*, **237**, 2613–2614.

Chan, C., Goldman, S., Ilstrup, D., Kunselman, A. and O'Neill, P. (1993). The pain drawing and Waddell's nonorganic physical signs in chronic low back pain. *Spine*, **18**, 1717–1722.

Chatman, A., Hyams, S., Neel, J. et al. (1997). The patient-specific functional scale: measurement properties in patients with knee dysfunction. *Phys. Ther.*, **77**, 820–829.

Chow, R.K., Harrison, J.E., Brown, C.F. and Hajek, V. (1986). Physical fitness effect on bone mass in post menopausal women. *Arch. Phys. Med. Rehabil.*, **67**, 231.

Co, Y., Eaton, S. and Maxwell, M. (1993). The relationship between the St Thomas and Oswestry disability scores and the severity of low back pain. *J. Manip. Physiol. Ther.*, **16**, 14–18.

Coman, W.B. (1986). Dizziness related to ENT conditons. In: *Modern Manual Therapy of the Vertebral Column*, ed. G. Grieve, pp. 303–314. London: Churchill Livingstone.

Coscia, M., Leipzig, T. and Cooper, D. (1994). Acute cauda equina syndrome. *Spine*, **19**, 475–478.

Dalton, P.A. and Jull, G. (1989). The distribution and characteristics of neck-arm pain in patients with and without a neurological deficit. *Aust. J. Physiother.*, **35**, 3–8.

Daniel, D.M., Stone, M.L., Sachs, R. and Malcolm, L. (1985). Instrumented measurement of anterior knee laxity in patients with acute anterior cruciate ligament disruption. *Am. J. Sports Med.*, **13**, 401–407.

de Jong, P.T.V.M., de Jong, J.M.B.V., Cohen, B. and Jongkees, L.B.W. (1977). Ataxia and nystagmus induced by injection of local anesthetics in the neck. *Ann. Neurol.*, **1**, 240–246.

Delitto, A., Erhard, R. and Bowling, R. (1995). A treatment-based classification approach to low back syndrome: identifying and staging patients for conservative treatment. *Phys. Ther.*, **75**, 470–489.

Deyo, R. and Centor, R. (1986). Assessing the responsiveness of functional scales to clinical change: an analogy to diagnostic test performance. *J. Chron. Dis.*, **39**, 897–906.

Deyo, R. and Diehl, A. (1988). Cancer as a cause of back pain. Frequency, clinical presentation and diagnostic strategies. *J. Gen. Intern. Med.*, **3**, 230–238.

Deyo, R., Rainville, J. and Kent, D. (1992). What can the history and physical examination tell us about low back pain? *J.A.M.A.*, **268**, 760–765.

Dreyfuss, P., Tibiletti, C. and Dreyer, S. (1994). Thoracic zygapophyseal joint pain patterns: a study in normal volunteers. *Spine*, **19**, 807–811.

Dudgeon, D., Raubertas, R. and Rosenthal, S. (1993). The short-form McGill pain questionnaire in chronic cancer pain. *J. Pain Symptom Manage.*, **8**, 191–195.

Evans, P. (1980). The healing process at cellular level: a review. *Physiotherapy*, **66**, 256–259.

Fairbank, J., Davies, J., Couper, J. and O'Brien, J. (1980). The Oswestry Low Back Pain Disability Questionnaire. *Physiotherapy*, **66**, 271–273.

Feagin, J.A. and Curl, W.W. (1976). Isolated tear of the anterior cruciate ligament: 5 year follow-up study. *Am. J. Sports Med.*, **4**, 95–100.

Feinstein, B., Langton, J.N.K., Jameson, R.M. and Schiller, F. (1954). Experiments on pain referred from deep somatic tissues. *J. Bone Joint Surg.*, **36**, 981–997.

Fernbach, J., Langer, F. and Gross, A. (1976). The significance of low back pain in older adults. *Can. Med. Assoc. J.*, **115**, 898–900.

Fox, E. and Melzack, R. (1976). Trancutaneous electrical stimulation and acupuncture: comparison of treatment for low back pain. *Pain*, **2**, 141–148.

French, S. (1988). History taking in the physiotherapy assessment. *Physiotherapy*, **74**, 158–160.

Frost, H., Klaber-Moffett, J., Moser, J. and Fairbank, J. (1995). Randomised controlled trial for evaluation of fitness programme for patients with chronic low back pain. *Br. Med. J.*, **310**, 151–154.

Gatchel, R., Polatin, P. and Kinney, R. (1995). Predicting outcome of chronic back pain using predictors of psychopathology– a prospective analysis. *Health Psychol.*, **14**, 415–420.

Gebhart, G.J. and Ness, T.J. (1991). Central mechanisms of visceral pain. *Can. J. Physiol. Pharmacol.*, **69**, 627–634.

Geisser, M., Robinson, M., Keefe, F. and Weiner, M. (1994). Catastrophizing, depression and the sensory, affective and evaluative aspects of chronic pain. *Pain*, **59**, 79–83.

Gibson, T., Grahame, R., Harkness, J., Woo, P., Blagrave, P. and Hills, R. (1985). Controlled comparison of short wave diathermy treatment with osteopathic treatment in non specific low back pain. *Lancet*, **June**, 1258–1260.

Goldberg, M.E., Eggers, H.M. and Gouras, P. (1991). The ocular motor system. In: *Principles of Neural Science*, 3rd edn, ed. E.R. Kandel, J.H. Schwartz and T.M. Jessell, pp. 660–678. Connecticut: Prentice Hall.

Gracely, R., McGrath, P. and Dubner, R. (1978a). Ratio scales of sensory and affective verbal pain descriptors. *Pain*, **5**, 5–18.

Gracely, R., McGrath, P. and Dubner, R. (1978b). Validity and sensitivity of ratio scales of sensory and affective verbal pain descriptors: manipulation of affect by diazepam. *Pain*, **5**, 19–29.

Gran, J.T. (1985). An epidemiological survey of the signs and symptoms of ankylosing spondylitis. *Clin. Rheumatol.*, **4**, 161–169.

Grieve, G.P. (1986). Bony and soft-tissue anomalies of the vertebral column. In: *Modern Manual Therapy of the Vertebral Column*, ed. G.P. Grieve, pp. 3–20. London: Churchill Livingstone.

Gronblad, M., Lukinman, A. and Konttinen, Y. (1990). Chronic low back pain: intercorrelation of repeated measures for pain and disability. *Scand. J. Rehabil. Med.*, **22**, 73–77.

Gronblad, M., Hupli, M., Wennerstrand, P. et al. (1993). Intercorrelation and test–retest reliability of the Pain Disability Index (PDI) and the Oswestry Disability Questionnaire (ODQ) and their correlation with pain intensity in low back pain patients. *Clin. J. Pain*, **9**, 189–195.

Gronblad, M., Hurri, H. and Kouri, J. (1997). Relationships between spinal mobility, physical performance tests, pain intensity and disability assessments in chronic low back pain patients. *Scand. J. Rehabil. Med.*, **29**, 17–24.

Haggman, S., Maher, C. and Refshauge, K.M. (2004). Screening for depression by first contact physical therapists managing low back pain. *Physical Therapy* (accepted March 2004).

Hains, F., Waalen, J. and Mior, S. (1998). Psychometric properties of the neck disability index. *J. Manip. Physiol. Ther.*, **21**, 75–80.

Hathaway, S.R. and McKinley, J.C. (1943). *Minnesota Multiphasic Personality Inventory Revised*. Minneapolis, MN: University of Minnesota Press.

Helfet, A.J. and Gruebel, L. (1978). *Disorders of the Lumbar Spine*. Philadelphia, PA: J.B. Lippincott.

Indahl, A., Velund, L. and Reikeraas, O. (1995). Good prognosis for low back pain when left untampered. A randomised clinical trial. *Spine*, **20**, 473–477.

Jensen, M., Karoly, P. and Braver, S. (1986). The measurement of clinical pain intensity: a comparison of six methods. *Pain*, **27**, 117–126.

Jensen, M., Karoly, P., O'Riordan, E., Bland, F. and Burns, R. (1989). The subjective experience of acute pain. An assessment of the utility of 10 indices. *Clin. J. Pain*, **5**, 153–159.

Jensen, M., Strom, S., Turner, J. and Romano, J. (1992). Validity of the Sickness Impact Profile Roland Scale as a measure of dysfunction in chronic pain patients. *Pain*, **50**, 157–162.

Jensen, M., Turner, J. and Romano, J. (1994). Correlates of improvement in multidisciplinary treatment of chronic pain. *J. Consult. Clin. Psych.*, **62**, 172–179.

Jensen, M., Turner, J., Romano, J. and Fisher, L. (1999). Comparative reliability and validity of chronic pain intensity measures. *Pain*, **83**, 157–162.

Kannangara, S. and Shenstone, B. (1988). Seronegative spondyloarthropathies. A distinct group of disorders. *Curr. Ther.*, **April**, 77–100.

Karas, R., McIntosh, G., Hall, H., Wilson, L. and Melles, T. (1997). The relationship between nonorganic signs and centralisation of symptoms in the prediction of return to work for patients with low back pain. *Phys. Ther.*, **77**, 354–360.

Kelly, J.P. (1991). The sense of balance. In: *Principles of Neural Science*, ed. E.R. Kandell, J.H. Schwartz and T.M. Jessel, pp. 500–511. Connecticut: Prentice-Hall.

Kendall, N., Linton, S. and Main, C. (1997). *Guide to Assessing Psychosocial Yellow Flags in Acute Low Back Pain: Risk Factors for Long Term Disability and Work Loss*. Wellington: Accident Rehabilitation and Compensation Insurance Corporation of New Zealand and the National Health Committee.

Kopec, J., Esdaile, J., Abrahamowicz, M. et al. (1995). The Quebec back pain disability scale. Measurement properties. *Spine*, **20**, 341–352.

Kremer, E., Atkinson, J.H. and Ignelzi, R.J. (1981). Measurement of pain: patient preference does not confound pain measurement. *Pain*, **10**, 241–248.

Kremer, E., Atkinson, J. and Kremer, A. (1983). The language of pain: affective descriptors of pain are a better predictor of psychological disturbance than pattern of sensory and affective descriptors. *Pain*, **16**, 185–192.

Lancourt, J. and Kettelhut, M. (1992). Predicting return to work for lower back pain patients receiving worker's compensation. *Spine*, **17**, 629–640.

le Blanc, F., Cruess, R., Dupuis, M., Rossignol, M., Spitzer, W. and Dauphinee, S. (1987). Scientific approach to the assessment and management of activity-related spinal disorders. *Spine*, **12** (7 suppl.), 20.

Lewis, T. (1942). *Pain*. London: Macmillan.

Lindstrom, I., Ohlund, C., Eek, C. et al. (1992). The effect of graded activity on patients with subacute low back pain: a randomised prospective clinical study with an operant-conditioning behavioural approach. *Phys. Ther.* **72**, 279–293.

Linton, S. and Gotestam, K. (1983). A clinical comparison of 2 pain scales: correlation, remembering chronic pain, and a measure of compliance. *Pain*, **17**, 57–65.

Maher, C., Latimer, J. and Refshauge, K.M. (2001). *Atlas of Clinical Tests and Measures for Low Back Pain*. Sydney: Manipulative Physiotherapists Association of Australia.

Maitland, G.D. (1964). *Vertebral Manipulation*, 1st edn. London: Butterworths.

Maitland, G.D. (1986). *Vertebral Manipulation*, 5th edn. London: Butterworths.

Malmivaara, A., Hakkinen, U., Aro, T. et al. (1995). The treatment of acute low back pain. Bed rest, exercise or normal activity? *N. Engl. J. Med.*, **332**, 351–355.

Margolis, R., Tait, R. and Krause, S. (1986). A rating system for use with patient pain drawings. *Pain*, **24**, 57–65.

Margolis, R., Chibnall, J. and Tait, R. (1988). Test–retest reliability of the pain drawing instrument. *Pain*, **33**, 49–51.

Martire, J.R. (1987). The role of nuclear medicine bone scans in evaluating pain in athletic injuries. In: *Clinics in Sports Medicine*, pp. 713–738. Philadelphia, PA: W.B. Saunders.

McCombe, P., Fairbank, J., Cockersole, B. and Pynsent, P. (1989). Reproducibility of physical signs in low back pain. *Spine*, **14**, 908–918.

McCreary, C., Turner, J. and Dawson, E. (1981). Principal dimensions of the pain experience and psychological disturbance in chronic low back pain patients. *Pain*, **11**, 85–92.

McCulloch, J.A. and Waddell, G. (1980). Variation of the lumbosacral myotomes with bony segmental anomalies. *J. Bone Joint Surg.*, **62B**, 475–480.

McKenzie, R.A. (1981). *The Lumbar Spine – Mechanical Diagnosis and Therapy*. New Zealand: Upper Hutt, Spinal Publications.

McKinney, L. (1989). Early mobilization and outcome in acute sprains of the neck. *Br. Med. J.*, **299**, 1006–1008.

McKinney, L.A., Dornan, J.O. and Ryan, M. (1989). The role of physiotherapy in the management of acute neck sprains following road-traffic accidents. *Arch. Emerg. Med.*, **6**, 27–33.

Meade, T., Dyer, S., Browne, W., Townsend, J. and Frank, A. (1990). Low back pain of mechanical origin: randomised comparison of chiropractic and hospital outpatient treatment. *Br. Med. J.*, **300**, 1431–1437.

Melzack, R. (1975). The McGill pain questionnaire: major properties and scoring methods. *Pain*, **1**, 277–299.

Melzack, R. (1987). The short-form McGill Pain Questionnaire. *Pain*, **30**, 191–197.

Mense, S. (1993). Nociception from skeletal muscle in relation to clinical muscle pain. *Pain*, **54**, 241–289.

Mooney, V. and Robertson, J. (1976). The facet syndrome. *Clin. Orthop. Rel. Res.*, **115**, 149–156.

Nicholas, M.K., Wilson, P.H. and Goyen, J. (1992). Comparison of cognitive-behavioural group treatment and an alternative non-psychological treatment for chronic low back pain. *Pain*, **48**, 339–347.

O'Connor, M.I. and Currier, B.L. (1992). Metastatic bone disease: metastatic disease of the spine. *Orthopedics*, **15**, 611–620.

Ohlund, C., Lindstrom, I., Areskoug, B. et al. (1994). Pain behavior in industrial subacute low back pain. Part 1. Reliability: concurrent and predictive validity of pain behavior assessments. *Pain*, **58**, 201–209.

Ohnaus, E. and Adler, R. (1975). Methodological problems in the measurement of pain: a comparison between verbal rating scale and the visual analogue scale. *Pain*, **1**, 379–384.

Pengel, L.H.M., Refshauge, K.M. and Maher, C.G. (2004). Responsiveness of pain, disability and physical impairment outcomes in subjects with low back pain. *Spine*, **29** (in press).

Pocock, N.A., Eisman, J.A., Yeates, M.G., Sambrook, P.N. and Eberls, S. (1986). Physical fitness is a major determinant of femoral neck and lumbar spine bone mineral density. *J. Clin. Invest.*, **78**, 618–621.

Polatin, P., Cox, B., Gatchel, R. and Mayer, T. (1997). A prospective study of Waddell signs in patients with chronic low back pain. When they may not be predictive. *Spine*, **22**, 1618–1621.

Price, D., McGrath, P., Rafii, A. and Buckingham, B. (1983). The validation of visual analogue scales as ratio scale measures for chronic and experimental pain. *Pain*, **17**, 45–56.

Ransford, A., Cairns, D. and Mooney, V. (1976). The pain drawing as an aid to the psychologic evaluation of patients with low back pain. *Spine*, **1**, 127–134.

Refshauge, K.M. (1994). Rotation: a valid premanipulative dizziness test? Does it predict safe manipulation? *J. Manip. Physiol. Ther.*, **17**, 15–19.

Riddle, D. and Stratford, P. (1998). Use of generic versus region-specific functional status measures on patients with cervical spine disorders. *Phys. Ther.*, **78**, 951–963.

Roland, M. and Fairbank, J. (2000). The Roland–Morris Disability Questionnaire and the Oswestry Disability Questionnaire. *Spine*, **25**, 3115–3124.

Roland, M. and Morris, R. (1983). A study of the natural history of back pain. *Spine*, **8**, 141–150.

Ross, R. and LaStayo, P. (1997). Clinical assessment of pain. In: *Assessment in Occupational Therapy and Physical Therapy*, ed. J. van Deusen and D. Brunt. Philadelphia: W.B. Saunders.

Rowell, L.B. (1986). *Human Circulation Regulation During Physical Stress*. New York: Oxford University Press.

Rushmer, R.F. (1976). *Cardiovascular Dynamics*, 4th edn, pp. 217–245. Philadelphia: W.B. Saunders.

Sadowska-Wroblewska, M., Filipowicz, A., Garwolinska, H., Michalski, J., Rusiniak, B. and Wroblewska, T. (1983). Clinical symptoms and signs useful in the early diagnosis of ankylosing spondylitis. *Clin. Rheumatol.*, **2**, 37–43.

Scalzitti, D. (1997). Screening for psychological factors in patients with low back problems: Waddell's nonorganic signs. *Phys. Ther.*, **77**, 306–312.

Schaible, H.-G. and Grubb, B.D. (1993). Afferent and spinal mechanisms of joint pain. *Pain*, **55**, 5–54.

Schumacher, H.R. (1988). *Primer on the Rheumatic Diseases*, 9th edn. Atlanta: Arthritis Foundation.

Scott, J. and Huskisson, E. (1976). Graphic representation of pain. *Pain*, **2**, 175–184.

Scrimshaw, S. and Maher, C. (2001). Responsiveness of visual analogue and McGill pain scale measures. *J. Manip. Physiol. Ther.*, **24**, 501–504.

Sheldon, H. (1984). *Boyd's Introduction to the Study of Disease*, 9th edn, pp. 131–157. Philadelphia: Lea and Febiger.

Simmonds, M., Olson, S., Jones, S. et al. (1998). Psychometric characteristics and clinical usefulness of physical performance tests in patients with low back pain. *Spine*, **23**, 2412–2421.

Spector, T.D. and Sambrook, P.N. (1993). Steroid osteoporosis. *Br. Med. J.*, **307**, 519–520.

Stratford, P., Binkley, J., Solomon, P. et al. (1994). Assessing change over time in patients with low back pain. *Phys. Ther.*, **74**, 528–533.

Stratford, P., Gill, C., Westaway, M. and Binkley, J. (1995). Assessing disability and change on individual patients: a report of a patient specific measure. *Physiother. Can.*, **47**, 258–263.

Stratford, P., Binkley, J. and Riddle, D. (1996). Health status measures: strategies and analytic methods for assessing change scores. *Phys. Ther.*, **76**, 1109–1123.

Stratford, P., Riddle, D., Binkley, J., Spadoni, G., Westaway, M. and Padfield, B. (1999). Using the Neck Disability Index to make decisions concerning individual patients. *Physiother. Can.*, **spring**, 107–119.

Strong, J., Ashton, R., Cramond, T. and Chant, D. (1990). Pain intensity, attitude and function in back pain patients. *Aust. Occup. Ther. J.*, **37**, 179–183.

Sunderland, S. (1978). *Nerve and Nerve Injuries*, 2nd edn. London: Churchill Livingstone.

Toole, J.F. and Tucker, S.H. (1960). Influence of head position upon cerebral circulation. *Arch. Neurol.*, **2**, 616–623.

Turner, J. and Clancy, S. (1986). Strategies for coping with chronic low back pain: relationship to pain and disability. *Pain*, **24**, 355–364.

van der Linden, S., Valkenburg, H.A. and Cats, A. (1984). Evaluation of diagnostic criteria for ankylosing spondylitis. A proposal for modification of the New York criteria. *Arthr. Rheum.*, **27**, 361–368.

Vernon, H. and Mior, S. (1991). The Neck Disability Index: a study of reliability and validity. *J. Manip. Physiol. Ther.*, **14**, 409–415.

Vlaeyen, J., Kole-Snijders, A., Rotteveel, A., Ruesink, R. and Heuts, P. (1995a). The role of fear of movement/(re)injury in pain disability. *J. Occup. Rehabil.*, **5**, 235–252.

Vlaeyen, J., Kole-Snijders, A., Boersen, R. and van Eek, H. (1995b). Fear of movement/(re)injury in chronic low back pain and its relation to behavioural performance. *Pain*, **62**, 363–372.

Waddell, G., McCulloch, J., Kummel, E. and Venner, R. (1980). Nonorganic physical signs in low-back pain. *Spine*, **5**, 117–125.

Waddell, G., Main, C.J., Morris, E.W. et al. (1982). Normality and reliability in the clinical assessment of backache. *Br. Med. J.*, **284**, 1519–1523.

Waddell, G., Pilowsky, I. and Bond, M. (1989). Clinical assessment and interpretation of abnormal illness behaviour in low back pain. *Pain*, **39**, 41–53.

Waddell, G., Newton, M., Somerville, D. and Main, C. (1995). A fear-avoidance beliefs questionnaire (FABQ) and the role of fear avoidance beliefs in chronic low back pain and disability. *Pain*, **52**, 157–168.

Waddell, G., Feder, G., McIntosh, A., Lewis, M. and Hutchison, A. (1996). *Low Back Pain Evidence Review*. London: Royal College of General Practitioners.

Werneke, M., Harris, D. and Lichter, R. (1993). Clinical effectiveness of behavioural signs for screening chronic low back pain patients in a work-oriented physical rehabilitation program. *Spine*, **18**, 2412–2418.

Westaway, M., Stratford, P. and Binkley, J. (1998). The patient-specific functional scale: validation of its use in persons with neck dysfunction. *J. Orthop. Sports Phys. Ther.*, **27**, 331–338.

Wheeler, A., Goolkasian, P., Baird, A. and Darden, B. (1999). Development of the Neck Pain and Disability Scale. Item analysis, face, and criterion-related disability. *Spine*, **24**, 1290–1294.

Whooley, M., Avins, A., Miranda, J. and Browner, W. (1997). Case-finding instruments for depression. Two questions are as good as many. *J. Gen. Intern. Med.*, **12**, 439–445.

Williams, P.R. and Warwick, R. (eds) (1980). *Gray's Anatomy*, 36th edn. London: Churchill Livingstone.

Zusman, M. (1986). The absolute visual analogue scale (AVAS) as a measure of pain intensity. *Aust. J. Physiother.*, **32**, 244–246.

Chapter 6

The physical examination

K.M. Refshauge and J. Latimer

INTRODUCTION

In this chapter several aspects of the physical examination are reviewed, including selection of tests to perform, how to perform common tests, reliability and validity of the tests and how to interpret the test findings. Our legal responsibilities as health professionals are also presented.

As discussed in Chapter 5, the first important decision to make is about diagnosis, i.e. whether the patient's condition is suitable for physiotherapy, or is likely to be specific or serious pathology requiring other intervention. If the condition is likely to respond well to physiotherapy, treatment is selected based on the findings from the physical examination as well as from the history.

To select relevant tests, we need to know the purpose of the test, and of the examination as a whole. In general terms, the purposes of the physical examination are to:

- confirm or reject the diagnoses formed from the history. That is, the physical examination is based on the findings from the history
- identify outcomes to establish goals and for monitoring progress
- select the most appropriate treatment.

Because it is not necessary (and, indeed, probably unwise) to perform all of the possible tests on a patient, only tests that assist with making decisions about diagnosis or management should be performed. Selection of tests is becoming more difficult, because the enormous growth in knowledge over the last few decades has led to new theories about diagnosis and treatment, and new test procedures have been designed to examine many of these new theories. Most such tests are comprehensively described in a wide variety of books (Grieve, 1984; Maitland, 1986; Magee, 1987, Richardson et al., 1999). Only those tests commonly used by physiotherapists to make diagnostic or treatment decisions have been chosen for discussion here. For example, passive accessory motion is described because physiotherapists use information from these tests to predict whether the patient will benefit from treatment by mobilization or manipulation, to determine the specific region to be treated and to select the treatment technique to apply. In contrast, doctors rarely assess passive motion of the spine as this is not useful in forming a medical diagnosis or

selecting medical intervention, such as medication or advice. Thus, testing is generally confined to those procedures relevant to ideas about diagnosis and overall management.

CONSENT

Before any physical testing is performed valid consent should be obtained from the patient. A health professional should not, legally, touch or treat a patient without the patient's valid consent, irrespective of how unwise you think the patient's refusal may be (Giesen, 1988). The ideals behind the obtaining of valid consent are that the decision about whether or not to accept intervention is the patient's decision, not the health professional's, and that every person has the right to decide what is done to his or her own body (Giesen, 1988). In many countries the basic human right of self-determination is constitutionally protected.

Valid consent consists of four parts:

1. Consent must be voluntarily given.
2. The consent should cover the act performed.
3. The person giving the consent must be legally competent to do so. If the patient is unable to give consent, as is the case with children, a relative can give consent on the patient's behalf.
4. The consent must be informed to some degree. This means that the patient should be given enough information to make a considered decision (O'Sullivan, 1983).

It is important that physiotherapists understand their legal responsibilities. Further information about aspects of law that affect health professionals can be found in O'Sullivan (1983), Siegler et al. (1987), Buckley (1988) or Giesen (1988).

DIAGNOSTIC RESPONSIBILITY

The reason for including this section on diagnostic responsibility is that physiotherapists are responsible for recognizing signs and symptoms that indicate concern (often referred to as red or yellow flags). This is becoming an increasingly important part of our practice. Situations where important signs or symptoms were not recognized by the treating practitioner are presented in Table 6.1. All of these patients were treated for at least 2 weeks with various procedures including mobilization,

Table 6.1   Illustrations of misdiagnosis with serious consequences

Physiotherapist's diagnosis and basis for treatment	Treatment given	Actual cause of symptoms and consequences of lack of recognition
Tension headache	Mobilization of upper cervical spine	Severe headache from cervical aneurysm, resulting in stroke
Non-specific mechanical low back pain	Mobilization of lumbar spine	Osteoid osteoma. Appropriate management implemented after progression of disease
Sacroiliac joint dysfunction with 'functional' overlay	Short-wave diathermy, interferential, traction, mobilization, bedrest	Neuroma in spinal canal. Surgical removal
Non-specific neck pain with referral to arm and hand	Mobilization of cervical spine	Osteosarcoma of humerus

Feldenkrais techniques, relaxation, manipulation and injection of local anaesthetic into trapezius muscle. In no case did the treating practitioners recognize cardinal signs of serious pathology that required referral to an appropriate medical practitioner, *not* treatment with manual techniques. Three patients suffered serious consequences from the inappropriate treatment.

As first-contact practitioners, physiotherapists have specific legal and ethical responsibilities. These responsibilities include providing a high standard of care for all patients. To provide a high standard of care physiotherapists need to remain current in their knowledge and skills. This involves awareness of recent research findings, and incorporation of these findings into clinical practice. Physiotherapists must also recognize the limitations both of their own practice, and of treatment options available to them. This means that physiotherapists need to recognize when to send patients for further investigation or management and who will be the most relevant practitioner for referral. Sometimes, the most relevant practitioner might be another physiotherapist with particular expertise.

THE GENERAL TESTING PROTOCOL: LOOK, FEEL AND MOVE

In all fields of physical medicine, diagnoses (either clinical diagnoses based on the patient's signs and symptoms or pathological diagnoses) and appropriate treatment are identified by the overall protocol of look, feel and move. This is particularly apt for the practice of physiotherapy, since we rarely use invasive procedures. For all patients, therefore, at least some aspects of observation, palpation and movement testing will be performed.

This overall protocol appears to be effective and efficient. Additional procedures can be used to test for specific pathologies or dysfunction. However, the salient features of many musculoskeletal disorders and resultant functional deficits can be identified using the above protocol, resulting in accurate diagnosis and selection of appropriate management regimens.

The physical examination is therefore primarily aimed at confirming diagnoses suggested by the history and identifying the most appropriate treatment regimens. Some further information may also be gained about prognosis and factors contributing to the condition. Musculoskeletal conditions of the spine presenting to physiotherapists are often of non-specific pathology. In these cases, the clinical diagnosis is of great importance. Once the general functional deficit is established (e.g. inability to put on shoes and socks, walk or climb stairs) specific aspects of function are tested. If there are red flags present, further investigations will be required to confirm the specific pathology.

PRINCIPLES OF THE PHYSICAL EXAMINATION

The physical examination includes the following routine tests:

- observation
- active movements with more stressful procedures applied when applicable
- palpation.

In addition, when relevant, the following tests are also performed to determine function of specific structures:

- passive motion testing of vertebral segments
- tension in neuromeningeal structures
- neural conduction
- vertebrobasilar sufficiency
- extensibility and strength of muscles
- muscle performance.

Further tests can be performed, including various aspects of function or movement control, such as proprioception (for review see McCloskey, 1978), coordinated muscle activity and muscle activation levels.

Results of all tests performed are correlated with information previously gathered in the history and with results of preceding physical tests. The physiotherapist is looking for consistent patterns of signs and symptoms (Barrows and Feltovich, 1987). If signs and symptoms are inconsistent, it is important to re-evaluate the data.

The physical examination is performed systematically. This is because routines optimize efficiency; however, routines should not be performed thoughtlessly. If the purpose of each test is clearly understood, the results can be interpreted in light of results of other tests and ideas about diagnosis and treatment. By understanding this process, only appropriate information will be collected.

SAFETY AND COMFORT OF PATIENTS

During testing all reasonable care must be taken to ensure the comfort and safety of the patient. Comfort can be maximized by carrying out relevant tests in one position before moving on to the next position. This means, for example, that all relevant tests are performed in standing (or walking, etc.) before tests in sitting, and then tests in supine, side-lying and finally prone. This also optimizes efficiency. In each position, active movements are usually tested before passive movements, because this allows the patient to control the movement if there is any pain. When testing passive movements, the physiotherapist can then take into account the range of movement available and the amount of pain experienced by the patient during the movement. For example, active rotation of the lumbar spine would be tested before

either passive rotation movements or rotation positioning of the lumbar spine.

The order of application of test procedures is important for some tests but not for others. Those tests with implications for further testing (such as the neurological examination) are usually performed early in the examination. Also, general tests are usually performed before specific tests so that, for example, active cervical spine rotation would be assessed prior to rotation at individual intervertebral segments.

The vigour of the physical examination is determined by the irritability of the condition (how easily symptoms are provoked and the severity and persistence of symptoms). If an examination is too gentle, the presenting problem may not be identified, as anatomical structures may not have been sufficiently stressed. On the other hand, an examination that is too vigorous may exacerbate the presenting symptoms to an extent where no more testing is possible, and insufficient information has been gained. If the condition is irritable, then the physiotherapist should modify the physical examination in some way, to prevent exacerbating the symptoms needlessly. Usually the number of tests performed under these circumstances is limited, so the most useful tests must be identified, that is, those tests that give important information about the pathological or clinical diagnosis and about treatment.

In patients with irritable conditions it is still usually possible to perform most tests, including observation, all active movements (to initial onset or increase of pain), neurological tests (sensation and reflexes, and generally muscle power), tension tests, gentle palpation and passive motion tests (again, performed gently, to first onset or increase in pain). Specific structures, such as muscles, would be tested when the information is crucial to management decisions. If, however, management would not change with the results of a relevant test procedure, the physiotherapist may decide to perform these tests on subsequent treatment occasions when pain has settled.

MEASUREMENT

By performing various tests in the physical examination, physiotherapists are actually conducting a series of measurements on the patient (see Ch. 4). All test procedures included in the physical examination should therefore be performed in a reproducible (standardized) manner, with appropriate adaptations for the individual patient. Since the results of our physical tests provide the basis for many diagnostic and management decisions, and are used as outcome measures to monitor progress, we must be confident about the results. You will notice therefore, in the physical examination tests, that information about the reliability and validity of these tests is provided to help you determine how useful the test results are likely to be.

The variables that are measured depend on the test performed, but may include function, range of movement, pain response, muscle strength and sensory loss. Some factors may be difficult to measure such as abnormalities found on observation or small changes perceived on passive motion testing, while other factors, such as range of movement or muscle strength, may be easier to measure accurately. Rarely do we formally measure the outcome of all tests performed. In general the variables that should be accurately measured during the physical examination are:

1. Those related to the patient's main concern. For example, if a patient is attending physiotherapy because cervical spine pain and stiffness have reduced the patient's ability to rotate when reversing the car, cervical rotation should be measured, and reversing the car, using the Patient Specific Functional Scale.

2. The variables that should change with intervention. For example, if passive mobilizations are applied to the talocrural joint to increase range of motion and decrease swelling after ankle sprain, then dorsiflexion range and swelling should be measured.

Thus, appropriate variables should be measured, and they should be measured in a reliable and, where possible, valid way. See Maher et al. (2001) for a comprehensive and detailed description and analysis of measurement techniques for the lumbar spine and throughout this chapter. Such care in measurement ensures that the measurement obtained is useful, with minimal error (see Ch. 4). Measurement of specific test results is further addressed by the various authors who have contributed sections to this chapter.

The remainder of this chapter outlines the test procedures used most frequently in the physical examination, describing the background to the tests, many of the test procedures themselves, the indications for testing, the interpretation of test results and the implications for treatment. Further reading for each section is located at the end of the chapter.

Observation

M. Goodsell and K.M. Refshauge

Using the protocol of look, feel and move (and further investigate when necessary), the first procedure in the physical examination is to observe the patient. Physiotherapists informally and formally observe patients and the affected parts of the body before touching or moving them.

The *purpose* of observing the patient is to gain general information about functional deficits and about other abnormalities, such as posture, that might be manifestations of the presenting disorder. It is often suggested that size or shape of spinal curvature in each region of the spine may contribute to the patient's presenting problem. The validity of associating spinal alignment with the presence of symptoms is generally poor. The size of those spinal curves that have been investigated is not related to the onset or presence of pain (Dieck et al., 1985; Refshauge et al., 1995; Levangie, 1999), even in pregnancy (Bullock et al., 1987; Franklin and Conner-Kerr, 1998), except in the cervical spine where a more forward head position has been associated with the presence of headache (Griegel-Morris et al., 1992; Watson and Trott, 1993).

Observation of posture in the clinic raises other questions, such as whether patients adopt their habitual sitting or standing posture while being formally observed by the physiotherapist, and also whether habitual standing or sitting posture reflects positions actually adopted during work or leisure activities. Therefore, it is important to correlate the information gained from formal observation with the information gained informally when the patient was first greeted, was questioned during the history and during any functional testing.

Although physiotherapists systematically observe patients as part of the physical examination, we have already informally noted the patient's demeanour, the ease of movement and the body part apparently affected by the time the patient enters the examination cubicle. When taking the history, we also note any positions of discomfort, for example, whether patients prefer to sit or stand, whether they hold their arm against their body, or whether they keep one leg extended while sitting. The difficulty experienced during undressing gives us some information about the functional deficit as well as the movements that may provoke symptoms.

It is essential to explain to the patient the reason for undressing, i.e. to expose the region for examination, as many people feel uncomfortable when scantily clad, particularly in the presence of a stranger, and with the possibility of other people entering the examination cubicle. Therefore, we must offer patients a gown and the presence of a chaperone if desired. The physical examination then commences with a formal observation of the patient and the affected part.

TEST PROCEDURE

Formal observation of the patient includes gaining a general impression of the overall posture of the patient and checking for any specific asymmetries or abnormalities. Following this general check, it is usual to inspect the part more closely.

General postural overview

The patient is observed in standing (lumbar and thoracic spines) or in sitting (cervical spine) with the relevant region exposed. This means wearing underwear with no footwear for lumbar and thoracic spines, but the lower body can remain clothed for cervical and upper thoracic spines.

For all regions of the spine, the physiotherapist notes:

- muscle wasting (e.g. gastrocnemius, quadriceps, supraspinatus)
- swelling
- scars

- skin changes
- bony alignment (e.g. spondylolisthesis may be evident by an anterior displacement at the level of the affected vertebra)
- asymmetry (e.g. unequal skin creases at the waist)
- positional deformities (e.g. winged scapula).

For lumbar and thoracic spine the physiotherapist also notes:

- leg-length discrepancies
- size of spinal curvature (thoracic kyphosis and lumbar lordosis)
- scoliosis (rotational deformity)
- sciatic scoliosis/list (antalgic position of lateral flexion without compensatory rotation: a reversible lateral flexion posture).

For the cervical and upper thoracic spines, with the patient seated, the physiotherapist notes:

- size of cervical lordosis
- size of kyphosis at cervicothoracic junction
- lateral flexion or rotation deformities (e.g. wry neck)
- shoulder height discrepancies.

PROCEDURE

To gain this information efficiently, the physiotherapist usually observes posterior, anterior and lateral views of the patient. From the posterior aspect observation consists of:

- spinal alignment
- shoulder height
- scapular position
- level of posterior superior iliac spines (indicating level of pelvis)
- height of iliac crests (level and rotation, indicating position of pelvis)
- equality of gluteal folds
- height of knee creases
- calcaneal angle (equal, and not excessively pronated or supinated)
- muscle bulk (e.g. gluteus maximus, gastrocnemius).

From the lateral aspect observation consists of:

- head position (poke neck/forward head position)

- thoracic kyphosis (size and length. Long thoracic curvature may indicate Scheuermann's disease)
- rotation of ribcage (associated with scoliosis)
- lumbar lordosis
- genu recurvatum.

From the anterior aspect observation consists of:

- head position (wry neck, asymmetry in rotation or lateral flexion)
- shoulder height
- waist curves (increased asymmetry in structural and postural scoliosis)
- height of anterior superior iliac spines (indicating level of pelvis)
- patellar height and position
- forefoot position.

Relevant abnormalities or asymmetries should be measured if the physiotherapist intends to alter them. Some features are difficult to measure, e.g. skin changes or muscle wasting. Other features are easier to measure, such as true leg length, which can be measured using a tape measure from the anterior superior iliac spine to the medial malleolus (see Grieve (1986) or Magee (1987) for further information). Magnitude of spinal curves is also easily measured using a flexible ruler or photography, both of which have a demonstrated high reliability (Hart and Rose, 1986; Refshauge et al., 1994a). Other features are possible, although difficult, to measure, such as patellar position or calcaneal tilt, and results must therefore be interpreted cautiously.

INTERPRETATION OF INFORMATION

Information about abnormalities and asymmetries is used for decisions about pathology, factors contributing to the presenting problem, selection of further assessment procedures and treatment selection. Some examples of abnormalities that might indicate pathology in the affected area include:

- Scars: indicate either past trauma or surgery, both of which must be investigated for relevant past history (such as laminectomy, fusion) and for mobility of scar tissue during palpation.

- Skin colour: indicates state of the circulation (whether blood supply is adequate, such as in heart conditions or in thoracic outlet syndrome).

A blueish tinge suggests anoxia, and redness indicates inflammation or infection. Skin colour may also indicate the state of the patient's general health, sympathetic changes, bruising and the presence of other diseases.

- Substantial muscle wasting may indicate partial denervation at any point along the course of a nerve prior to entry to the muscle. With musculoskeletal conditions of the spine, the nerve compromise may be at the level of the nerve root or spinal nerve (see The neurological examination, later in this chapter).

- Winging of the scapula generally indicates reduced conduction in the long thoracic nerve. Serratus anterior, the affected muscle, is deep and therefore wasting will probably not be evident.

- A 'step' in the low lumbar spine may indicate spondylolisthesis, where the affected vertebra has slipped forward, taking with it the attached superior vertebra, giving the appearance of a step.

Asymmetries of posture may be directly related to the onset of symptoms. Such asymmetrical postures may be adopted as positions of pain relief, as in the case of an acute wry neck deformity in the cervical region, or a reduced lumbar lordosis or sciatic scoliosis in the lumbar region. In some cases such positions may suggest particular pathology, for example, sciatic scoliosis is thought to be associated with intervertebral disc pathology (McKenzie, 1981), although this clinical association has not been substantiated and pain-producing intervertebral disc pathology is probably difficult to differentiate from other sources of pain (Twomey, 1992). It seems that other postural features, for example size of spinal curvature, are observed because it is known that maintaining awkward or end-of-range positions for long periods causes pain (Harms-Ringdahl and Ekholm, 1986; Braun and Amundson, 1989). Extremes of spinal curvature are sometimes likened to end-of-range positions. Since tissues adapt to applied stress, it is speculated that adaptations such as muscle shortening occur in response to stresses applied in postures maintained for prolonged periods, such as an increased lumbar lordosis. It is possible that altered range of movement, coinciding with postural abnormalities, may alter function or movement patterns, resulting in increased stress in the tissues. The tissues may be unable to sustain the magnitude or type of this resultant stress. These hypotheses are tentative, however, because there is little evidence to support them.

Postural asymmetries are not clearly indicative of disorders. The size of lumbar lordosis has been shown not to be predictive of onset of pain or related to presence of pain (Dieck et al., 1985; Levangie, 1999), even in pregnancy, despite significant postural changes (Bullock et al., 1987; Franklin and Conner-Kerr, 1998). The thoracic spine has not been investigated except in pregnancy. The cervical spine has been the subject of few studies, but preliminary work suggests that cervical spine posture may not be related to pain in the cervical spine or trapezius region (Refshauge et al., 1995). On the other hand, people with frequent headaches have been shown to have a more forward head position than people with infrequent or no incidence of headache (Watson and Trott, 1993). There is also a wide range of normal postural variation, and asymmetries are common (During et al., 1985; Raine and Twomey, 1994). Therefore the physiotherapist must decide whether observed asymmetries or other abnormalities are related to the patient's presenting symptoms. This cannot always be clearly established, but as a general rule, if the symptoms improve when the patient's posture is altered, then the asymmetry or alignment can be considered to be one of the factors related to the patient's symptoms. For example, using a lumbar roll to alter sitting posture by increasing the lumbar lordosis in sitting has been shown to reduce some patients' symptoms (Williams et al., 1991). In this case some characteristic of the lordosis in sitting can be assumed to be associated with back and leg symptoms. However, it is not possible to demonstrate such an association when the patient has no symptoms at rest or when the symptoms are not easily provoked. In these circumstances the physiotherapist might choose to intervene to change posture and to evaluate the effect of intervention on symptoms over a period of time.

Other features of alignment of body segments such as that caused by inequality of leg length or magnitude of foot pronation have been raised as possible contributors to spinal pain. The association between mild leg-length inequality and pain is unclear, although it seems that a small discrepancy (up to 20 mm) is not associated with spinal pain (Pope et al., 1985; Soukka et al., 1991). This does not mean that unequal leg length is never related to spinal pain, but a relationship should be established in individual patients before intervening. A relationship can be explored by inserting a temporary orthotic into the patient's shoe, and noting any change in symptoms during functional activities, e.g. walking or running. If the pain decreases after equalizing leg length, it can be assumed that the symptoms were related to the inequality. The relevance of foot pronation to spinal or leg pain is also unclear. Although often described (McConnell, 1986), such a relationship has never been demonstrated when the magnitude of pronation is compared between symptomatic and asymptomatic states (see data in Gerrard, 1989).

Information about posture is still evolving. At present perceived postural abnormalities are difficult to interpret since normative data are not extensive, some postural characteristics may change with age (Milne and Lauder, 1974), although other characteristics may not alter with increasing age (Griegel-Morris et al., 1992). There is a wide variation in normal (i.e. asymptomatic) postures, slight asymmetries are common (e.g. few people appear to have equal shoulder height), and, as yet, 'ideal' posture has not been determined, nor established as desirable. In addition, surface contours do not appear to mirror bony vertebral alignment (Refshauge et al., 1994b) and therefore conclusions about magnitude of spinal curvature cannot easily be drawn from observation of surface contours. Thus the presence of any postural abnormalities must be interpreted with caution, and cannot be viewed in isolation. Rather, the information should be compared with the total clinical picture of signs and symptoms.

IMPLICATIONS FOR THE PHYSICAL EXAMINATION AND TREATMENT

Few postural asymmetries or abnormalities are definitively associated with spinal pain. Nevertheless they may form part of a recognizable pattern of signs and symptoms, indicating specific pathology.

Specific abnormalities, such as scars, signs of decreased nerve conduction (muscle wasting) or skin changes are usually further tested in the physical examination. Signs of reduced nerve conduction indicate that a neurological examination is required, scars should be palpated and signs of circulatory disturbance (skin changes) tested by feeling strength of pulses and, when indicated, performing tests for thoracic outlet syndrome (Magee, 1992).

Observed asymmetries or abnormalities in postural alignment might be further explored to determine whether they are associated with symptoms. This association may be investigated by facilitating a more 'ideal' alignment (e.g. correcting a sciatic scoliosis, facilitating chin retraction or altering pelvic tilt) and noting the effect on symptoms. For example, if chin retraction increases symptoms in a patient who has marked chin protraction, this suggests that the posture is antalgic, whereas if chin retraction decreases symptoms, this suggests that intervention to alter the position of chin protraction may be of benefit. A relationship between the patient's symptoms and any abnormal features should thus be established before intervening to change these features. When the physiotherapist chooses to intervene to change posture it is important to measure changes in the variable of interest, for example either pain or postural alignment. There has been surprisingly little investigation of the effect of intervention designed to alter posture either in terms of symptom relief or in changing the relevant postural characteristics. The few studies available suggest that the use of a lumbar support changed the intensity and area of back and leg pain (Williams et al., 1991), but that exercises may not alter forward position of the head on the neck (Feldman et al., 1994) in a healthy population.

Observation is useful for gaining an overall impression of the patient's alignment and general posture, as well as gaining some specific information about abnormalities that may be related to the presenting disorder. This information should be evaluated carefully, interpreted with caution and followed up with other tests during the physical examination.

Active movement testing

K.M. Refshauge

The purpose of active movement testing is to reproduce the patient's pain and/or measure range of movement limitation, to gain general information to formulate the clinical diagnosis and treatment. In addition, the patient's response to active movements can be used to verify whether or not the patient has a mechanical problem. During active movement testing, the physiotherapist determines the movements most affected, in what way these movements are affected, the effect of pain on movement and the range of movement available. From this information, baseline measures are made for reassessment so that it can be clearly established whether the patient's movement impairment has improved following treatment.

It is sometimes suggested that the results of active movement testing may indicate the anatomical structures involved in the disorder because those structures stressed during a specific movement may be responsible for symptoms reproduced during that movement. This seems possible in principle, based on a mechanical model of reasoning, but is probably more useful in the periphery than in the spine. The fact that the tissues involved in non-specific mechanical spinal pain have not been identified cautions against placing too much weight on such hypotheses, whereas in the periphery specific tissues may be more readily identified as injured. For example, a torn anterior talofibular ligament will usually cause pain when stressed in plantarflexion and inversion. Finally, the results of active movement testing also aid in treatment selection. For example, the most affected movement(s) may be used to increase the treatment dose for non-irritable conditions and the direction of movement that eases symptoms may be used for irritable conditions.

PROCEDURES FOR TESTING ACTIVE MOVEMENTS

This section is directed towards active movement testing in the spine, but the principles apply equally well to the periphery. Active movements are generally tested following the formal observation of the patient. All physiological movements (flexion, extension, lateral flexion and rotation) are examined systematically. The testing procedure for each movement should be standardized to enable accurate reassessment following treatment and prior to the next treatment session.

ORDER OF TESTING

Although all movement directions are usually assessed, on rare occasions for irritable conditions it may not be possible to test all movements. In such cases, it is important to examine the movement direction that appears to be related to the greatest functional deficit. This movement is usually, but not necessarily, the most symptomatic movement. This movement may also involve combinations of single-plane movements. The most affected movement direction(s) will have been established in the history when discussing activities that provoke symptoms.

A routine sequence of active movement testing is normally followed; however, the normal sequence may be altered when there is doubt about the patient's ability to complete testing because of an irritable condition. A patient may complain of difficulty in removing shoes and socks because of severe lumbar pain, for example. This may indicate that flexion is the main problem and therefore flexion should be among the first movements examined. More commonly, however, the therapist conducts a standard assessment sequence (often this sequence consists of flexion followed by extension, side flexion to each side and rotation to each side) but the patient's symptoms are closely monitored to identify immediately any exacerbation. In the case of patients with non-irritable conditions, the patient should be able to perform a comprehensive assessment of active movements without requiring a change in the normal sequence of testing.

INSTRUCTIONS

Clear and appropriate explanations to the patient are essential in achieving adequate testing of active movements. First, the patient is questioned about pain at rest. If pain is present before testing proceeds, the intensity should be noted and carefully monitored throughout the examination. Further instructions should reflect the irritability of the condition. If the condition is not easily exacerbated (is not irritable), the patient is asked to move as far as possible through range of movement. The physiotherapist then identifies the limit of movement in terms of both what prevents further movement (e.g. pain, stiffness), and the range of movement available. If the symptoms seem to be easily provoked, the patient is instructed only to move until the initial onset of pain, or in patients with resting pain, until the first increase in the resting pain occurs.

EVALUATION OF ACTIVE MOVEMENTS

Overall range of movement, or range to the first onset of pain in the case of irritable conditions, is measured. The intensity of pain provoked when performing the most symptomatic movement(s) is rated, e.g. on a visual analogue scale, as this may be the impairment that the physiotherapist aims to change. The shape of the spinal curves during movement is also observed because this may give information about areas of the spine where movement is either decreased or increased, although the reliability and validity of such observations are likely to be poor. Symmetry of movement is noted in unilateral movements where comparisons with

the contralateral side are possible, and the quality of the movement may give information about ease of movement and antalgic deviations. Information about range, pain, spinal curves and asymmetry is further investigated during the physical examination using, for example, passive motion testing.

Active movement testing of the cervical and upper thoracic spine

Active movements are examined with the patient seated on a stool or on the end of a treatment plinth (Figs 6.A5–6.A7). Chairs with backs are generally avoided since the back support may encourage slumping. It is also useful for the therapist to observe the natural sitting posture of a patient, to implicate posture in the patient's presentation (McKenzie, 1981). Nevertheless, the lumbar lordosis should be maintained during active movement testing to standardize the start position because the posture of the lumbar and thoracic spines may affect the range of cervical movement observed. Thus the starting (or neutral) position should be with the patient looking ahead, and sitting comfortably upright with the lumbar lordosis maintained. Unilateral movements, e.g. side flexion and rotation, are compared with movement to the contralateral side.

Active movement testing of the mid and low thoracic spine

Active movements of the thoracic spine can be assessed either in sitting or in standing, although the lumbar spine moves with the thoracic spine in these positions. In sitting, however, thoracic spine rather than lumbar spine movement seems to be better emphasized. In sitting, the habitual lumbar lordosis should be maintained to prevent a starting position of thoracic and lumbar spine flexion. Patients cross their arms across the chest, to standardize the starting position and to enable the spine to be moved as a unit, thereby minimizing uncontrolled movement of the shoulders and scapulae. Flexion, extension, lateral flexion and rotation can all be examined using this standardized starting position.

Alternatively, differentiation between low cervical and upper thoracic spinal regions may be required. Movement can be emphasized at the thoracic spine while limiting movement at the cervical spine by placing the hands behind the neck with the elbows together at the front. Movements into flexion and extension and side flexion will occur at the thoracic spine with little occurring at the cervical spine.

Active movement testing of the lumbar spine

Active movements of the lumbar spine are examined with the patient standing, with the possible exception of rotation. The region to be examined should be clearly exposed, to enable viewing movement of the intervertebral segments. The patient should not be wearing shoes because high heels or uneven wear of the heels or soles may alter the starting position of the spine and may not be comparable on repeat visits. In addition, shoes add variability to any tape measurements of finger to floor distance. For flexion, extension and lateral flexion patients slide their hands down their legs. Rotation is often examined in sitting to enhance stability and, as for the thoracic spine, it is convenient for patients to cross their arms across the chest. The starting position should again be standardized, and unilateral movements compared with movement to the contralateral side.

As well as observing active movements, the physiotherapist may observe activities described by the patient in the history as provoking symptoms. For this reason, a physiotherapist may well examine thoracic movements in standing, or all lumbar movements in sitting, to improve the likelihood of reproducing symptoms. Examples of activities that commonly aggravate symptoms and that can easily be assessed and measured in the clinical context include walking, stair climbing, rising from sitting or putting on shoes. All these activities can be adequately measured (see section on Motor performance: evaluation and measurement, later in this chapter).

MEASUREMENT

The most affected movement(s) should be measured carefully. There are many methods that are simple to use, are widely available and provide reliable measurements. These measurement methods include tape measure for flexion, extension and lateral flexion of all spinal regions (Hsieh and Yeung, 1986; Beattie et al., 1987; Perret et al., 2001) and, for cervical spine rotation, the spondylometer for flexion and extension in the lumbar spine (Twomey and Taylor, 1979) and the cervical range of motion (CROM) measuring device for cervical spine movements (Youdas et al., 1991; Garrett et al., 1993). These measurement methods have a demonstrated high reliability, although only the spondylometer and the attraction–distraction use of the tape measure in the lumbar spine are likely to make valid measurements of spinal motion. Rotation is difficult to measure in the lumbar spine, so the therapist should watch this but measure another affected movement with a reliable method. However, increase in overall range of movement (e.g. reaching the feet to put on trousers) is a more likely aim of treatment than increase in lumbar spine motion in isolation. Therefore, measuring overall movement such as fingertips to floor for lumbar spine flexion probably adequately reflects the aim of treatment. These measurement methods are illustrated in Figures 6.A1–6.A4 for the lumbar spine, and Figures 6.A5–6.A7 for the cervical spine in the Appendix at the end of this chapter, with an accompanying evaluation.

APPLYING FURTHER STRESS TO ACTIVE MOVEMENTS

If symptoms have not been provoked by active movement testing, or have not been provoked to the desired extent or full symptom distribution (in the case of non-irritable conditions only) further stress may be applied to the movements. The purposes of further stressing active movements are to determine whether the movement is completely asymptomatic, to plan treatment if the movement is not symptom-free, and to monitor progress.

Overpressure is the most common procedure, and is performed by applying gentle pressure at the end of range. The aim of applying overpressure is to observe the effect on symptoms of further stressing the movement at end of range. If no symptoms are reproduced on overpressure it is generally considered that the movement is symptom-free and 'normal' (Maitland, 1986).

Combined movements are also commonly used to further stress active movements that are slightly symptomatic or have been reported as symptomatic in the history (Edwards, 1987). Although the concept of combining physiological movements in examination and treatment arose from knowledge of coupled movements (Edwards, 1987), combined movements do not necessarily replicate coupled movements (see Ch. 2 for further discussion).

When combining active movements, the most affected movement is usually performed first, and then the next most symptomatic movement is superimposed. If, for example, the patient complained of cervical spine pain when throwing the ball in the air in preparation for a tennis serve, and only slight pain was reproduced on cervical spine extension during active movement testing, the physiotherapist might decide to further stress extension by superimposing movements in other planes (rotation or lateral flexion). It would be usual to ask the patient to extend the cervical spine, and then while maintaining extension at the point of symptom onset to add rotation to the cervical spine. If this were painfree, lateral flexion instead of rotation might be added to the extension. A detailed description of combined movements appears in other musculoskeletal textbooks and therefore will not be discussed here (Grieve, 1984; Maitland, 1986; Edwards, 1987, 1988).

Repeated movements, i.e. performing several movements in quick succession in the same direction, may also be tested. This is particularly relevant when repetitive activity has been reported as symptomatic, or when the physiotherapist anticipates that repeated active movements may be used as a treatment strategy. It has been suggested that repeated movements may decrease pain in some spinal conditions, increase pain in some and have no effect in others. McKenzie (1981) describes this approach in detail.

Sustained movements or positions may be assessed if they are reported as provocative during the history. For example, lumbar spine flexion may be sustained if sitting is painful, or cervical spine flexion sustained if reading, writing and watching television are provocative activities. It is more efficient (less time-consuming) to reassess dynamic activities, so movements are generally sustained only in the absence of provocative dynamic activities.

IMPLICATIONS FOR TREATMENT

Information from active movement testing is used in several ways, but mainly for treatment decisions and as baseline measurements for reassessment, and occasionally for diagnostic information. The ease of symptom provocation, the severity of symptoms provoked and the movement restriction manifested are all determined from active movement testing. The results of active movement testing (which movement is affected, how it is affected and the extent to which it is affected) assists in determining the treatment technique and the vigour or dose of treatment.

Ease of symptom provocation is elicited from the history. This information is then compared with the patient's ability to move during movement testing. Usually severe pain results in marked movement restriction, whereas mild pain results in minor movement restriction. Therefore, if a patient has very severe pain, but active movements are largely unaffected, suspicion would be aroused about the nature of the disorder, because the condition could be due to more serious pathology.

Positions or movements to avoid and positions of comfort may also be identified for patients with irritable conditions that are mechanical. If a condition is irritable, the first goal of treatment is pain relief. It is therefore important to identify those movements that exacerbate symptoms, and any movements or positions that may relieve symptoms. If there are any movements or positions that relieve symptoms, these may be used as a treatment, or may be used to position the patient during application of an alternative treatment strategy.

For non-irritable conditions, however, the most provocative direction of movement is often used for treatment or for positioning during treatment to increase the force or intensity of the treatment dose. Results of further testing, such as passive motion testing, and tension tests are also compared with the results of the active movement tests to identify and monitor consistency of patterns of signs and symptoms.

TESTING ACTIVE MOVEMENTS IN OTHER JOINTS THAT POTENTIALLY CONTRIBUTE TO THE SYMPTOMS

Patients often present with pain radiating over several joints and other somatic structures. All potentially injured structures are tested during the physical examination. This includes structures located under the pain distribution, or that could refer pain in the presenting distribution. It is mostly not possible or efficient to examine thoroughly all regions in a single visit, so screening tests are used to determine the potential contribution of anatomical structure(s) or regions to the patient's presenting problem. If a screening procedure reproduces the patient's symptoms, then that structure(s) or region must be examined more specifically and thoroughly. If no symptoms are reproduced, then the structure or region is generally excluded from further consideration, depending on the value of the tests (see Ch. 4).

Joints potentially referring pain or lying beneath the pain pattern are generally tested using active movements, with further stress applied as necessary (such as overpressure) to exclude the contribution of that joint to the pain pattern. In all cases, the patient is asked to move the joint through its full active range, and if the movement is symptom-free, overpressure is applied.

It is important to test these joints in such a way that only the joint of interest is maximally stressed, and not other structures that potentially contribute to the symptoms, because these tests should differentiate one source of pain from another. For example, if pain potentially originating in the lumbar spine crosses the sacroiliac joint (SIJ) and hip joint and the history suggests that the hip or SIJ is a possible source of the symptoms, then the lumbar spine, hip and SIJ must all be tested. If pain is reproduced during a test procedure, but all three regions have been equally stressed, a judgement cannot be made about the most likely source of symptoms, and where to direct further examination and treatment.

Test procedures

To determine whether joints underlying the pain pattern are contributing to the symptoms, the following tests are performed. When relevant, e.g. in the periphery, the tests are compared with the non-affected side. Occasionally, it might be necessary to test the joint in a more stressful position to provoke symptoms.

Sacroiliac joint

Since there are no active movements specific to the SIJ, the SIJ is tested by palpation and passive motion testing. The initial screening procedure is to distract and compress the joint by pushing the iliac crests apart (compression of SIJ) and pushing them together (distraction of SIJ) in the frontal plane with the patient in supine. The value of these tests is discussed in the section on Passive motion tests, later in this chapter.

Hip

The hip is positioned in flexion (approximately 90° if this range is available with the knee flexed) and internal and external rotation are tested. This test stresses the hip joint more than the lumbar spine or SIJ. Hip flexion with adduction can also be tested, if required, remembering that the SIJ may also be stressed with this test.

Shoulder

The shoulder is commonly involved in cervical spine disorders. The shoulder movements of flexion and abduction are tested with overpressure, and more planes of movement are tested if required. Quadrant is not usually performed as the initial test procedure. If it is necessary to examine the joint further, then quadrant (described in Maitland, 1986) or any other procedures may be appropriate.

Ankle

Usually, dorsiflexion and plantarflexion with overpressure are tested in the ankle. Dorsiflexion should be tested with knee flexion, otherwise the test is only an assessment of calf muscle length.

Knee, elbow and wrist

These joints are all tested initially using flexion and extension with overpressure. Additional movements may be tested, e.g. in the elbow and forearm supination/pronation, and in the wrist ulnar and radial deviation.

These tests are preliminary examination tests to determine if the articular complex is contributing to symptoms. If these tests reproduce symptoms further examination should be directed at these structures.

Testing adequacy of cerebral blood flow (vertebrobasilar insufficiency)

K.M. Refshauge and R. Boland

All patients who present with cervical spine disorders are routinely questioned in the history about whether they suffer from dizziness, because dizziness can be an early symptom of inadequate cerebral blood flow (see Ch. 5). It is particularly important for physiotherapists to establish the cause of the dizziness because a few physiotherapy techniques also compromise blood flow (e.g. end-of-range rotation) or carry risk of serious complications (e.g. neck manipulation). However, dizziness is a non-specific symptom that is extremely common, affecting ~30% of older persons, and has a wide variety of causes (Tinetti et al., 2000; Sloane et al., 2001).

Dizziness has been classified into four major subtypes to assist with differential diagnosis. These subtypes include vertigo, presyncope, disequilibrium and other dizziness types (Sloane et al., 2001). Vertigo is a sensation of the outer world revolving about the patient or the patient moving in space (typically spinning). Vertigo is a symptom of vestibular disorders (Simon et al., 1998). Presyncope is a sensation of lightheadedness and is often described as an impending faint. Presyncope is episodic and usually results from diffuse temporary cerebral ischaemia (Sloane et al., 2001). Disequilibrium is a sense of imbalance arising from the legs and trunk but does not involve sensations in the head. If experienced in isolation, these symptoms of disequilibrium are generally attributed to neuromuscular problems. Other types of dizziness are typically described with some vagueness because the patient may have difficulty describing the sensation. Such dizziness is most often caused by psychological disturbances, and is often accompanied by other somatic symptoms, such as headache and abdominal pain (Drachman, 1998).

Dizziness is, therefore, a symptom of many common clinical presentations including disturbances of the vestibular system, postural hypotension, Ménière's disease and cervical vertigo. Of particular concern to physiotherapists is dizziness caused by vertebrobasilar insufficiency (VBI), because there is the potential for causing critical occlusion of cerebral blood flow when using some common therapeutic procedures for the cervical spine. Such procedures include combining extension with rotation and manipulation of the cervical spine, both of which can cause critical occlusion, with serious consequences, such as hemiplegia, 'locked-in' syndrome or, in extreme cases, death (Schellhas et al., 1980; Horn, 1983; Patijn, 1991). When examining the cervical spine, therefore, the presence of VBI must be identified as it will contraindicate certain examination and treatment procedures (e.g. cervical spine quadrant, manipulation) and will indicate caution when applying others (e.g. end-of-range rotation manoeuvres, traction, and probably passive treatments in rotation and/or extension of the cervical spine). Differential diagnosis must be attempted through careful questioning and physical testing. Nevertheless, when dizziness is the only presenting symptom it may be impossible to make a definitive diagnosis (Lord, 1986; Grant, 1988).

VERTEBROBASILAR INSUFFICIENCY

The vertebrobasilar system provides approximately 20% of intracranial blood supply, the carotid system providing the remainder (Lord, 1986; Zwiebel, 1986). The cranial structures supplied by the vertebrobasilar system include the occipital cortex, the brainstem from the midbrain to the upper spinal cord and the cerebellar hemispheres. This territory includes numerous motor and sensory tracts, the reticular formation, cranial nerves III–XII and their nuclei, including vestibular nuclei (Fisher et al., 1961; Lord, 1986). VBI occurs when either focal or overall blood volume is reduced to a level causing ischaemia (generally thought to require reduction by approximately 50%: Stopford, 1916; Hardesty et al., 1963; Lord, 1986). Symptoms are caused by ischaemia in the structures supplied by the vertebrobasilar system (Thiel, 1991). Thus, a great variety of symptoms are possible. Dizziness is the most common (in

45% of patients with transient ischaemic attacks of the vertebrobasilar system), and usually the first symptom (Fisher et al., 1961; Fujita et al., 1995), and ataxia is the second most common symptom (Lord, 1986). Ataxia alone may be difficult to differentiate from disequilibrium or dizziness induced by vertigo or muscular weakness on the basis of the history. Other symptoms of VBI include diplopia (double vision), paralysis of gaze towards the side of the lesion, dysphagia, dysarthria, impaired trigeminal sensation (snout paraesthesia/anaesthesia) and drop attacks (in which the patient suddenly falls to the ground and may remain conscious). Drop attack is thought to be strongly indicative of VBI, but the ischaemic lesion responsible has not been clearly identified. However, evidence from autopsy examination suggests that drop attacks result from ischaemia of corticospinal tracts in the pons and medulla (Lord, 1986).

The vertebral arteries (VAs) are of concern to physiotherapists because their intimate relationship with the cervical spine as they pass through the formina intertransversarii makes them vulnerable to injury during certain therapeutic procedures such as sustained rotation or manipulation (Fig. 6.1; Williams and Warwick, 1980; Lord, 1986). Blood flow through the VAs is normally reduced during cervical spine extension and/or rotation

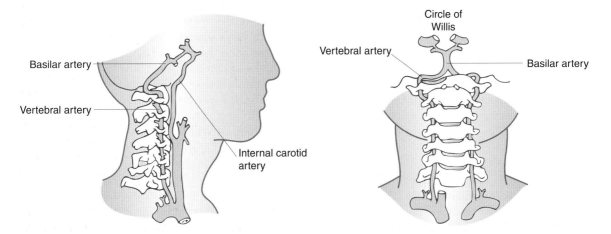

Figure 6.1   Intracranial arteries; (a) lateral view and (b) anteroposterior view. The four parts of the vertebral arteries are shown, including the entry of the arteries into the cervical spine at approximately C6, the course through the transverse foramina of the cervical vertebra, the 180° turn across C1 and the intracranial union with the basilar artery before joining the circle of Willis.

(Stevens, 1991; Refshauge, 1994), in patients with dizziness (Thiel et al., 1994) and potentially in patients with degeneration of the cervical spine (Olszewski et al., 1994). It is possible that symptoms occur when vascular anomalies or pathology cause further compromise, although anomalies in the vertebrobasilar system are extremely common (Loeb and Meyer, 1965; Lord, 1986) and are normally overcome by competent collateral adaptations within the circulatory system (Mishkin and Schreiber, 1974; Lord, 1986). It appears that symptoms arise when there is an acute change in the vertebrobasilar system, such as from traumatic damage to the artery lumen, or compromised blood flow from sustained cervical spine rotation and/or extension (Okawarra and Nibbelink, 1974). The position of cervical spine rotation may result from either moving the head on a stable body or moving the body while the head remains stable, resulting in relative cervical rotation.

Various extrinsic pathologies or anomalies have been shown to impinge on the external walls of the VA and thereby narrow the lumen. These extrinsic disorders and anomalies include:

1. Osteophytes, especially of the uncovertebral joints and zygapophyseal joints, forcing the VA to deviate around them

2. Common anomalies in the vertebrobasilar system include the VA originating from the posterior aspect of the subclavian artery (a common phenomenon; Lord, 1986), the VA passing through the longus colli or the anterior scalene muscles, and the presence of a bony ring (normally present in 30% of cadavers) instead of the occipitoatlantal membrane normally encircling the vertebral artery as it crosses the superior aspect of C1. All of these anomalies may result in occlusion on contralateral rotation of the cervical spine

3. The artery may pass beneath bands of cervical fascia, causing constriction on rotation (Lord, 1986).

There is no evidence that such disorders actually increase the risk of either critical reduction in cerebral blood flow or traumatic injury to the VA during vigorous procedures. There is some evidence, however, that other factors increase the potential hazard from manipulation, including asymmetry of the VAs (Lyness and Wagman, 1974), previous VA injury (Frumkin and Baloh, 1990) and previous ischaemic symptoms (Kanshepolski et al., 1972). Other risk factors, such as smoking, contraceptive use and hypertension, do not appear to increase the risk of complications following manipulation (Haldeman et al., 2002). For review see Mann and Refshauge (2001).

DIFFERENTIAL DIAGNOSIS OF VBI

Of the many conditions that cause symptoms of dizziness, those most likely to present to physiotherapists, or to coexist with musculoskeletal disorders of the spine, are postural (orthostatic) hypotension, Ménière's disease, vestibular dysfunction and cervical vertigo. Some of these are also the most difficult to differentiate from VBI. In fact, if dizziness is the only presenting symptom, it may not be possible to differentiate vestibular disorders or cervical vertigo from VBI. Some conditions that can present with dizziness include:

1. Orthostatic hypotension: symptoms of feeling faint or lightheaded are caused by a sudden decrease in cerebral blood flow from altered blood pressure when changing posture. Therefore dizziness is experienced during postural changes from a low to high position, such as getting out of bed. However dizziness is not caused by cervical spine movements (Burton, 1965; Rowell, 1986), so postural hypotension can usually be clearly differentiated from VBI.

2. Ménière's disease: this disease affects the endolymph in the labyrinth. Symptoms include fluctuating hearing loss associated with tinnitus, a feeling of pressure in the ears, episodic vertigo or dizziness, and nausea and vomiting. Although not usually difficult to distinguish from VBI, definitive diagnosis is made by audiometry (Coman, 1986).

3. Vestibular dysfunction: symptoms are caused by dysfunction anywhere in the vestibular system, such as in the semicircular canals. When fluid in the affected canal is disturbed, such as by movement of the head, hairs specific to that canal are moved (Kelly, 1991) and a rotating or

turning sensation is experienced, commonly termed vertigo. The particular movements affected will depend on the canal affected, but may include flexion or lateral flexion (unlike dizziness caused by VBI, which may be worsened with extension and rotation: Coman, 1986). The vestibular system can also be disordered as the result of ischaemia affecting the vestibular nuclei or altered afferent input from cervical spine structures (de Jong et al., 1977). Since the vertebrobasilar system supplies both the brainstem and the vestibular nuclei, it is sometimes difficult to distinguish between vestibular or labyrinth disorders, and VBI (brainstem) disorders (Coman, 1986). Pathological nystagmus is a cardinal feature of vestibular disorders, but may also be caused by VBI (causing ischaemia in the vestibular system: Lord, 1986; Goldberg et al., 1991).

4. Cervical vertigo: symptoms include ataxia and dizziness, and arise from abnormal afferent impulses from deep cervical spine structures, particularly muscles, zygapophyseal joints and the posterior longitudinal ligament (de Jong et al., 1977; Abrahams, 1981). In laboratory-induced cervical vertigo, symptoms are thought to be mediated through the vestibular nuclei, occurring on movement of the head. It may therefore be difficult to distinguish cervical vertigo from lesions of the vestibular system or from VBI (de Jong et al., 1977). Differential diagnosis is generally made retrospectively, after symptoms have responded to cervical spine treatment.

Differentiation of the cause of dizziness is generally based on the behaviour of dizziness, and therefore may be established in the history. Frequency and duration of dizzy episodes may assist in determining the cause of symptoms: in cervical vertigo, the episode usually lasts for seconds only; in Ménière's disease, episodes last for hours; in acute vestibular failure episodes may last for weeks (Coman, 1986; Sloane et al., 2001). In VBI, duration of episodes probably depends on magnitude of provocation, and therefore may result in transient episodes lasting from seconds to weeks, or may result in permanent impairment. If patients complain of dizziness, they should be tested in the physical examination to confirm the

suspected diagnosis. Testing must be performed with extreme caution to avoid exacerbating potentially dangerous pathology.

INDICATIONS FOR VA TESTING

In 1988 the Australian Physiotherapy Association approved a test protocol for premanipulative testing that was revised in 2000. The new clinical guidelines for premanipulative procedures for the cervical spine (Magarey et al., 2000) are outlined below and are performed in an attempt to enhance safety during manipulation. The standard tests are performed whenever a patient complains of dizziness, but particularly when:

1. patients present with cervical symptoms (pain including headache and/or stiffness) and dizziness, where the behaviour and history of the dizziness and other symptoms appear to be related to movements of the cervical spine

2. dizziness or symptoms of VBI are provoked during cervical spine treatment

3. symptoms of VBI are experienced following treatment

4. the physiotherapist proposes using a technique that could compromise the VA (e.g. manipulation), even in individuals who have not experienced symptoms of VBI. VA testing is routinely performed before every cervical spine manipulation.

VA tests should be performed after examination of active movements, but probably before examination of positions combining extension and rotation. Performing active movements before VA tests provides information about available range of movement and pain reproduction, allowing appropriate performance of extension and rotation during VA testing. VA tests are also performed before sustained positions (where applicable) as positive test results will contraindicate the use of these procedures.

TEST PROCEDURES

Standard tests

Tests are performed in sitting and/or supine lying positions (as appropriate for each patient). Both positions are not usually necessary. Minimum testing recommended includes:

- sustained end-range cervical rotation to the left and right
- the position or movement that provokes symptoms, as described by the patient (Magarey et al., 2000).

Sustained extension and rotation combined with extension to left and right were part of the original protocol, but are now considered optional. Each test position is maintained at end of range for a minimum of 10 s unless symptoms are provoked, in which case the head is immediately returned to the neutral position. 'On return to neutral from the sustained position, a period of at least 10 s should be allowed before proceeding with the next examination procedure' (Magarey et al., 2000).

During each test and after each test position has been released, the patient should be questioned about the onset of dizziness. Patients should also keep their eyes open during testing to allow identification of nystagmus (Coman, 1986). Latent responses can occur after release of test positions (Grant, 1988).

Additional tests performed when patients present with dizziness not provoked by standard testing, including:

- cervical extension
- cervical rotation combined with extension
- the simulated manipulation position (prior to manipulation)
- quick movement of the head through the available range of movement when the patient relates dizziness to quick movements of the head rather than head postures or positions (Magarey et al., 2000).

Where dizziness is provoked on rotation, either during sustained postures or repetitive motion, these tests may be further explored to differentiate dizziness arising from the vestibular apparatus of the inner ear from that caused by neck movement. These tests consist of:

- head held still, sustained trunk rotation to left and right, and could also include
- head held still, repetitive trunk rotation to left and right (Magarey et al., 2000).

Positions are sustained for a minimum of 10 s, but released if symptoms are provoked. Positive results in these tests suggest that dizziness is not caused by a vestibular disorder. However, instead of performing these tests to differentiate vestibular from vascular dizziness, it may be more prudent to refer the patient for appropriate investigation.

Issues related to these tests are debated more fully in the *Australian Journal of Physiotherapy* Forum (AJP Forum, 2001).

VA TESTING IN THE PRESENCE OF AN IRRITABLE CONDITION

It may be difficult to perform any or all of the test procedures in a patient with an irritable condition or alternatively, in a patient with significantly limited range because of pain or age-related factors. Irritable conditions are characterized by the range of movement being markedly restricted by pain. This may therefore preclude sustaining any cervical spine positions, particularly at the end of range. Since vigorous end-of-range procedures (provocative for VBI) would not normally be used to treat irritable conditions, it is generally safe to treat such conditions using gentle manoeuvres in the absence of knowledge of VA test results. Testing must be performed, however, when range of movement has increased, and the physiotherapist intends to use more vigorous procedures, including passive mobilization techniques in end-of-range rotation or extension positions. It would therefore also be considered unwise to manipulate acute wry neck, since full VA testing is impossible, and these tests are considered mandatory before manipulation.

MANIPULATION

Manipulation of the cervical spine has resulted in many severe accidents; reports appearing in the literature primarily record incidence of Wallenberg's syndrome, 'locked-in' syndrome and death (Terrett, 1987; Patijn, 1991). Since the consequences can be grave, all precautions must be taken to ensure the procedure is made as safe as possible. Generally, the reported deaths seem to have been due to single or multiple large-range generalized rotation manipulations of the cervical spine. There is anecdotal evidence from the many unreported cases that it is poor clinical reasoning rather than poor technique that is responsible for many of the complications.

VA testing is therefore routinely performed before every cervical spine manipulation, even in the absence of reports of dizziness. This does not ensure safety of the manipulation since the ability of the arteries to withstand externally applied forces at high velocities has not been tested, but it does ensure adequate vertebrobasilar or collateral circulation in provocative positions, important in the event of VA occlusion. When manipulation of the cervical spine is planned, therefore, patients are placed in the position of manipulation in addition to the standard test positions. Testing before every cervical spine manipulation consists of positioning the patient in either sitting or supine lying, and reapplying the testing protocol described earlier. In addition the following is investigated:

- simulated manipulation position. The patient's head and neck are held in the manipulation position as a sustained premanipulative procedure.

The manipulation position is sustained for 10 s, but immediately released if symptoms are reproduced. Latent responses may occur following release of a test position.

When using manipulative procedures, consideration should be given to issues of informed consent (see the Introduction to this chapter, and Magarey et al., 2000 for further explanation, and for suggested information given to patients). Informed consent should be gained before any procedure, but the potential risks associated with cervical spine manipulation demand particular stringency in clearly gaining and recording valid consent. Results of all tests undertaken should also be accurately recorded.

INTERPRETATION OF TEST RESULTS

If any of the test results are positive, it is initially assumed for reasons of safety that VBI is the cause. Although reliability and validity of the tests have not been extensively investigated, there is information to suggest that the VA test procedures may identify position-induced VBI. Several cadaver studies demonstrated reduced fluid flow (sometimes becoming absent) through contralateral vertebral and internal carotid arteries in combined extension and rotation (Tissington Tatlow and Bammer, 1957; Toole and Tucker, 1960) and flow was further reduced by the addition of cervical spine traction (Tissington Tatlow and Bammer, 1957). *In vivo* studies have demonstrated decreased blood flow in extension and rotation (Schmitt, 1991; Refshauge, 1994), altered flow occurring as early as 45° range of rotation (Stevens, 1991; Refshauge, 1994; Thiel et al., 1994; Haynes, 1995, 1996). Therefore, current information suggests that the tests may be valid in terms of compromising blood flow, but that the high number of false-positive and false-negative test results suggest poor discriminability of the test (Bolton et al., 1989; Rivett et al., 1999).

Sensitivity of the tests has undergone preliminary investigation by Hutchinson (1989), who determined that:

1. The most sensitive tests were combined extension and rotation in the sitting position and rotation in the supine position. The use of the sustained manipulation position was relatively insensitive.

2. The patient's haemodynamic status changes with increasing range of motion, a negative test result sometimes becoming positive; therefore repeat testing is essential before each provocative treatment occasion.

Current understanding of the tests suggests that they are probably valid for detecting position-induced dizziness, the most sensitive tests being combined rotation and extension in sitting, and rotation in supine, but false-positive and negative results can occur. Results must therefore be interpreted with caution, the severity of consequences dictating that it is prudent to err conservatively. On the basis of current knowledge, these tests appear to be the most reasonable available for testing adequate cerebral blood flow, but they give no information about the safety of the actual high-velocity/high-force technique defined as manipulation.

IMPLICATIONS FOR TREATMENT

Positive results during or after any of the test or other examination procedures contraindicate examination of the quadrant position (Maitland, 1986), any procedure that provokes dizziness and treatment with cervical manipulation. When patients complain of dizziness that is not reproduced during testing, it is generally considered wise initially to avoid potentially provocative treatments such as manipulation or any procedure that provokes dizziness, until symptoms respond and the nature of the dizziness is clarified. Precautions and constant questioning about dizziness and associated symptoms must accompany forceful application of mobilization, rotation and traction procedures. Traction combined with rotation is best avoided. Patients with suspected VBI who have not reported their symptoms to their medical practitioner should be referred for confirmation and further investigation if appropriate.

The issues regarding the relative benefits versus risk are not discussed here; however, a comprehensive discussion of these can be found in Refshauge et al. (2002).

TENSION TESTS

For many decades intervertebral disc pathology (disc protrusion in particular) was considered the main cause of low back pain, and the straight leg raise (SLR) test was strongly associated with identifying disc protrusions (Charnley, 1951). The SLR therefore became an important procedure, and was generally tested routinely in patients with low back pain. This convention has persevered, despite the current view that disc pathology is not a major cause of low back pain. Many tension tests have now been described that are appropriate for testing in patients presenting with spinal pain. This suggests that the interpretation of results of tension testing has broadened considerably from the original purpose of detecting disc pathology.

Tension tests are widely used by physiotherapists and medical practitioners to examine the response to movement of nerve, its surrounding connective tissue and the associated vessels (Maitland, 1986;

Butler, 1991). As neural tissues are moved through their tissue beds during the procedures, it is thought, and has been demonstrated, that tension is transmitted within the neural tissues (Breig and Troup, 1979; Lewis et al., 1998; Kleinrensink et al., 2000). It should be remembered, however, that the mechanism of pain production is complex and may not be directly attributed to tension. Thus, 'tension test' is a term of convenience, not of diagnosis, and in some cases may be deceptive. One group has found that decreased compliance during SLR correlated with onset of hamstring muscle activity in asymptomatic and symptomatic (with LBP) subjects, and that this did not change with the addition of sensitizing movements (Hall et al., 1998). Other problems associated with the terminology of 'tension tests' are summarized elsewhere (Shacklock, 1995).

Information gained from tension tests differs from what is derived from the neurological examination (see The neurological examination section, later in this chapter). In the neurological examination, the therapist tests conduction properties of a nerve, whereas tension tests are used to assess how neural tissue transmits tension, and moves relative to surrounding tissues. The two forms of examination, however, should be considered together during the diagnostic triage of patients. For instance, patients with low back pain and signs of both nerve irritation, such as reduced SLR causing leg pain, and neurological changes from nerve root compromise can be confidently triaged into the nerve root category, rather than the category of simple low back pain (Waddell, 1998).

The tension tests most frequently described on historical bases are SLR (Charnley, 1951), prone knee bend (PKB: Dyck, 1976) and passive neck flexion (PNF: Brudzinski, 1909; cited in O'Connell, 1946). Additionally, the upper-limb tension test (ULTT: Elvey, 1983) and slump test (Maitland, 1978, 1979, 1985) have gained wider exposure and acceptance in the medical literature, despite still being predominantly used by physiotherapists. Tension tests are still widely used by medical practitioners mainly to determine the contribution of neuromeningeal structures to a patient's symptoms, whereas physiotherapists also use these tests as treatment procedures, and to monitor a patient's progress after treatment.

Aim of the tests

Like other tests in the physical examination, the therapist applies tension tests to provoke the particular symptoms that the patient has reported, and measures range to the onset of pain (P1), or to the limit of the patient's pain tolerance (P2). The area of pain and range to either P1 or P2 can then be assessed to determine whether a positive response has been elicited. Except for PNF, which is a spinal movement that is performed in the sagittal plane, every tension test involves comparison of spinal or peripheral joint movements between sides, so range and pain responses can be compared between right and left. Therefore, a subject's response can be defined according to the following criteria:

- Does the test reproduce the patient's symptoms?
- Is there a difference in range of movement between right and left sides?
- Are reproduced symptoms in a location too remote to be due to local structures moved during the test?

The significance of the first two criteria should be familiar to all physiotherapists. Most physical tests are deemed positive if they reproduce the subject's specific pain at an earlier point in range (or within a defined time, such as in Phalen's test for carpal tunnel syndrome: Gellman et al. (1986)) than the contralateral side. The definition of a positive test is addressed below for each tension test. The third criterion however, is an application of clinical reasoning principles that can improve decisions arising from examination results. For instance, a therapist can have increased confidence in the results of an SLR test if ankle dorsiflexion is performed with the hip held in 45° of flexion, and the subject reports an increase in, or onset of, upper thigh and buttock pain. No structure around the ankle or in the lower leg that is moved during dorsiflexion can be strongly implicated in pain production in this scenario, except for the sciatic nerve and its lumbosacral roots. Even if one proposed that movement of the fascial covering of the calf muscles exerted tension on the fascia of the posterior thigh (Williams et al., 1989), it is still more logical to ascribe pain production to a known powerful pain provocateur such as the sciatic

nerve roots. Thus, therapists should compare the site of pain reproduction with structures moved during the stimulus movement, and consider these issues when analysing the patient response. In this example, fascial involvement could be further discounted by direct palpation of the thigh and buttock. Consider how less confident a therapist might be about neuromeningeal involvement if the same dorsiflexion manoeuvre during SLR reproduced a patient's popliteal or calf pain instead?

Mechanism of pain production

Nociceptive responses do not usually occur when normal spinal nerves and nerve roots are stretched or compressed (Howe et al., 1977). Ectopic and nociceptive impulses are only generated if the nerves have been structurally damaged, increasing their sensitivity to stimulation. Some authors have demonstrated how minor mechanical stimulation of damaged nerve roots and spinal nerves will generate painful or nociceptive discharge (Smyth and Wright, 1958; Howe et al., 1977). The issue of whether tension underlies the mechanism of pain production when nerve is strained is controversial. It has been argued that, within the spinal canal, tension is the pathologically significant force and Breig describes the close relationship between pressure and tension, and the way in which application of a compressive force may concomitantly increase axial tension over a small area (Breig, 1978). It should also be noted that trauma to a nerve (such as following compression injury or other chronic damage) results in the neural tissues becoming stiffer during the repair phase (Beel et al., 1984). Thus, not only may pain be reproduced during tension testing, but reduced compliance of neural tissue may also limit movement.

Indications for testing

Tension tests are not performed as a matter of routine but rather, because the test has been implicated by the patient's presentation. Consequently, a tension test is indicated for any of the usual reasons why a therapist examines potential structural sources of symptoms:

- It underlies the area of pain.
- It can refer to the area of pain.

- It is a 'special structure' that should be tested separately because it might be implicated in the subject's presentation (e.g. as for the cruciate ligament in reports of instability around the knee, or the vertebrobasilar system in reports of vertigo/dizziness).

Thus, certain tests might always be performed for certain clinical presentations because one of the above practice guidelines applies. For instance, in the discussion below, SLR should always be examined in patients complaining of low back pain, especially if this is associated with posterior leg symptoms, since the lumbosacral roots are structures that can refer to the area of symptoms. Therapists should ensure that they could justify any test procedure according to one of these criteria, not simply because the test is a routine one.

Based on knowledge of the structures stressed by each test procedure, and on expected patterns of symptom reproduction, it would appear logical that:

- PNF and SLR are performed in patients with low back pain (Maitland, 1986; Butler, 1991)
- PKB is tested when the patient has pain in the lumbar spine and anterior thigh, (the dermatomes corresponding to the roots of the femoral nerve (Estridge et al., 1982).

The more stressful procedures of ULTT and slump should be considered separately to the above procedures. They are considered more stressful for certain anatomical regions, and probably have larger potential for aggravating patients presenting with significant discomfort or acute neurological signs (Elvey, 1986; Butler, 1991). This could be because both tests take longer to perform, so painful tissues are stressed for longer. In addition or alternatively, both tests involve adding spinal movements to limb joint movements, thus neural tissues are stressed from both cephalad and caudad directions. For reasons of safety, therefore, these procedures should be performed only:

- after the individual components of the test have been examined
- when patients are non-irritable
- when neurological findings have been examined on a sufficient number of occasions

and verified to be negative or positive and stable or positive and improving.

Specifically, slump should be performed when:

- a patient has lumbar spine and posterior leg pain
- it is thought that neuromeningeal structures could be a source of symptoms, but SLR and PNF have not sufficiently reproduced symptoms in the same radiation or intensity as reported
- the patient complains of symptoms reproduced in positions similar to slump, such as in long sitting (with the straight leg outstretched), e.g. when reading in bed, or getting into or out of a car.

ULTT should be performed when a patient has cervical spine and arm pain, and:

- it is thought that neuromeningeal structures could be the cause of the patient's upper limb symptoms, for example the patient describes symptom provocation during activities similar to the ULTT position
- the physical examination of the cervical spine and shoulder has not sufficiently reproduced symptoms in the same radiation or intensity as reported.

What is a positive response?

The term 'positive' is generally used in orthopaedic medicine to describe a response that suggests the presence of pathology, although physiotherapists have broadened the term to encompass any symptom-producing manoeuvre. The rationale for this is probably historical, and arose because physiotherapists use tests that reproduce symptoms as treatment techniques, unlike medical practitioners. One example is the use by physiotherapists of passive accessory intervertebral movements for acute and subacute low back pain. These techniques are used to localize the source of symptoms, while not defining a specific pathology, before mobilizing the most comparable level as a treatment technique. Physiotherapists are therefore interested in any response during performance of tension tests, and the point in range in which they occur is noted. Nevertheless, when interpreting the results of tension tests, physiotherapists' definition of a positive response should be consistent with that understood in orthopaedic medicine, but allow for our further use of the techniques as treatment interventions, for instance, such as using slump stretches as treatment techniques for grade 1 tears of the hamstrings group (Kornberg and Lew, 1989). Using these guidelines, the term 'positive' should not only be consistent with the three criteria described above under 'Aim of the tests', but also account for specific test results, as described below.

Test procedures and interpretation of test results

Straight leg raise

The SLR produces tension and movement in the sciatic nerve, and the spinal nerves and nerve roots (SN/NR) that contribute to it (L4–S3) (Goddard and Reid, 1965).

Standard test procedure For examination of SLR the patient lies supine and completely relaxed. The test should initially be standardized, because data from a number of studies indicate that error during SLR can be reduced if the procedure is standardized between occasions of testing (Dixon and Keating, 2000). The starting position is with the hip in neutral abduction/adduction and neutral rotation, the head unsupported (no pillow is necessary unless pain demands one) and the ankle relaxed. The physiotherapist supports the ankle posteriorly (this usually forces the ankle into some plantarflexion) and the anterior aspect of the knee superior to the patella (Fig. 6.A8). The leg is then elevated passively into hip flexion, while knee extension is maintained (Breig and Troup, 1979). This standard procedure can be reliably reproduced using symptomatic patients (Boland and Adams, 2000), and range of hip flexion can be measured using a tape measure or goniometer (Hsieh et al., 1983) or pendulometer (Boland and Adams, 2000). The procedure is illustrated in Figure 6.A8 in the Appendix at the end of this chapter.

Sensitizing procedures Neuromeningeal structures may be further stressed by using sensitizing manoeuvres. Sensitizing manoeuvres aim to stress further neural connective tissue whilst only minimally stressing other tissues that could produce the patient's symptoms (Breig and Troup, 1979;

Boland and Adams, 2000). The commonest sensitizing procedure for SLR is ankle dorsiflexion. Hip flexion is reduced slightly (usually by approximately 5°) until symptoms reproduced during SLR disappear. Dorsiflexion of the ankle is then added while the position of hip flexion is held (Breig and Troup, 1979).

Current opinion holds that the addition of ankle dorsiflexion to SLR increases tension in the sciatic nerve and its contributing SN/NR, while not significantly increasing tension in other lumbar spine structures or in the hamstrings muscle group. An increase in pain with the addition of dorsiflexion is therefore thought to indicate an abnormal response to tension in the neuromeningeal structures. When relevant, PNF, hip adduction or hip internal rotation can be added to SLR in the same way, with the intention of further increasing tension (Breig and Troup, 1979). The addition of ankle dorsiflexion to SLR has been shown to reduce range of hip flexion to onset of symptoms in a symptomatic sample, without compromising high reliability (Boland and Adams, 2000).

Positive response A positive response is considered to be reproduction of leg symptoms early in range of hip movement (<30–45° hip flexion), especially when compared with the other side, though reproduction of lumbar pain should be viewed as significant too. Troup categorized a positive response as being within a range of 15–45° of hip flexion, implying that early reproduction of symptoms might not be from neuromeningeal causes (Troup, 1981). This is supported by other research demonstrating that pelvic movement occurs within 9° of SLR being commenced (Bohannon et al., 1985). A positive SLR can be caused by various pathologies, but the most frequently cited is that of a space-occupying lesion (usually a fragment or herniation of intervertebral disc: Charnley (1951); Smyth and Wright (1958); MacNab (1971)). This may produce inflammatory changes in the nerve causing an abnormal response to tension (Smyth and Wright, 1958; Howe et al., 1977). It should be noted, however, that the intervertebral disc is not the sole cause of decreased SLR. Any impediment to free movement of neural tissues within the intervertebral foramina, such as scarring or osteophytic changes associated with the Z-joint, may restrict SLR (see 'Diagnostic validity', below). Some authors have reported cases of restricted and painful SLR due to adhesion of spinal roots to the dural orifice in the absence of discal pathology (Lerman and Drasnin, 1975).

Passive neck flexion

PNF is thought to apply tension to the spinal cord and associated pain-sensitive dura, and the lumbar nerve roots (Breig and Marions, 1963; Maitland, 1986).

Standard test procedure   PNF is tested with the patient lying comfortably supported in supine. The physiotherapist carefully flexes the patient's cervical spine, ensuring control during the movement to avoid rotation and side flexion of the cervical spine. The cervical spine should be fully flexed (i.e. ensure upper cervical flexion also occurs) rather than causing an anterior shearing movement in the low cervical spine.

Sensitizing procedure   SLR can be combined with PNF in the same way as described during SLR above. PNF can be added before or after SLR is performed and may require a second therapist to help when the two procedures are combined. It should be noted that asking the patient *actively* to flex the cervical spine might result in lumbar flexion occurring (through rectus abdominis contraction), increasing the chances of false-positive test results for the *passive* neck flexion test.

Positive response   A positive response is reproduction of any lumbar or lower thoracic spine pain or perhaps leg pain (Butler, 1991). As when dorsiflexion is performed prior to SLR, a reduction of range of PNF when taken to P1 should be observed if SLR is performed prior to PNF as a sensitizing manoeuvre.

Prone knee bend

PKB produces tension in the femoral nerve and the SN/NR that contribute to it (L2–L4; Dyck (1976)).

Standard test procedure   PKB is tested with the patient lying comfortably relaxed in prone. The physiotherapist carefully flexes the knee to onset of symptoms or end of range (Fig. 6.A9). Initially the test is standardized, with the hip in neutral. Knee flexion can be measured with a goniometer, or a tape measure can be used to measure the distance from heel to buttock crease (see Fig. 6.A9, in Appendix at the end of this chapter).

Sensitizing procedure   Hip extension can be added as a sensitizing manoeuvre to increase tension in the femoral nerve and its contributing SN/NR (Dyck, 1976). Care should be taken to minimize lumbar spine rotation and extension. Interpretation of results from the addition of cervical flexion/extension to PKB is equivocal, with only minimal investigation of the procedure having occurred (Davidson, 1987), hence, the value of these additions to PKB is unclear.

A positive response   A positive response is reproduction of lumbar spine and anterior leg pain early in range of knee flexion (<60–90° knee flexion), particularly when compared with the contralateral side. Symptoms reproduced further into range could be due to other factors, for instance, anterior thigh pain might be a response to stretch of rectus femoris or anterior tilt of the pelvis inducing lumbosacral movement. A positive PKB is thought to arise from pathology such as a space-occupying lesion affecting the SN/NR associated with the femoral nerve (Dyck, 1976; Estridge et al., 1982).

Slump

The slump test is thought to apply more tension to neuromeningeal structures than SLR, PNF or a combination of these two tests in supine (Maitland, 1978, 1979, 1985). Slump is tested with the patient seated comfortably on the end of a plinth. The therapist should stand on the symptomatic side for patients with unilateral symptoms. This allows better control of the painful side. The standard protocol for examining slump is:

- Active flexion of the thoracic spine by the patient, while the head is kept erect and the sacrum vertical. Overpressure is applied to thoracic flexion, and maintained throughout the remainder of the procedure.

- Active flexion of cervical spine is performed. Overpressure is applied and maintained.

- The *asymptomatic* knee is actively extended.

- Dorsiflexion is applied.

- The patient is asked to extend the cervical spine, and the effect on symptoms is noted.

- The patient is asked to attempt further knee extension, while the cervical spine is in the neutral or extended position, and the therapist notes whether further knee extension is possible.

- The procedure is then applied to the other side starting with cervical spine flexion again. Knee extension, ankle dorsiflexion, cervical spine extension and finally knee extension are repeated on the *symptomatic* side (Maitland, 1985).

At each step, symptoms are noted before adding the next step of the protocol. Results from testing the symptomatic side are compared with those of the asymptomatic side, according to the three criteria described earlier.

A positive response An abnormal response to slump testing in the lumbosacral/sciatic neuromeningeal structures is indicated by:

- reproduction of symptoms (especially when in a location remote from the joint being moved) when the spine is fully flexed and the leg fully extended, followed by a decrease in symptoms with cervical extension
- an increase in knee extension and/or ankle dorsiflexion with cervical extension
- a difference in range of knee extension/ankle dorsiflexion between sides.

High intertherapist agreement for identifying positive slump has been demonstrated using the first two criteria (Philip et al., 1989) using a sample of subjects with low back pain with or without leg symptoms. It should be noted that not all studies have described the third criterion for confirming a positive slump test (Philip et al., 1989; Turl and George, 1998). However, well-known authors (Butler, 1991) also suggest that ranges of knee extension should be symmetrical between sides. An inability of even an asymptomatic subject to achieve full knee extension in the slump position, with the cervical spine in either extension or flexion, should be considered normal (Johnson and Chiarello, 1997).

Upper–limb tension test

The ULTT is thought to increase stress in the cervical spine neuromeningeal structures including mid-low cervical SN/NR (C5–T1), brachial plexus and peripheral nerves (Selvaratnam et al., 1989; Kleinrensink et al., 2000). The standard test is performed with the patient lying comfortably in supine, the use of a flat pillow, and consists of the following steps:

- shoulder depression
- glenohumeral abduction behind the coronal plane (i.e. slight extension)
- glenohumeral external rotation
- forearm supination
- elbow extension
- wrist and finger extension
- contralateral cervical lateral flexion (Elvey, 1983; Kenneally, 1985; Selvaratnam et al., 1994)
- wrist and finger extension is withdrawn by moving these into flexion.

The last step described above is open to debate. It has usually been recommended that the final movement should be ipsilateral cervical lateral flexion. The aim of this manoeuvre is to relax tension in neuromeningeal structures, and note the patient's pain response. However, this final procedure of adding and then withdrawing the same cervical movement is inconsistent with the logic applied at the end of the slump test, when neck extension is performed after ankle dorsiflexion, and before knee extension. A similar sequence of adding and withdrawing movements from 'opposite ends' of the cervicobrachial neuromeningeal tree should be applied during the ULTT to clarify any relationship between symptoms and neuromeningeal structures. Thus, the last step described above is recommended, instead of ipsilateral cervical lateral flexion or stopping the test after adding contralateral lateral flexion.

A positive response An abnormal response to testing cervicobrachial neuromeningeal structures using the above protocol is indicated by:

- reproduction of symptoms in response to contralateral lateral flexion of the cervical spine, with the elbow and wrist joints held stable (e.g. at P1)

- reduction of symptoms when the wrist and fingers are flexed
- observed difference in range of movement between sides in any of the components when taken to pain onset (Elvey, 1983; Selvaratnam et al., 1994).

Many variations of the ULTT have been described (see Butler, 1991). The rationale underlying these variations is that tension can be altered in the cervical neuromeningeal tissues by changing the position of limb segments, before applying spinal movements or tension in the reverse order. Additionally, it is speculated that some variations are specific for different peripheral nerves, and these have been shown to alter the test response (Elvey, 1979, 1981; Yaxley and Jull, 1993; Grant et al., 1995). The validity of these assumptions remains to be confirmed by further quality investigations; however, it is doubtful that the ULTT can be used specifically to stress or strain specific cords of the brachial plexus, or specific cervical roots (Kleinrensink et al., 2000). Nevertheless, for a full exploration of the various tests, see Butler (1991), and for their underlying theory, see Butler (1991) and Shacklock (1995). Butler (1991) also presents alternative handling procedures for each technique. It should be emphasized, however, that whichever form of ULTT is used, interpretation of test results will depend on how effectively the operator stabilizes each limb segment, before adding the next movement to the test.

Diagnostic issues

Slump and ULTT procedures have not been investigated as thoroughly as SLR. Since they are probably more stressful procedures, it is unlikely that they would be used to identify serious pathology in the presence of significant pain. Therefore, these tests probably do not have the same diagnostic significance as SLR, PNF and PKB.

Diagnostic validity

Straight leg raise

The SLR was originally described to differentiate hip from sciatic symptoms, a purpose for which it is still used today. Over time, the diagnostic utility of the SLR has been frequently debated. Charnley's (1951) widely held view that a severely restricted SLR indicated the presence of a protruding disc has been challenged by several authors (Fahrni, 1966; Lerman and Drasnin, 1975). In fact, this observation gave rise to the slump tests (Maitland, 1978, 1979). It has been subsequently demonstrated that some patients with SLR restricted to 35° or less have no disc pathology at surgery, but rather a nerve root adherent to the disc or intradural adhesions of specific nerve roots (Fahrni, 1966; MacNab, 1971). Hence, a severely restricted SLR should not be used in isolation to implicate the disc as the source of a patient's symptoms. Similarly, SLR is not diagnostically useful in determining whether the symptoms are due to intra- or extrathecal dural adhesions, intraneural pathology or venous congestion within the intervertebral foramen.

Conversely, a crossed SLR has been proposed as a possible diagnostic indicator of disc pathology. A crossed SLR occurs when SLR performed on the asymptomatic leg reproduces symptoms in the symptomatic leg. In some patient groups, this has been demonstrated to be a better diagnostic indicator of a space-occupying lesion than the standard SLR (Hudgins, 1979). Thus, the standard SLR does appear to increase tension in neuromeningeal structures and cause pain in sensitized neural tissues. It is therefore valid, but does not appear to have high sensitivity or specificity.

Passive neck flexion

The PNF test was originally advocated as a test for meningitis (Brudzinski (1909), cited in O'Connell (1946)) prior to Breig and Marions (1963) describing the cephalad movement of the lumbar nerve roots and dura during the manoeuvre. PNF has not been further investigated, therefore little is known of its diagnostic validity for lumbar space-occupying lesions.

Prone knee bend

The PKB test, first described by Wasserman (1918), is probably the least useful of the tension tests and, like PNF, has not been rigorously investigated. The test was devised as an aid in diagnosing upper lumbar disc lesions. Most authors agree that symptom reproduction may be from increased tension in nerve roots (Estridge et al., 1982; Dyck, 1984). Since the upper lumbar nerve roots are probably subjected to the most tension during PKB, it is expected that anterior thigh pain will be reproduced during the test. Christodoulides, however, argues that the L4 nerve root is most affected, and therefore that posterolateral thigh pain should be reproduced, although there is no further supporting evidence for this view (Christodoulides, 1989). The usual assumption is that PKB is performed to reproduce anterior thigh pain, although the test gives little information about cause of the symptoms. This controversy highlights the limitations of using PKB for diagnosis.

Slump

The slump test was devised to identify sources of leg symptoms other than pathology of the intervertebral disc or within the intervertebral foramina (Maitland, 1978, 1979, 1985). Some evidence exists for the theoretical basis underlying the slump test. The addition of cervical flexion during slump reduces range of knee extension compared with knee extension performed with cervical extension (Fidel et al., 1996). Pain induced in the posterior thighs of asymptomatic subjects during slump with cervical flexion has been shown to decrease in response to cervical extension (Lew and Briggs, 1997).

Upper–limb tension test

The ULTT as originally described was thought to stress the ulnar nerve more than other peripheral nerves, as well as more proximal neuromeningeal tissue (Elvey, 1979). Later this view was modified (Elvey, 1983), and the current standard test procedure is thought to stress the median nerve more than other peripheral nerves (Kenneally, 1985; Butler, 1991). Butler (1991) has further described variations that he believes impose stress on other nerves of the brachial plexus. Variations have been applied during investigations into effects of occupation on response to the test (Grant et al., 1995) and treatment effects for conditions such as carpal tunnel syndrome (Tal-Akabi and Rushton, 2000).

Normative responses have been reported for the standard ULTT procedure (Kenneally, 1985;

Rubenach, 1985; Bell, 1987; Landers, 1987), and for a variation hypothesized to affect the radial nerve (Kenneally, 1985; Rubenach, 1985; Bell, 1987; Landers, 1987; Yaxley and Jull, 1993). From this information, and from comparison with the response when testing the patient's asymptomatic arm, it is possible to identify an abnormal response (Grant et al., 1995). Until further investigations are completed, it is not possible either to establish clearly the location of pathology or to identify the type of pathology. It seems possible, however, to distinguish pain caused by tension in upper limb neuromeningeal tissues from pain caused by other somatic structures (Quillen and Rouillier, 1982; Simionato et al., 1988; Selvaratnam et al., 1994).

Discriminative validity

During the performance of each of the tension tests, many structures are moved and stressed. For example, during SLR, other lumbar structures, the SIJ, hip and hamstrings are also stressed. In fact, SLR is also a test of hamstrings length (Gajdosik et al., 1993) and putting hamstrings on maximal tension as during SLR, without adding ankle dorsiflexion, would be expected to reproduce pain from a hamstrings lesion. Testing of PNF also stresses the cervical and upper thoracic spines in flexion, so range to pain onset must be considered, as should the site where pain is produced by the test. The slump test stresses all of the above structures, as well as the low thoracic spine and lower limb joints. PKB affects the knee, hip, and various muscle groups, in addition to the femoral nerve. The ULTT stresses cervical spine and shoulder structures, and the elbow, wrist and finger joints. All these issues infer that most of the tension tests would have relatively poor discriminative validity.

Discriminative validity has been investigated for SLR and ULTT. While not statistically analysed, SLR, without the addition of sensitizing manoeuvres, appears to have high sensitivity and low specificity (Fahrni, 1966; MacNab, 1971; Hudgins, 1979). ULTT appears to be able to discriminate between neurogenic and other somatic sources of symptoms in one well-conducted trial (Selvaratnam et al., 1994). It is clearly difficult, however, to interpret results of tension tests in isolation without other information from the history and physical tests.

Nevertheless, addition of sensitizing manoeuvres probably enhances the discriminative capacity of the tests. If a sensitizing manoeuvre increases symptoms, it is generally believed that neuromeningeal tissue is responsible for the symptoms, since other structures may not be further stressed. Since the tests have limited diagnostic value, it is again advised that results of the tension tests should be correlated with the full clinical presentation.

Implications for measurement

Like most test procedures in manual medicine, a positive response to a tension test in itself does not necessarily indicate specific pathology. It indicates a heightened responsiveness of the neuromeningeal tree to movement. In contrast to a positive neurological examination, a positive tension test does not constitute a contraindication or precaution to any management strategy. Instead, the implications of heightened sensitivity to movement should be carefully considered and a positive tension test should be correlated with the findings of the rest of the history and physical examination. A safe and valid clinical reasoning position to proceed from is that a positive response to a carefully performed tension test (including any sensitizing manoeuvre) indicates neuromeningeal involvement in the patient's symptoms. From this position, the therapist should consider whether the positive test should be used as a reassessment sign and/or a treatment technique.

Some tension tests have been tested for reliability using procedures and measurement tools that are directly transferable to the clinic. This applies to slump (Philip et al., 1989) and SLR (Boland and Adams, 2000) and, to a lesser extent, for ULTT. However, the procedures for measuring PKB and PNF with a tape measure or inclinometer are simple and likely to be reproducible. Measuring ULTT, however, requires special instrumentation (Selvaratnam et al., 1994) or two operators (Grant et al., 1995). Thus, PNF and PKB are probably appropriate for reassessment, but caution should be exercised if ULTT is used, unless appropriate instrumentation is used or multiple operators are involved.

Implications for treatment

Each of the tension tests can also be applied as a treatment technique. Usually one element of the test is selected, e.g. elbow extension in the ULTT position, or ankle dorsiflexion in the SLR or slump position. This is either repeated using a rhythmic oscillatory physiological procedure as a mobilizing technique, or is sustained for a gentle stretch. To be consistent with other manual therapy techniques, it is appropriate to use a tension test procedure as a treatment when it is the most provocative physical test (i.e. reproduces symptoms maximally during the physical examination), the condition is not irritable and especially when there is no other physical finding. Tension test procedures are infrequently used as the technique of choice at the first treatment session. Responses to treatment using these techniques can vary, occasionally markedly increasing symptoms (Butler, 1991). It is therefore recommended, particularly for the novice, that the patient's signs and symptoms are clearly understood before using a tension test procedure as a treatment technique. Additionally, the underlying pathology must also be considered.

One study (Scrimshaw and Maher, 2001) evaluated the role of SLR stretches, as advocated by Fahrni (1966) in the management of patients who had undergone lumbar discectomy. The addition of SLR stretches to the usual postoperative regimen had no effect on outcome, and interestingly, no difference was observed in range of SLR between treatment and control groups. This study casts doubt on whether neural mobilization as a therapy has any effect on this type of problem; however, others (Kornberg and Lew, 1989) have found that slump stretches were effective as an adjunctive treatment for managing grade 1 hamstrings group tears in Australian football players. Another study found that ULTT and carpal mobilization had similar effects in reducing symptoms (compared with no intervention) of carpal tunnel syndrome in a sample of patients (Tal-Akabi and Rushton, 2000). These conflicting data indicate that therapists must be cautious in applying tension tests as treatments, and that more quality randomized controlled trials with different clinical conditions and samples are required to verify the effectiveness of tension tests as treatments.

Proposed mode of action

Given the current knowledge of tissue mechanics, including hysteresis and creep (Fung, 1981; Herbert, 1988; Bogduk and Twomey, 1991), and the fact that neural tissue behaves in a similar manner to other biological tissues (Sunderland and Bradley, 1961a, b) it is difficult to see how stretching neural tissue could have other than short-term reversible mechanical effects. Butler (1991) has provided several possible explanations for the prolonged treatment effects observed. He hypothesized that the effects could be mediated by dispersion of intraneural oedema, lengthening of neural tissue, improved intraneural blood supply or improved axonal transport. While each of these proposed mechanisms is sustainable from a theoretical viewpoint, there is little evidence that any of them actually occurs.

Dose

In pharmacological practice therapeutic doses of pharmaceutical agents can be clearly established; however, in the area of neural treatment techniques and indeed manual therapy in general, physiotherapists rely on personal experience, anecdotal evidence and recommendations from experienced clinicians when deciding treatment dose (Grieve, 1984; Maitland, 1986; Butler, 1991). There are no data clarifying the relationship between symptoms and dose, and since the mode of effect is unclear, it is difficult to propose appropriate dosages when applying tension tests. The usual dose on the first treatment occasion may be to perform the technique (e.g. ankle dorsiflexion in the slump position) for approximately 30 s. If the patient's signs and symptoms improve, this dose may be repeated. It is recommended that the patient's signs and symptoms be closely monitored during the first treatment session. Treatment can be repeated until reassessment signs stabilize between repetitions. The therapist should measure other variables, such as active movements or neurological signs to compare improvement across a number of variables.

Reassessment following treatment and prior to the second treatment occasion will clarify the response and enable modification of dosage as required.

Conclusion

Tension tests have been the subject of increased interest in recent years, particularly with the development of the ULTT and its several variations. These tests are useful in clinical practice, but it should be noted that development has outpaced rigorous investigation into reliability, validity and clinical effectiveness of the tests. Tension tests are useful adjuncts to other examination procedures. They are stressful and are probably relatively selective for neuromeningeal tissues, though not necessarily to specific nerves for all tests. Since so many pathologies provoke normally painless neural tissues to induce pain in response to neural movement, however, tension tests have low specificity. Thus, tension tests cannot be interpreted in isolation to formulate pathological diagnoses. Physiotherapists, however, can compare results of tension tests with findings from the history and the physical examination to refine clinical diagnoses and treatment options. To be most useful, the tests must be performed in a reproducible manner.

It is likely that the novice will have difficulty interpreting findings from the tension tests. Many anatomical structures are exposed to various stresses during testing, and many varied pathologies may induce a painful response. It is therefore recommended that novices use tension tests as treatment procedures only in the absence of other treatment possibilities, until they are clear about the nature of the patient's disorder, and can predict the likely response to treatment. Any treatment consisting of a tension test that results in a response inconsistent with what was predicted, particularly if that response is one where the patient's symptoms and signs worsen, should be carefully re-evaluated before it is repeated. At the very least, dose should be revised and the hypothesized pathology confirmed.

The neurological examination
K.M. Refshauge and E.M. Gass

Many patients with spinal conditions have pain or other symptoms referred into the limb. In such cases physiotherapists perform neurological tests to determine whether conduction properties in the relevant parts of the nervous system are normal. The results of these tests are diagnostically important and have implications for both assessment and treatment (Rydevick et al., 1989). These tests are also used to monitor progress of the patient's condition. The parts of the nervous system of particular interest when dealing with spinal musculoskeletal conditions are the spinal nerve, nerve root, spinal cord and the cauda equina (Figs 6.2–6.4).

SPINAL NERVE/NERVE ROOT

Conduction in the SN/NR complex is tested when symptoms are suspected to arise from compromise of these structures. Compromise of the SN/NR can result from:

1. mechanical compromise of the nerve resulting in intraneural oedema which would in turn cause pressure on axons (Hoyland et al., 1989)
2. compromise of the blood vessels associated with the SN/NR, causing ischaemia (Hoyland et al., 1989)
3. traction injuries
4. friction fibrosis (Sunderland, 1978).

It is difficult, if not impossible, to distinguish clinically between compromise of a spinal nerve and nerve root. Many authors refer only to compromise of nerve roots (Helfet and Gruebel, 1978), but others include the spinal nerve, as symptoms are often the same, and pathology in the intervertebral foramen is frequently postulated as a potential site of nerve compromise (McNab, 1972; Hoyland et al., 1989). Therefore, the complex is referred to as

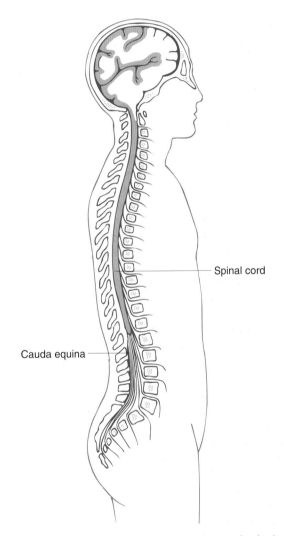

Figure 6.2 Location of spinal cord and cauda equina in the spinal canal.

SN/NR in this text, and is tested as an anatomical complex. Integrity of SN/NR is tested by determining the presence of a dermatomal distribution of altered sensation and/or a myotomal pattern of

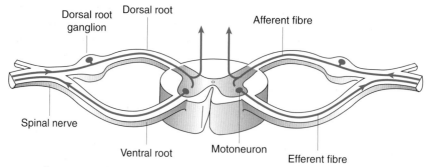

Figure 6.3 Diagrammatic representation of a section of the spinal cord, with afferents entering posteriorly and ascending through tracts to various intracranial centres, and efferent information exiting the spinal cord anteriorly.

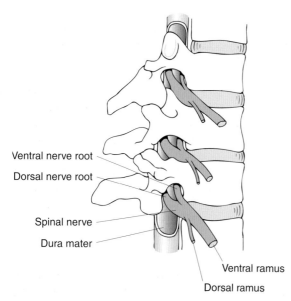

Figure 6.4 Dorsal and ventral roots exiting the spinal canal, uniting in the intervertebral foramen to form the spinal nerve, and dividing into ventral and dorsal rami after exit from the foramen.

motor weakness and/or decreased reflex response. A dermatome is the area of skin supplied by a single spinal nerve, and a myotome is the muscle supplied by (or largely supplied by) a single spinal nerve (Osol, 1972).

Indications for testing

Testing of the SN/NR complex should be undertaken when symptoms are present that could originate from compromise of this complex, including:

1. pain in a dermatomal distribution (for dermatomal maps, see Williams and Warwick, 1980)
2. pain referred from the lumbar spine past the buttock, or from the cervical spine referred beyond the point of the shoulder
3. altered sensation (e.g. paraesthesia, anaesthesia) in the limb (lower extremity for the lumbar spine, upper extremity for the cervical spine)
4. pain in the lower extremity that may be related to a lumbar spine condition, or in the upper extremity that may be related to a cervical spine condition
5. complaints of weakness in a limb.

Test procedures

Compromise of SN/NR can affect neural conduction, and therefore result in reduction in one or more of the following: sensation, reflexes, muscle power. These modalities are therefore tested to determine the presence of a neurological deficit.

Testing of sensation

Physiotherapists commonly test response to light touch and pinprick as these sensations are carried by the large-diameter group II afferent fibres to the dorsal column. These large-diameter fibres are particularly vulnerable to compression (because they are located at the outer part of the nerve) and to ischaemia (because they require a greater supply of oxygen and nutrients to function normally than do small-diameter fibres). Therefore, altered conduction in group II afferents may be one of the first indicators of SN/NR compromise.

Testing consists of running cotton wool lightly around either both lower or both upper limbs simultaneously (i.e. across several dermatomes with each sweep), asking the patient to report any differences in sensation in one part of the limb or from one limb to the other. If areas of altered sensation are identified they are delineated using gentle pinprick. This pinprick should be sharp not painful, ensuring that the large group II fibres carrying non-noxious information are tested rather than the smaller group III or group IV, carrying noxious stimuli (Kandell et al., 1991). Areas of sensory change are recorded (generally on a body chart) and compared with dermatomal areas of innervation (Bickerstaff, 1980) to determine first, whether there is SN/NR compromise, and second, the affected level, i.e. the segmental level corresponding to the dermatome.

Several other aspects of sensation could be tested, for example:

1. Two-point discrimination, testing the integrity of the dorsal column and lemniscal systems (Foreman and Croft, 1988), although it has been suggested that this test is not sensitive to SN/NR compromise (Gelberman et al., 1983).

2. Vibration, testing integrity of group II fibres, dorsal column and medial lemniscal systems (Kandell et al., 1991). This test appears to be sensitive to SN/NR compromise (Gelberman et al., 1983).

3. Temperature sensibility, testing the integrity of the lateral spinothalamic tract of the spinal cord (Kandell et al., 1991) and the group III fibres (Barr, 1974). Extremes of temperature, however, are perceived as painful stimuli.

4. Proprioception, testing skin and joint receptors, muscle spindles, group I and II fibres, and dorsal column and medial lemniscus systems (Foreman and Croft, 1988).

These other sensory modalities are not routinely tested. The purpose of sensation testing is to use efficient testing procedures to detect SN/NR compromise and the affected level, rather than differential diagnosis of affected spinal tract. Light touch and pinprick, testing large-diameter fibres, are currently the most appropriate to achieve this purpose.

Testing of reflexes

There are four types of reflex that can be tested in the peripheral nervous system: deep tendon reflexes, superficial, visceral and pathological (Foreman and Croft, 1988). Deep tendon reflexes are tested by physiotherapists to determine the presence and segmental level of SN/NR compromise. An intact deep tendon reflex requires integrity of the stretch reflex arc (Lance and McLeod, 1975).

The stretch reflex is elicited by briskly striking the tendon with a tendon hammer while the muscle is on slight stretch and the patient is relaxed. The number of times the reflex is elicited is arbitrary, the test being repeated until the examiner is satisfied that the response can be interpreted. The response is compared with the other side and with the known range of normal (Skre, 1972). A decreased or absent reflex may indicate a compromise of the corresponding SN/NR or peripheral nerve, and an increased response may indicate a lesion in the central nervous system (CNS: see under Central nervous system, later in this chapter).

Testing of muscle strength

Muscles are tested for isometric strength to determine whether nerve conduction is affected. The muscles tested are innervated or largely innervated by a single SN/NR and therefore represent myotomes. Myotomes C5–T1 are tested in the cervical spine and L2–S2 for the lumbar spine.

There are no clearly defined myotomes in the upper cervical spine (above C4), most muscles in this region being innervated by multiple segments (Williams and Warwick, 1980). Occasionally muscle power is tested in the upper cervical spine. The results, however, must be interpreted with caution since weakness will not indicate involvement of a single SN/NR. Note that when testing the mid-low cervical spine SN/NR, C4 is not tested. Although trapezius is often reported as a myotome for C4 (Maitland, 1986; Magee, 1987), trapezius receives its motor supply from cranial nerve XI (spinal accessory nerve), although the C4 derma-tome overlies the upper trapezius region (Williams and Warwick, 1980). Muscle strength is not tested in the thoracic spine since segmentally innervated muscles (intercostal muscles) are not accessible for this type of testing. In the lumbar spine, L1 is not tested because there is no corresponding myotome, muscles in this region also being sup-plied by several segmental levels.

Myotomes are generally tested using maximum voluntary isometric contraction. This practice is sup-ported by some authors who suggest that decreases in strength may only be detected on maximum sustained or repeated contractions (Lieberman et al., 1983), while others claim that resisted contraction through a range of motion may be more sensitive (Bickerstaff, 1980). The presence of pain may reduce the strength of contraction. If weakness appears to be caused by pain on contraction, results must be interpreted in light of this. It is therefore important to interpret findings from the other neurological tests, and not rely on findings of painful weakness in isolation. The most valid and sensitive method of testing myotomes therefore remains somewhat controversial. The current practice of testing max-imum voluntary isometric contraction will proba-bly continue in use until another clinically viable method is demonstrated to be more appropriate. Muscle power can be measured using a hand-held dynamometer, weights or numerous mechanical devices, such as the Cybex or Kincom (Gaines and Talbot, 1999).

Interpretation of test results

Our interpretation of neurological findings is influ-enced by the reliability and validity of the tests, as well as by the rest of the clinical presentation.

Sensation

Standardization of the test procedure will enhance reliability. During testing a stimulus of constant intensity should be applied (Sunderland, 1978). This pressure must also be appropriate: if intensity is too gentle, only the exquisitely sensitive hair fol-licles may be stimulated rather than all light touch receptors, perhaps reducing the response. One way to standardize pressure during testing pinprick

sensation is to hold the pinhead between the index finger and thumb. As the pinhead is pressed into the skin, the pads of the adjacent finger and thumb pads limit and standardize the pin pressure between tests. This is a practical application of a method described by Sunderland (1978).

Identification of the spinal segmental level involved from the area of sensory loss probably does not have high discriminative validity. Der-matomal maps of segmental sensation vary between individuals (Skre, 1972) and between the right and left limb of the same individual, this difference not being related to limb dominance (De Palma and Rothman, 1970; Weiss et al., 1985). Some of this variation may be attributed to bony and neural anomalies (McCulloch and Waddell, 1980; Neidre and McNab, 1983; Young et al., 1983). Dermatomes are also known to overlap; however, dermatomes vary in a minor way, overlapping rather than varying in a completely random man-ner. Therefore, although a single affected level may be difficult to identify with certainty, it is probable that the SN/NR compromised can be isolated to two possible levels. It may be import-ant, however, to identify the anatomical location of the compromise, which may not be at the level of exit of the SN/NR, particularly in the lumbar spine (Kortelainen et al., 1985).

Reflexes

Reflexes, like sensation, are subject to large normal variation. It is not uncommon for normal hyper- or hyporeflexia to occur and there may be some nor-mal difference between right and left (Luhan, 1968). There is also an apparent reduction in magnitude of response with increasing age (Skre, 1972; Bowditch et al., 1996), indicating that hyporeflexia in the elderly, either unilateral or bilateral, may be an insignificant finding. In fact, bilateral absence of ankle reflexes has been found in 5% of people aged between 40 and 50 years, increasing to bilat-eral absence in 80% of people older than 80 years of age (Bowditch et al., 1996). Unilateral absence of reflex is less common (5% of those aged between 40 and 60 years, and ~10% in those aged over 60 years: Bowditch et al., 1996).

The reflex arc is influenced by converging input. The CNS can directly influence the alpha and gamma motor neurons, and it is thought that skin and joint receptors could also have an effect (Appelberg et al., 1983), suggesting that both the CNS and other somatic structures could affect the reflex response. The effects of this may be demonstrated when using reinforcement (Jendrassic's manoeuvre), when contraction of a muscle distant from the site of the reflex can increase the response (Lance and McLeod, 1975). Hagbath et al. (1975) suggest that slight muscle contraction gives a more reliably enhanced response than does Jendrassic's manoeuvre. To enhance reliability of response, testing should be standardized considering particularly the amount and direction of applied force. Therefore, reliability of reflex testing is probably improved if the patient is tested in lying while relaxed. The effect of any manoeuvre to augment a reflex can then be assessed.

As a result of the variability associated with reflex testing, it is prudent to note only large discrepancies or asymmetry of the stretch reflex when interpreting reflex response and compare these findings with the overall clinical picture (Lance and McLeod, 1975).

Muscle strength

Interpretation of muscle testing is complicated by several factors. Myotomes overlap with variations between individuals, perhaps due to anomalies in the bony or neural system. This reduces specificity of myotomal identification. Overlap of myotomes also maintains innervation to a muscle when conduction from one spinal segment is interrupted, if other contributing segments are uninterrupted. In addition, there appears to be a compensatory mechanism that may occur in patients with chronic SN/NR compromise, whereby the motor units still conducting nerve impulses increase their firing frequency and collateral axon sprouting reinnervates denervated muscles, resulting in little or no apparent strength deficit (Bohannon and Gajdosik, 1987). The muscle could therefore have approximately normal strength.

Testing muscles manually is known to have low sensitivity (Gelberman et al., 1983), demonstrating that altered strength is not detected until there is a substantial reduction (approximately 30%) in motor action potentials. This indicates that a large asymmetry may be present, yet not evident on muscle testing (Bohannon and Gajdosik, 1987).

Muscles also exhibit a length–tension relationship, generating different forces at different lengths, therefore joint position must be standardized for testing. To enhance the probability of detecting abnormalities, it is important to standardize the test procedure, including position of both patient and tester, hand position, external cues and dominance of the physiotherapist's resisting arm. Manual muscle testing appears to be reliable when using a dynamometer (Bohannon, 1986). Use of mechanical devices may allow detection of small changes; however, small changes need to be interpreted with caution, being aware of normal limb differences.

Conclusion

These neurological tests considered independently do not have high reliability or high specificity and sensitivity; however, the tests are rarely considered in isolation. All three tests (or two in the absence of a relevant reflex) are performed and the results considered in the context of the total clinical picture, e.g. the patient's age, the area and quality of symptoms, mode of onset, provocative movements and comparison with the other side and known normal ranges. It appears, therefore, that a decreased response in only one neurological test may not be as diagnostically significant as a decreased response in two or three tests. This is particularly true when the finding from neurological testing is indicative of a segmental level different from that suggested by the area of pain.

Neurological deficit and other somatic structures

There is no doubt that altered sensation, loss of motor power and reflex changes can be caused by SN/NR compromise (Helfet and Gruebel, 1978). However, it may be possible that neurological changes could be caused by a disturbance of somatic structures other than nerve, particularly where there is an isolated neurological deficit with no other supportive clinical findings. To date this has not been clearly demonstrated and remains hypothetical based on theory and clinical observation.

Compromise of normal SN/NR does not cause pain (McNab, 1972; Loeser, 1985), therefore, a neurological deficit can occur without pain. Under certain conditions, however, compromise of the nerve root may cause pain. Such conditions include previous damage to the nerve root, intraneural oedema causing axon compression and ischaemia from radicular artery compression (McNab, 1972; Olmarker et al., 1989; Rydevick et al., 1989). This pain should be accompanied by neurological deficit (Bogduk, 1987) since the function of large-diameter sensory and motor afferents is affected by compromise before the small-diameter nociceptive afferents (groups III and IV) within the SN/NR complex (Sunderland, 1978). Therefore, the absence of a neurological deficit, even when pain appears to be dermatomally distributed, may indicate that SN/NR is unlikely to be involved in symptom production, although the possibility that a dermatomal distribution of pain could precede onset of neurological deficit from compromise of a SN/NR cannot be discounted.

The diagnostic decision is less clear when a dermatomal area of pain is accompanied by an isolated neurological deficit, such as a small area of sensory change, or a slightly altered reflex, or equivocal alteration in muscle power. It is possible that such a deficit is due to altered afferent input from somatic structures converging at spinal cord level, from altered facilitation in C3–C4 propriospinal neurons (Burke et al., 1992a, b) or from descending control from higher centres. Such neurophysiological phenomena occur, but evidence of their clinical manifestation is still only hypothesized. Again, the possibility that these findings indicate a developing neurological disorder cannot be discounted.

There is scant, but consistent, clinical evidence that somatic structures other than nerve may cause neurological deficit. Resolution of neurological deficit (normalized reflex) has been observed after injection of Xylocaine into the zygapophyseal joints (Mooney and Robertson, 1976). This study has often been criticized for the volume of injection material (2–5 ml) used which would not only fill the zygapophyseal joint capsule but also disseminate into surrounding tissues (McCall et al., 1979). Nevertheless, if SN/NR compression had been the cause of the decreased reflex due to direct compression or intraneural oedema, it seems unlikely that introducing more fluid to the region (further increasing pressure) would restore the reflex. The Xylocaine may have affected the joint receptors, which could affect the alpha and gamma motor neurons (Appelberg et al., 1983) and thus the reflex arc. It is perhaps possible, therefore, that somatic structures may cause changes in deep tendon reflexes. Normalized muscle strength has also been observed immediately after traction (Knutsson et al., 1988).

In general, a decrease in response to neurological testing indicates the possibility of SN/NR compromise. In fact, if there is a decrease in at least two tests, it should be assumed that SN/NR compromise is the cause. This situation is less clear where pain is accompanied by a small decrease in response to one neurological test, with no other clinical evidence suggestive of SN/NR compromise. It seems possible in this case, that besides representing an early stage of a neurological disorder, the isolated neurological deficit in the presence of an inconsistent clinical picture is caused by somatic structures other than neural structures.

Implications for further testing and treatment

In the presence of a clinical picture indicative of definitive or potential SN/NR compromise, physical tests that are thought to reduce the size of the intervertebral foramen, increase the compromise of the nerve or increase intraneural inflammation should be avoided. These tests include passive accessory movements and possibly oscillatory passive physiological movements. Treatments aimed at increasing the size of the intervertebral foramen are generally recommended (Maitland, 1986). Such treatments are thought to include sustained traction, rotation and perhaps lateral flexion away from the affected side. Other treatments may be used when the neurological deficit is chronic and/or stable (i.e. response has not changed to testing over approximately 1–2 weeks), when the deficit is unrelated to the presenting problem (and would not be affected by treatment of the presenting problem) and when the therapist is certain that the deficit is not caused by relevant neural structures (usually not on the first day presenting for treatment). In these latter instances, the treatment most appropriate to the presenting problem (e.g. oscillatory techniques) may be implemented, but the neurological deficit must be constantly monitored to ensure no further decrement.

CENTRAL NERVOUS SYSTEM (SPINAL CORD)

The CNS is comprised of all parts of the nervous system proximal to the anterior horn cell in the spinal cord. Disorders of the CNS, termed upper motor neuron lesions (UMNL), can therefore arise from lesions anywhere in this part of the nervous system, for example in the brain (e.g. hemiplegia, brain trauma) or in the spinal cord (e.g. rheumatoid arthritis in the cervical spine, causing displacement of C1 on C2, compressing the spinal cord at this level), or both the brain and the spinal cord (e.g. multiple sclerosis). It is important for physiotherapists to determine whether pathology exists locally in the painful region of the spine, because sometimes this pathology can be serious and contraindicate manual treatments in this region. On the other hand, a UMNL affecting the brain, such as stroke, does not have implications for local treatment of musculoskeletal disorders of the spine. Physiotherapists therefore need to determine whether there is upper motor neuron involvement in the disorder, the cause of the UMNL and the location of the pathology.

Indications for testing

Testing of the CNS is not routine, being performed only as indicated. Tests to identify UMNL will be incorporated into the neurological examination in the presence of:

1. ataxia, i.e. the loss of full control of movement (sometimes people describe vertigo or dizziness as unsteadiness of gait, but this is not ataxia)

2. bilateral non-dermatomal distribution of symptoms in the lower extremities for the lumbar spine, and in the upper as well as lower extremities for the cervical spine (symptoms may initially manifest unilaterally, and as the condition worsens, become bilateral, therefore, an early presentation may not appear typical)

3. findings on SN/NR testing suggestive of UMNL, such as exaggerated tendon reflexes including overflow (i.e. one tendon reflex also elicits response in another muscle) or bilateral non-dermatomal distribution of sensory changes.

Test procedures

Procedures to identify UMNL would usually be performed in addition to the tests for sensation, reflexes and muscle strength described in the SN/NR section, above. The procedures below performed by physiotherapists identify a general UMNL only, and are:

- testing for the presence of clonus
- testing the Babinski reflex
- sensation, reflex and muscle strength testing as part of the SN/NR test.

Other tests can be performed, but do not appear to give additional information useful for management of the musculoskeletal condition. Additional tests include: Chaddock sign, Gordon reflex, Schoffer's reflex, Hoffmann's sign, as well as many others (described in Kandell et al., 1991).

Testing for the presence of clonus

Rationale Clonus is the term used to describe the abnormal, rhythmic, repetitive reflex twitches elicited when tension is suddenly applied to a muscle or muscle group and maintained (Zimmerman, 1978). The phenomenon is observed when pathological changes in the CNS, probably affecting the corticospinal tract, lead to a facilitation of the spinal stretch reflexes (Bannister, 1992).

The stretch reflex can be thought of as a dynamic closed loop functioning to regulate muscle length, particularly in the presence of perturbations (Zimmerman, 1978). Pathological CNS changes can increase the gain of the dynamic closed loop leading to situations of instability and overcompensation, manifested as undesirable oscillations of muscle contraction/relaxation following the sudden change in muscle length.

Clonus may therefore be observed in many muscles and may not need a specific test procedure as, in some patients, it may be demonstrated during reflex testing, or even while sitting with the feet on the floor. More commonly, however, a specific test to elicit clonus is performed.

Test procedure Clonus can be tested in many muscle groups, but the ankle plantarflexors are usually tested. With the patient relaxed and well supported the physiotherapist applies a sudden dorsiflexion movement to the patient's ankle, thus applying a stretch to the plantarflexors. Dorsiflexion is maintained for a short time and the presence of clonus is detected by observation and palpation. The test is generally considered positive (abnormal) if clonus is present (more than five reflex twitches).

Testing for the presence of Babinski reflex (extensor plantar reflex)

Rationale After the first year of life, a normal response to a firm scratch along the lateral aspect of the foot is plantarflexion of the toes with dorsiflexion of the foot and possibly some contraction of other leg muscles such as tensor fascia latae (Bannister, 1992). In 1896 Babinski suggested that in the presence of any UMNL, commonly a corticospinal tract lesion, the normal plantar reflex is replaced by an abnormal upward extensor movement of the great toe. With a UMNL the local plantar reflexes (extensor reflex) to the toes are lost and the flexion reflex dominates so that blunt scratch stimulation to the sole of the foot not only evokes flexion of the ankle and leg but also dorsiflexion of the toes (Bouchier and Morris, 1982). The abnormal extensor plantar reflex is part of widespread nociceptive reflex activity of the whole lower limb. When fully demonstrated the reflex includes flexion of hip, knee and ankle joints, dorsiflexion of the great toe and abduction or fanning of the other toes with dorsiflexion. This abnormal response is not normally present and therefore indicates the presence of a UMNL.

Test procedure The patient should be relaxed and well supported. The physiotherapist gently keeps the patient's foot stable while firmly scratching the outer surface of the sole with a blunt object (such as the end of the percussion hammer). The manoeuvre should start at the heel, continue along the lateral aspect of the sole and curve medially at the forefoot, terminating beneath the first metatarsophalangeal joint. Care should be taken to provide neither a painful nor a light and ticklish stimulus

as strong withdrawal of the foot and leg will make test interpretation difficult. The physiotherapist should observe the big toe carefully, because the decision about a positive test response predominantly rests upon accurate observation of movement of the big toe and, to a lesser extent, the other four toes.

The test is positive or abnormal if the big toe dorsiflexes. The other toes may also dorsiflex and fan outwards in abduction. Response of the big toe is the most important, and if no response is elicited (no movement of the big toe into either dorsiflexion or plantarflexion) the test should be repeated more firmly.

Positive Babinski test is often described as an 'upgoing toe' and gives a general indication of the presence of a UMNL. The term 'upgoing toe' is preferable to terms involving flexion and extension which can be confusing.

Testing reflex response

Rationale In the presence of compromise of SN/NR conduction, reflex response is decreased. An increased response, however, may indicate a UMNL, as the gamma efferent system supplying the ends of the muscle spindles is regulated by inhibitory descending motor pathways (Lance and McLeod, 1975). Thus, any block to this inhibitory regulation may cause hyperreflexic responses.

Test procedure Reflexes are tested during the SN/NR examination, described earlier. If an increased response is identified during this examination, reflexes in the untested extremities are investigated. For example, a person with spinal cord compromise due to local pathology in the lumbar spine may have an increased response in L3–L4 and S1–S2 reflexes, while the upper-extremity reflexes may remain normal. On the other hand, if the spinal cord compromise is due to cervical spine pathology, both upper- and lower-extremity reflex responses would be increased. In other words, reflexes below the level of the lesion will be increased.

Interpretation of test results

The tests used to identify a UMNL have not been subjected to rigorous investigation of their reliability or validity. Nevertheless, they are in widespread use amongst all health personnel managing patients with neurological disorders. Information is available about reflex testing, indicating that reflexes vary within and between individuals and may decrease in size of response with increasing age (Skre, 1972). It is also known that some clonus may be present normally in the elderly, although the response is usually less than three beats (Skre, 1972). A clonus response can also be elicited in normal asymptomatic young people, if the plantarflexors are stretched at a particular point in range of movement. It seems, however, that a positive Babinski response is rarely present in a normal population. Therefore, in the presence of equivocal findings, such as the presence of clonus in the absence of positive results in the other two tests, a diagnosis of UMNL is not clearly established. As with other examination procedures, the presence of a positive response in all three tests is required for definitive diagnosis of a UMNL, although hyperreflexia is probably most heavily weighted.

Implications for treatment

The clinical significance of the presence of a UMNL must be determined in conjunction with the patient's medical practitioner. Since the purpose of the tests is to identify contraindications or precautions to manual therapy treatment for spinal pain, it is the cause of the UMNL and location of any pathology that is of concern. Manual therapy can be used safely to treat spinal pain in the presence of a UMNL if the cause of the UMNL is distant from, and unrelated to, the cause of the spinal pain (e.g. hemiplegia or brain injury). Manual therapy would be contraindicated, however, for treating cervical spine pain in the presence of severe rheumatoid arthritis causing compression of the spinal cord. It is recommended, therefore, that when a physiotherapist suspects an undiagnosed UMNL, contact is made with the relevant medical practitioner to establish the cause definitively. The suitability of manual therapy can then be determined.

CAUDA EQUINA (LUMBOSACROCOCCYGEAL SN/NR)

The cauda equina is anatomically composed of the ventral and dorsal nerve roots from lumbar, sacral and coccygeal spinal cord segments (Williams and Warwick, 1980). In adults, the lumbar, sacral and coccygeal segments of the spinal cord lie in the region between the 10th thoracic vertebra and the first lumbar vertebra. The nerve roots descend from the spinal segment of origin to their point of exit from the vertebral canal as segmental spinal nerves. Since this arrangement of obliquely descending nerve roots within the spinal canal resembles a horse's tail, it is termed the cauda equina. A lesion of the cauda equina may therefore interrupt conduction in several nerve roots, resulting in diffuse leg pain and signs and symptoms consistent with every level affected (Coscia et al., 1994). In musculoskeletal physiotherapy clinical practice, the principal concern is compromise of S2 SN/NR because this segmental level supplies the bladder, rectum and male sexual organs. Persistent compromise of S2 SN/NR may lead to necrosis of the roots, causing permanent loss of function of bladder and bowel, resulting in permanent disturbances in micturition and defecation (Coscia et al., 1994). It is therefore imperative that such a disorder is immediately recognized.

Micturition

The main structures involved in micturition are the urinary bladder and internal sphincter, composed of smooth muscle, and the external sphincter, composed of skeletal muscle. The smooth muscle of the bladder and internal sphincter are usually innervated by T11–L2 sympathetic nerves and S1–S2 parasympathetic nerves (Shefchyk, 2002). The sympathetic preganglionic fibres synapse in the coeliac and mesenteric ganglia, becoming postganglionic hypogastric nerves, while the parasympathetic preganglionic nerves reach the bladder. The skeletal muscle of the external sphincter is supplied by the pudendal nerve, composed of spinal segments S2–S4.

Micturition is a spinal reflex under voluntary control. It occurs when mechanoreceptors in the bladder wall are stimulated, causing excitation of the micturition centre in the anterior pons (Thorn, 1977; Shefchyk, 2002). Descending output excites parasympathetic S1 and S2 neurons, causing contraction of the smooth muscle (expansion of the internal sphincter). Concurrently, skeletal muscle of the external sphincter is relaxed, allowing micturition.

It appears that the major role of the sympathetic nervous system in micturition is maintenance of smooth-muscle tone at the neck of the bladder to provide continence. In addition, sympathetic stimulation in males causes closure of the neck of the bladder during ejaculation (Janig, 1978; Shefchyk, 2002).

Defecation

The main structures involved in defecation are the internal sphincter (smooth muscle) and the external sphincter (skeletal muscle). Sympathetic preganglionic efferent fibres to the rectum originate in the lateral grey matter of lower thoracic and possibly upper lumbar spinal cord and synapse in the inferior mesenteric plexus before reaching the rectum (Kaiser and Ortega, 2002). Parasympathetic efferent fibres are distributed via pelvic splanchnic nerves probably originating from S1–S2. The skeletal muscle of the anal sphincter is supplied by the pudendal nerve (S2–S4). For review, see Kaiser and Ortega (2002).

Defecation, like micturition, is a spinal reflex under voluntary control. Sympathetic nerve supply to the internal sphincter is excitatory whereas parasympathetic and somatic are inhibitory. Reflex evacuation of the distended rectum occurs when there is a transected cord if sacral segments of the cord remain intact. For review, see Griffiths (2002) or Quinn and Shannon (2000).

Bladder and bowel dysfunction can result from neural lesions such as:

1. interruption to afferent nerves from bladder and rectum (e.g. tabes dorsalis)
2. interruption to both afferent and efferent nerves (e.g. diabetic neuropathy, tumours of cauda equina, sacral SN/NR compromise, traumatic cauda equina lesions)
3. disturbance to facilitatory and inhibitory pathways between sacral spinal cord and brain (e.g. tumours, spinal cord transection, multiple sclerosis).

Indications for testing cauda equina (S2 SN/NR)

Testing for conduction in S2 SN/NR is performed when the patient complains of recent onset of:

1. frequency of micturition (uncontrolled and urgent) or urinary retention. There may also be complaints of disturbances to defecation
2. paraesthesia and/or anaesthesia in the saddle area, i.e. the genital area and around the natal cleft.

Test procedures

The test procedure is the same as that described in the neurological examination for the SN/NR complex, above, but should include sensibility testing (light touch) of the saddle area. There are no further specific tests to identify a cauda equina lesion, or specifically, S2 SN/NR compromise, but neurological testing would determine the segmental level affected (in this case S2 dermatome and myotome).

Interpretation of test results

It is extremely important that the physiotherapist recognizes compromise of conduction in S2 SN/NR immediately (Coscia et al., 1994). Recognition of S2 SN/NR compromise is made from:

1. history – reports of disturbed micturition and symptoms of saddle paraesthesia/anaesthesia
2. decreased muscle power in S2 myotome (toe flexors, with possible involvement of multiple segments)
3. decreased sensibility in S2 dermatome (with possible involvement of multiple segments).

When cauda equina compromise is suspected, i.e. in the presence of history findings, with or without decreased muscle power or sensation in S2 distribution, the patient should immediately be referred back to the medical practitioner. These patients should not be treated, especially with manual therapy. Clinical judgement must be used to decide what information to provide to the patient at this stage. An explanation of the findings and possible implications should be conveyed but in a manner mindful of the fact that a definitive diagnosis has not yet been made.

Passive motion tests
J. Latimer and C.G. Maher

During the physical examination physiotherapists frequently perform assessment procedures that involve the manual application of forces to selected regions of the spine or periphery. These assessment procedures are commonly referred to as 'passive motion tests' and in the spine include tests of both passive accessory intervertebral movement or PAIVM and passive physiological intervertebral movement or PPIVM. During the performance of these tests the physiotherapist notes any report of symptoms by the patient and also makes a judgement about the quality of the movement produced, e.g. whether the movement feels stiffer than normal. This information is used to select patients suitable for manual therapy, to assist in establishing a clinical diagnosis, to select the region to be treated and the most appropriate treatment technique.

Prior to performing passive motion tests in patients with spinal pain, the physiotherapist will have observed the patient and performed active movement tests, tension tests and a neurological examination in patients with suspected neural compromise (e.g. spinal nerve or nerve root compromise). In patients with acute neurological signs the therapist may decide not to perform passive movement testing as the information gained from these tests will not help in isolating the symptomatic level, nor in selecting the best treatment. The neurological signs have already indicated the SN/NR involved and traction or sustained rotation is often the treatment of choice. Rarely are passive accessory mobilizations used to treat patients with acute nerve root compromise.

INDICATIONS (AND CONTRAINDICATIONS) FOR TESTING

Soft-tissue palpation may be performed for all patients with spinal pain. Passive motion testing however is only performed in patients with spinal pain when there is no known contraindication to the application of forces to the spine. Disease processes that affect the structural integrity of the vertebral column or conditions that may be exacerbated by movement of the spine are the two main concerns of the physiotherapist. Such contraindications may include malignancy involving the vertebral column, cauda equina compromise, recent fracture, active inflammatory or infective bone disease and acute SN/NR compromise. Special care should be taken when performing passive motion tests on patients with osteoporosis, spondylolysthesis and when assessing the cervical spine in patients with rheumatoid arthritis or vertebral artery signs/symptoms.

TEST PROCEDURES

Soft-tissue palpation

Before performing passive motion tests to the affected spinal region, the soft tissues are gently palpated to help gain the confidence of the patient, and to provide information regarding:

- temperature, sweating
- muscle spasm
- bony anomalies
- soft-tissue thickening, tightness, swelling (either paravertebrally or involving the interspinous space)
- pain.

Temperature and the presence of sweatiness are usually assessed using the backs of the fingers. Presence of increased skin temperature or sweating is a sign of inflammatory disease or involvement of the autonomic nervous system, and is sometimes used to assess the extent and recency of trauma to a joint. However, these signs are more useful for diseases affecting peripheral joints than the spine. In patients with non-specific spinal pain the presence of sweatiness may only provide information about the room temperature or the state of anxiety of the patient.

In the spine, muscle spasm and thickening or tightness of the paravertebral tissues is detected using the tips of the middle three fingers to palpate the area. Bony prominences and interspinous spaces are also palpated. During this examination the patient is also questioned about the reproduction of any symptoms. Because of the morphology of the spine it is generally not possible directly to palpate the structures that may be the source of symptoms and so the test cannot be used to identify the symptomatic structure.

Judgements made regarding the presence of muscle spasm or bony anomalies have been found to be relatively unreliable (Keating et al., 1990) and so some physiotherapists do not collect this information. However the test yields reliable information regarding pain and symptom reproduction (Keating et al., 1990; Maher and Adams, 1994). It is this aspect of the test that best helps indicate the vertebral levels to be tested using passive accessory and physiological tests (Phillips and Twomey, 1996). (It needs to be remembered, however, that a patient may present with referred tenderness and hence the site of dysfunction may be well removed from the tender or painful area.)

In the periphery, palpation of the symptomatic area is also performed prior to testing passive movements. Unlike the spine, this palpation may help identify the symptomatic structure, especially where the structure is readily accessible, for example, the medial collateral ligament of the knee or the supraspinatus tendon of the shoulder. Hence palpation in the periphery provides more diagnostically useful information than in the spine.

Passive motion testing

Following soft-tissue palpation the physiotherapist proceeds to test the passive motion of the symptomatic spinal region or peripheral joint. Detailed descriptions of how to perform these assessment procedures are available in many of the manual therapy texts (Kaltenborn, 1980; Grieve, 1984;

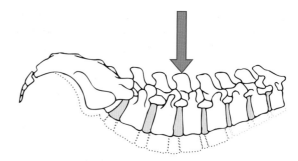

Figure 6.5 Posteroanterior pressure applied to the spinous process results in movement of the whole spine, even at levels quite distant to the site at which pressure is applied, although movement is emphasized at the level sustaining the force.

Maitland et al., 1986; Fig. 6.5) and therefore will not be described in detail here. Mechanical devices have been developed to measure more reliably the motion characteristics of the spine (Lee et al., 1995; Latimer et al., 1996a; Edmonston et al., 1998) but these are mainly used for research and will not be discussed here.

Passive accessory motion tests

There are two different types of information collected from passive accessory motion tests. The first is the patient's report of symptom behaviour in response to the test, while the second is the physiotherapist's perception of the quality of the movement that results from the forces applied during the test. The therapist makes a judgement regarding stiffness based on the amount of force applied and the amount of displacement that results. This stiffness is then compared with adjacent levels and the therapist's expectation of normal stiffness for that level, to determine whether abnormal stiffness is present. The patient is then reassessed to establish whether there has been any change in signs and symptoms. Because PAIVM testing and PAIVM treatment procedures are quite similar, improvement in the patient's condition following PAIVM testing is regarded by many physiotherapists as a good sign that PAIVM treatment will be successful.

Passive physiological intervertebral movement tests

To gain more specific information about the range of physiological movement available at various intervertebral segments, PPIVM techniques can be performed. Information gained from accessory movement testing of the spine is used to establish which levels to examine using PPIVM testing, although PPIVMs are also performed a few levels above and below the symptomatic spinal region. The results of active movement testing help select the physiological movements to be examined. For example, if a patient with low back pain is restricted in flexion and lateral flexion, these are the PPIVMs that are assessed. PPIVM techniques are primarily performed to identify intervertebral segments with restricted range of movement by comparison with the contralateral side and adjacent levels. It needs to be remembered, however, that different spinal levels will demonstrate varying ranges of motion, and that a unilateral movement restriction may affect movement of the contralateral side. Little information is gained from PPIVM testing in relation to symptoms. Following PPIVM testing the patient's signs and symptoms are reassessed and, if the patient appears improved, passive physiological mobilization techniques, such as rotation, flexion or lateral flexion, may be selected as a treatment.

Current use of passive motion tests

In the spine Passive motion tests are used by physiotherapists for a number of purposes in addition to establishing a clinical diagnosis and selecting treatment. The tests are also used to predict prognosis and to document patient recovery (Riddle, 1992). While these tests have been used for all of these purposes, current evidence would suggest that not all of these uses are in fact valid.

It is probably important to state first of all that passive motion tests are not useful in establishing a structural diagnosis to explain the patient's spinal pain. In fact current opinion is that it is not possible to make a structural diagnosis for the majority of patients with spinal pain even following a full clinical examination and the use of imaging and laboratory tests (Waddell et al., 1996). In the common case where a structural diagnosis cannot be made the patient is usually described as having non-specific spinal pain.

Caution needs to be employed when using the test results to document patient recovery.

Considerable evidence has shown that the patient's report of symptom provocation with the test is more reliable than the physiotherapist's perception of movement (Maher and Adams, 1994). It is probably more useful, therefore, to use information regarding the degree of symptoms reproduced on a passive motion test when deciding whether a patient has improved or not. Similarly the symptom response may be more helpful when selecting the region to be treated and the technique to apply. This point is taken up further under Interpretation of test results, below.

To date there is little experimental evidence to suggest that the presence of pain and/or movement abnormalities on passive motion tests is a prerequisite for a patient to benefit from manual therapy. DiFabio in 1992 reviewed the large number of clinical trials that have evaluated spinal manipulative therapy (SMT) to provide a profile of the type of patient that would respond to SMT. Interest-ingly, subjects with pain or reduced range on passive motion testing were not a feature of this group of patients, while factors related to the area and duration of pain and the presence of pending litigation were more indicative of whether a patient would improve following manipulation. Koes et al. (1993) came to a similar conclusion in a subgroup analysis of their manipulation clinical trial. These results suggest that passive motion tests may not help select patients likely to benefit from manipulation. Information from the history, such as central or bilateral low back pain of less than 1 month's duration and no pending litigation, best describes the patient likely to benefit from SMT.

Passive motion tests are probably of most value in helping to select a region to be treated and the technique to apply. The reproduction of symptoms, or the recognition of movement abnormalities such as abnormal stiffness during the performance of the test, is usually regarded as an indication that treatment should be directed to that spinal segment. The direction of application of the force may be inclined medially or laterally, and in a cephalad or caudad direction depending on which is most provocative in patients with non-irritable conditions, and least provocative in patients with irritable conditions. Frequently the manual test that revealed these findings would be used as the actual treatment technique. Improvement in the patient's signs and symptoms following a passive motion test is also regarded as a strong indication that the testing procedure should be used as a treatment at that level.

All this information must be considered in relation to the history findings. In this regard a useful guide is the concept of 'comparability' advocated by Maitland et al. (1986). This concept suggests that positive passive motion test results are only of clinical significance if they can logically be related to the patient's symptoms. For example, increased stiffness noted at T4 is not anatomically linked to a patient's buttock pain whereas tenderness and stiffness at L5 are anatomically related.

In summary, the decision to perform passive motion testing in patients with spinal disorders is based upon a proposed relationship between symptoms and abnormal passive movement or stiffness, and the hypothesized mechanism of action of mobilization and manipulation. The usefulness of passive motion testing in helping to isolate symptomatic structures, assisting in determining patient prognosis and predicting whether a patient is improving or not, has still to be investigated. It is unlikely that passive motion tests alone will provide this information, but they may prove useful when combined with information from other physical tests. These issues will be discussed further when examining the validity and reliability of passive motion testing.

In the periphery Passive motion testing is frequently performed on patients presenting with disorders of peripheral joints. In contrast to the spine, passive motion testing in the periphery can be used to help establish which structure is the source of symptoms. For example, in patients with knee pain and instability following an injury, there are a range of passive motion tests such as the Lachman test (Katz and Fingeroth, 1986), pivot shift and McMurray's test (Stratford and Binkley, 1995) that can be used to help establish what anatomical structure has been damaged. The Lachman and pivot shift tests investigate the integrity of the cruciate ligament, while the McMurray's test investigates the integrity of the menisci. Where possible, clinicians should consider the diagnostic accuracy of a test and also the pretest probability that the

condition is present when interpreting test results. For example, if based upon the history you believe a patient has a pretest probability of 50% that a knee condition is due to an anterior cruciate ligament (ACL) disruption, this converts to an odds ratio of 1:1. A positive Lachman test with a positive likelihood ratio (+LR) = 27 (Table 6.2) converts this pretest odds ratio to a posttest odds ratio of 27:1 or a posttest probability of 27/28 or approximately 96% that they have an ACL disruption. If the test is negative, the pretest odds ratio of 1:1 changes to a posttest odds ratio of 0.19:1 (negative likelihood ratio: −LR = 0.19) or a posttest probability of approximately 16%. For more detailed discussion of how to perform these analyses, see Chapter 4. The high diagnostic accuracy of the Lachman test combined with the high pretest probability of the condition make this test highly useful. In contrast, if the pretest probability of a

Table 6.2 Diagnostic accuracy of motion tests used in musculoskeletal physiotherapy

Condition to be detected	Physical examination test	+LR	−LR
Sacroiliac joint as a source of pain[a]	Gillet	1.3	0.8
	Thigh thrust	0.7	1.3
	Patrick's	0.8	1.9
	Mid sacral thrust	0.7	1.6
	Spring	1.2	0.7
	Sacral sulcus	1.0	0.6
Anterior cruciate ligament disruption[b]	Drawer test	8.2	0.62
	Lachman test	27	0.19
	Pivot shift test	51.7	0.18
Labral tear, glenohumeral joint[c]	Crank test	13	0.10
Meniscal tear[d]	McMurray test	7.3	0.74
	Apley compression	0.8	1.1
Carpal tunnel[e]	Tinel	1.1	0.9
	Phalen	1.3	0.8

+LR, positive likelihood ratio; −LR, negative likelihood ratio.
[a] Dreyfuss et al. (1996).
[b] Katz and Fingeroth (1986).
[c] Liu et al. (1996).
[d] Fowler and Lubliner (1989).
[e] Buch-Jaeger and Foucher (1994).

condition is very low or a test has low diagnostic accuracy (i.e. LR close to 1.0), testing will provide little useful information. Interestingly, if the pretest probability of a condition is very high, testing will also provide little additional information as it is already extremely likely that the patient has the condition.

Table 6.2 details the diagnostic accuracy of manual passive motion tests commonly used in musculoskeletal physiotherapy. The LRs for the Lachman and pivot shift tests are markedly different to 1.0 and so are useful tests to apply if there is uncertainty on diagnosis. In contrast an older test, the anterior drawer test, has a smaller LR and so a positive result to that test provides less information. When choosing between tests it makes sense to select the test with +LRs that are large and −LRs that are low.

Unfortunately, there are few data available about the sensitivity and specificity of passive motion tests of the spine. However there is some information available about SIJ tests. You can see from the LRs cited in Table 6.2 that they are all close to 1.0 and therefore unlikely to be useful in diagnosing the SIJ as a source of pain.

Similar to the situation with spinal pain, when a structural diagnosis cannot be made for a peripheral disorder and serious pathology such as cancer has been excluded as a source of symptoms, passive motion tests can be used as treatment procedures to decrease pain and increase range of movement. Where the pathology of the disorder has been clearly established these passive mobilization procedures may still be useful; however, they need to be applied with respect to the nature of the pathology present. For example, if the patient has an acute partial disruption of the medial collateral ligament, mobilization procedures have the potential to adversely affect the underlying pathology and would probably be avoided. In contrast these procedures are unlikely to affect the pathology of an osteoarthritic knee and can be safely used to address any associated pain or loss of range.

Kaltenborn (1980) has suggested an indirect method for determining the most appropriate direction in which to assess and treat peripheral joints. This method is mainly based on the work of MacConaill and Basmajian (1969) who theorized that the type of movement occurring between joint surfaces is primarily determined by the shape of the joint surfaces. MacConaill and Basmajian described joint surface movement as a combination of spin, slide and roll, a slide occurring when the same point on one surface contacts a new point on the opposing surface, and a roll occurring when equidistant points on two surfaces contact each other. They suggested that when a convex surface moves on a concave one the direction of the slide that accompanies the roll is in the opposite direction to that of the roll. Thus when the arm is moved into abduction Kaltenborn suggests that the convex humeral head not only rolls upwards but also slides downwards on the concave glenoid cavity. Therefore caudal gliding mobilization of the humeral head may be performed to improve abduction. Kaltenborn (1980) states that this indirect method of determining the direction of mobilization should be used when the patient has severe pain, the joint is very hypomobile or the examiner has insufficient expertise to feel the joint gliding movement.

Several studies (Poppen and Walker, 1976; Harryman et al., 1990, McClure and Flowers, 1992) have challenged this convex/concave rule of joint surface motion. It has been demonstrated that, during physiological movement, accessory movement occurs in the direction opposite to that predicted by the convex/concave rule (Poppen and Walker, 1976). It is most likely that the degree and direction of accessory motion are dependent on many factors other than the joint surface shape, including the external forces generated by the muscles and periarticular structures. It would appear sensible, therefore, that following a decision to include passive motion testing in the physical examination, all directions of passive motion be assessed.

INTERPRETATION OF TEST RESULTS

Reliability of passive motion tests

The degree to which we rely on the results of our passive motion tests in helping to select the treatment is dependent upon the amount of error involved in these clinical measurements. Measurements with large errors should not be used as the basis for important clinical decisions. This section will consider the error associated with these tests by reviewing the reliability and validity of these tests.

The reliability of manual assessment procedures is typically affected by the type of judgement made with the test. When the tests are used to make a judgement on factors such as joint range of motion, endfeel, compliance, the presence of muscle spasm, trigger points or bony anomalies, the tests yield results of poor to fair reliability. In contrast when the test is used to make judgements related to pain, the test yields results of good reliability (Keating et al., 1990; Maher and Adams, 1994). This result has been observed in the assessment of the cervical, thoracic and lumbar spine and the SIJ by physiotherapists, doctors, chiropractors and osteopaths (Maher and Latimer, 1992). Interestingly, while clinical experience does seem to result in higher intratester reliability, the more important interrater reliablity is not affected (Mior et al., 1990).

Much has been written about the poor interrater reliability of PAIVM testing (Matyas and Bach, 1985; Maher and Adams, 1994). Recently, attempts have been made at the University of Sydney to improve PAIVM assessment. Researchers have identified two groups of factors that affect posteroanterior (PA) stiffness measurement. The first group contains factors known to affect the physical stimulus value such as the surface on which the test is performed, the position of the patient at the time of the test, the subject's breathing pattern, the presence of spinal muscle activity and the frequency and magnitude of the stiffness testing oscillations used (e.g. see Shirley et al., 1999; Squires et al., 2001). The second group contains factors known to affect a clinician's perception of stiffness, although the physical stimulus remains unchanged (e.g. see Maher and Adams, 1996a, b; Maher et al., 2002). These include the grip used by the therapist when performing the test, whether the therapist performs the test with the eyes open or closed and the number of loading cycles used to make a stiffness judgement. Knowledge of these factors has resulted in the development of a reliable protocol for PA stiffness testing (Chiradejnant et al., 2002). Factors should be controlled as described below.

The patient should be tested:

- on the same plinth surface
- at the same stage in the respiratory cycle (e.g. while breath-holding at functional residual capacity).

The therapist should perform the test using:

- the same testing grip (i.e. either the pisiform or thumb grip)
- the same visual state (i.e. either with the eyes open or closed)
- a standardized testing force (e.g. applying a maximum testing force of 120 N)
- a standardized testing frequency (using a metronome)
- a standardized testing angle (e.g. applying the force perpendicular to the plinth surface)
- three loading cycles to make a stiffness judgement.

In the future this testing protocol may be further revised to suggest that clinicians compare the patient's lumbar stiffness to a reference spring of known stiffness before making their judgements. Such a method has been demonstrated to improve interrater reliability and accuracy significantly (Maher et al., 1998). Development of the reference spring is currently underway at the University of Sydney.

It is important to note that few tests used in health care have perfect reliability and in fact some important judgements made by health workers have surprisingly low reliability. For example, several studies (Sidor et al., 1993; Siebenrock and Gerber, 1993) have shown that shoulder fracture classification by orthopaedic surgeons and radiologists has similar reliability to manual PA stiffness assessment performed in a non-standardized manner. None of the physical assessment procedures used to examine the spine have perfect reliability but rather range from very good to poor reliability. Where instruments such as an inclinometer or flexible rule are used to measure the range of movement of the spine, very good reliability can be attained (Maher et al., 2001). Visual estimation of spinal range and posture can yield measurements of poor reliability, as can reflex and sensation testing and manual muscle testing. The reality is that all the information collected in the physical assessment contains some error and this should be reflected in how information is used to make clinical decisions. Against this background it seems sensible that measurements with a large error should not be used as the sole basis for important clinical decisions.

The results of the studies on the reliability of manual assessment procedures suggest that, if a clinical decision is to be made based upon a single test, the more reliable pain provocation tests should be used in preference to other manual tests. However a clinical decision is rarely made using the results of one test. Usually an overall impression is made based upon the results of a pool of tests. Unfortunately there have been few studies that have examined the reliability of judgements based upon the results of several tests.

One study, that of Cibulka et al. (1988), found that judgements on the presence or absence of SIJ dysfunction were highly reliable ($\kappa = 0.88$) when the physiotherapists based their judgement upon a number of SIJ mobility and alignment tests adopting a decision rule that required at least three of the four tests to be positive. This strategy may also be applied to other regions of the spine. For example, if passive motion tests are positive at both L4 and L5, but more of the passive motion tests are positive at L5, then treatment should be directed to L5. Further, tests that reproduce the patient's symptoms (which are more reliable and so contain less error) are probably an even stronger suggestion that treatment should be directed to that level.

Validity of passive motion tests

Several studies have examined the validity of manual assessment procedures. For the purposes of this text, however, only the validity of PAIVM testing will be considered. While Maitland (1986) describes the test as one of accessory intervertebral movement, the true nature of the movement produced by the test is somewhat different. While the tests do produce movement of the contact vertebra relative to its starting position, not all of this movement could be intervertebral movement. Lee and Moseley (1991) have measured PA movement of 15 mm of the contact vertebra when a PA force of 150 N is applied to L3. If this movement is purely intervertebral movement, i.e. movement of the tested level on its neighbour, then significant encroachment of the cauda equina would result, because the diameter of the lumber dural sac is of the same magnitude, being approximately 15 mm (Penning, 1992).

The spine is in fact a series of linked segments and so it is to be expected that when a PA force is applied to one lumbar vertebra, movement of the whole lumbar region would occur. Lee et al. (1996) have modelled the response of the spine to the application of 100 N of PA force applied to the L3 spinous process. The model predicts that this force would produce anterior translation of the target vertebra relative to adjacent vertebrae of less than 1 mm with approximately 1° of extension. Lee and Evans (1997) have confirmed that the magnitude of vertebral translation when a PA force is applied to the spine is extremely small. In this *in vivo* study, a series of radiographic measurements were made while applying a PA force of 150 N to L4. A mean extension of 1.2° and a translation of less than 0.2 mm at the L4–L5 segment resulted. Both these studies suggest that the magnitude of intervertebral movement occurring during PA pressure testing is very small and hence likely to be difficult to detect. Figure 6.5 represents spinal extension occurring in response to PA pressure.

It seems likely therefore that PAIVM tests cannot be validly used to make inferences about intervertebral motion. However this does not preclude the tests from being used to make a judgement of the stiffness of the complex movement that results from the PA pressure. Because the movement is complex and only marginally related to intervertebral movement it may be more useful to talk of 'tests of PA stiffness' rather than 'passive acessory intervertebral movement tests'.

It is also important to consider whether the passive accessory motion tests are useful in discriminating asymptomatic subjects from symptomatic subjects. Sturesson et al. (1989) investigated the range of motion of the SIJ in subjects with and without SIJ pain. The study used tantalum markers implanted in the sacrum and ilium and stereophotogrammetric analysis and found that the range of motion was in fact quite small, with sagittal rotation ranging from 0.8 to 3.9° and movement between joint surfaces ranging from 0.1 to 1.6 mm.

The study found that there was no difference in range of motion between the symptomatic and asymptomatic SIJs and so raises questions about the value of performing clinical SIJ mobility tests to screen patients for SIJ dysfunction.

In the lumbar spine it appears that, while the PA pressure test may not be able to discriminate between symptomatic and asymptomatic subjects when performed on one occasion, if the test is used to measure the same patient during two different pain states some change in PA stiffness may be detected (Latimer et al., 1996b). One study that measured PA stiffness in patients when they presented with significant back pain and again when their low back pain was 80% better found that PA stiffness decreased by 1.21 N/mm between tests 1 and 2. A group of sex- and age-matched subjects without back pain failed to change. The mean reduction in stiffness was approximately 8% of the original stiffness value; however some subjects decreased their stiffness by up to 37%. This magnitude of change would probably be detected manually.

Finally it is useful to consider whether these PAIVM tests, when compared with other tests used to identify which vertebral levels are symptomatic, give the same results. Jull et al. (1988) found that a manipulative physiotherapist using PAIVM testing was able to identify correctly all symptomatic zygapophyseal joints that had previously been identified using a radiologically controlled diagnostic block. The physiotherapist also used these manual tests to reproduce the patient's pain and it may have been this more reliable pain information rather than information about spinal compliance that contributed to the high success in identification. This suggestion is supported by Phillips and Twomey (1996) who compared a manipulative physiotherapist's diagnosis of the symptomatic level to the level established by a unilevel lumbar spinal block procedure. This study found that when the physiotherapist used the patient's verbal response during PAIVM testing to identify the symptomatic level there was 100% sensitivity in diagnosing the symptomatic level. In contrast, when the physiotherapist did not attend to the patient's verbal response but only to what the physiotherapist could feel during the performance of the test, sensitivity fell to 60%.

Considered together, these studies provide strong support for the suggestion that the verbal patient response is probably the most valuable piece of information to collect during PAIVM testing.

IMPLICATIONS FOR TREATMENT

Consideration of the reliability, validity and sensitivity of passive motion tests suggests that, at present, treatment decisions should be guided more by symptom reproduction than by the perceived quality of movement. The first treatment option should be to direct treatment to the most painful spinal level (unless of course that level is not anatomically capable of producing the patient's symptoms). If this treatment strategy is unsuccessful then the less reliable stiffness findings can be used to select the level to treat but the physiotherapist needs to acknowledge that the stiffness information is less reliable, i.e. more error-prone, and so time may be wasted directing treatment to the wrong level.

Because the most effective treatment dose is yet to be determined for manual treatments the appropriateness of dose can only be established through close monitoring of the patient's condition. Following each repetition of the mobilization the patient should be reassessed and the dosage altered accordingly. The duration of each repetition is best determined by the patient's pain response and the spinal compliance perceived by the therapist while performing the mobilization. If a patient with an irritable condition complains that the symptoms are worsening or the therapist perceives an increase in tissue compliance, then the mobilization should be halted and the patient reassessed. If during the mobilization there is an improvement or no change in the patient's status then the mobilization is usually continued for 30–45 s.

In patients with non-irritable conditions pain is often provoked while performing the mobilization. The mobilization is generally continued until the patient reports that the symptoms have significantly changed, the therapist perceives a change in stiffness or, in the absence of these factors, 45–60 s has elapsed. The number of repetitions to be performed is usually based on reassessment of signs and symptoms following one repetition of mobilization. Generally if the patient is continuing to improve the repetition should be repeated. However, when treating a patient on the first occasion, it is safest to adhere to the guidelines suggested by Maitland (1986). In this instance two repetitions are given to patients with irritable conditions, while patients with non-irritable conditions may be treated with three to four repetitions.

One parameter of treatment dose, the grade of movement, can be quantified reliably if defined in relation to range (Matyas and Bach, 1985) and the pain response rather than a perceived resistance curve. If this approach is adopted then the dose of treatment can be recorded and this allows meaningful communication between therapists.

CONCLUSION

Passive motion tests are widely used by physiotherapists to select patients likely to benefit from mobilization, to formulate a clinical diagnosis and to help select the region and the most appropriate form of treatment for patients with both spinal and peripheral musculoskeletal disorders. Many studies have examined the reliability of these tests; however the more difficult task of establishing validity has been largely avoided. Physiotherapists need to consider that decisions based on the patient's pain response to passive motion testing are likely to provide a more accurate guide to patient management.

Muscle testing

R. Herbert

This section will examine some principles underlying clinical testing of muscle strength and muscle length.

TESTING MUSCLE STRENGTH

Clinicians test muscle strength both to provide information for diagnosis, and to assess the effectiveness of intervention aimed at increasing muscle strength.

Diagnosis

People develop weakness for many different reasons. Sometimes the cause of the weakness may not be obvious from the person's history. Then a careful physical examination can provide clues, especially about the distribution of weakness, which can aid diagnosis.

Manual muscle testing is widely used for diagnostic purposes, probably because the simplicity of the test procedures means that many muscle groups can be tested in a short period of time. A number of different manual muscle-testing protocols are in wide clinical use (Lamb, 1985), but all use similar criteria to assign grades based on the ability of the muscles to contract through range and against gravity or manual resistance. Some protocols are designed to test individual muscles (Daniels and Worthingham, 1986), whereas others test muscle groups (Kendall et al., 1993). Although tests of individual muscles are desirable for diagnostic purposes, the validity of assumptions underlying procedures which profess to test individual muscles is dubious; in reality it is often difficult to differentiate the weakness of one muscle from weakness of other muscles from the same muscle group. For this reason, it would seem more appropriate to test muscle groups, rather than individual muscles.

Studies of the reliability of manual muscle testing suggest that test–retest and intertherapist reliability is moderate (see Lamb, 1985 for a brief review). Typically, when several therapists use manual muscle testing to measure the strength of the same patients they agree on 50 or 60% of their measures, and they agree to within one grade on more than 90% of their measures. Given this finding, and that some of the manual muscle test grades (especially grades III and IV) encompass an enormous range of strengths (Munsat, 1990), it would appear that manual muscle testing is only likely to be useful for detecting gross muscle weakness or for detecting large changes in muscle strength over time. This may be useful for diagnosing peripheral nerve lesions. Manual muscle testing is not sufficiently sensitive or reliable to detect subtle weakness or small changes in strength, so it is not a suitable tool for assessing the response to therapeutic interventions.

Muscle testing is used for another purpose which arguably also falls under the heading of diagnosis. Tests of muscle can help localize pain-causing lesions. In particular, muscle testing is often used to determine if a muscle is the source of a person's pain (Corrigan and Maitland, 1983). For example, if a person's history is indicative of a hamstring muscle tear, a therapist may choose to see if pain is elicited with a strong isometric knee flexor contraction. The rationale is that if the muscle or its tendon is a source of pain, muscle contraction will stress the injured tissues and reproduce the person's pain. Other pain-sensitive structures will experience relatively little stress, and therefore this strategy should not elicit pain if tissues other than the muscle are responsible for the person's pain. Clinicians (and even some academics) know, however, that there is a tendency for isometric tests of muscle to produce false positives, because muscle contraction may stress other (non-muscle) structures. In particular, strong muscle contractions compress joint surfaces and stress ligaments. Thus, when testing most populations, positive findings should be considered cautiously, but negative findings can be considered quite strong evidence that the tested muscles are not the source of pain.

Quantifying the effect of intervention

It can be useful to measure muscle strength to determine if training has been aimed at appropriate muscle groups and is appropriate in terms of intensity and achieving clients' goals. Also, measurements of muscle strength can be useful for motivating people to comply with training protocols in cases of prolonged rehabilitation.

Three criteria should be applied to determine the suitability of any strength test:

1. Reliability. The test must be sufficiently reliable to distinguish 'signal' from 'noise'. That is, it must be possible to be confident that observed changes which are of a clinically significant magnitude are not simply measurement error. Typically, with training, people can be expected to experience strength gains of 1–3% per day (McDonagh and Davies, 1984). This means that, if measurements of strength are to be made weekly, they must be able to detect reliably changes in strength of between about 4% and 20%. The reliability of many clinical strength measurement procedures has been reviewed by Mayhew and Rothstein (1985) and Bohannon (1990). Most instrumented measures of muscle strength have adequate reliability.

2. Validity. Validity refers to the degree to which useful inferences can be drawn from test measures. When physiotherapists test strength to monitor progression, their concern usually is to make inferences about the ability of muscles to produce tension for the performance of motor tasks. For example, measurements of knee extensor strength following knee reconstruction are really only of interest in so far as they tell us something about how well the person is able to use his or her knee extensor muscles for tasks such as running, jumping and kicking.

    There have been very few studies which directly tackle the issue of the degree to which measures of muscle strength provide information about the ability of muscles to generate tension during the performance of motor tasks. One study which provides some insights to this issue simply looked at the relationship between a number of different measures (e.g. isokinetic, hydraulic and free-weight measures) of bench-press strength (Hortobagyi et al., 1989). This study found that, after measurement errors were accounted for, there was a moderate correlation between different measures of strength.

That is, people who performed well on one measure often, but not always, performed well on other measures of strength. To the extent that the different tests agreed they could be said to be measuring the same thing, but there was not perfect agreement between tests. This means that proficiency in one test may partly reflect a specific proficiency at the type of muscle contraction required for that test, rather than in some generalizable strength parameter.

There are still not enough data to be certain about the degree of generality which can be attached to most currently used measures of strength. However, it is probably reasonable to conclude provisionally that any reliable measure of muscle strength will provide some measure of functional strength (i.e. people with muscle weakness will tend to perform poorly on most measures of the strength of their weak muscles). However, the more closely the testing conditions resemble the task of interest, the more valid the test is likely to be (i.e., the more likely inferences about the ability of the muscles to generate tension during the performance of those tasks). The implication is that, in so far as is practical, testing procedures should employ muscle contractions that resemble (in terms of joint angles, joint angular velocities and postures) the strength-limited tasks of interest.

3. Practicalities. Some measuring tools are quick and easy to use, whereas others are time-consuming and useful for testing only a few muscle groups. The former are obviously preferred.

There are many procedures used by clinical therapists for measuring muscle strength. The next section briefly discusses the reliability, validity and practicalities of four of the most widely used procedures for measuring muscle strength: hand-held dynamometers, isokinetics, manual muscle testing and functional tests.

Hand–held dynamometers

The available literature suggests that hand-held dynamometers provide a highly reliable way of measuring isometric strength (for review, see Bohannon, 1990). The exception is when the subject being tested is capable of producing such large forces that the tester has difficulty keeping the dynamometer still (Bohannon, 1990). Hand-held dynamometers are suitable for measuring the strength of most large peripheral muscle groups, and some specialized hand-held dynamometers are available for testing smaller peripheral muscle groups, such as the muscles of the hand.

The appeal of these devices is that they can provide a highly reliable measure of isometric muscle strength with little more difficulty than manual muscle testing. The major drawback is that they can only be used to measure isometric strength, and (as discussed above, under the heading of validity) it is not clear how well inferences can be made from tests of this type to the ability of muscle to generate tension for task performance.

In the author's opinion, the reliability and ease of use of hand-held dynamometers make them the tool of choice for a wide range of clinical situations in which it is necessary to measure muscle strength.

Isokinetics

Isokinetic testing machines enable the measurement of torque produced by muscles as they perform constant-velocity contractions. These devices have become very popular as testing tools. Perhaps the most useful feature of isokinetic machines is their high reliability – typically, test–retest reliability is sufficiently high that measured changes of as a little as 10% can be confidently considered to be real changes in strength, rather than measurement error (for review, see Mayhew and Rothstein, 1985).

Despite their popularity, however, isokinetic machines have some distinct disadvantages. At a technical level, isokinetic torque measures are prone to a number of artifacts (particularly inertial artifacts caused by unwanted accelerations of the limb during testing; Winter et al., 1981; Sapega et al., 1982; Herzog, 1988), although these can now be dealt with reasonably satisfactorily with features such as preloading (e.g. Gravel et al., 1988; for a fuller discussion of these issues the reader is referred to Mayhew and Rothstein, 1985). More significantly, it can be argued that isokinetic testing conditions are far removed from the way in which muscles are required to contract for the performance of everyday tasks, and that therefore isokinetic tests may provide a less valid test of the ability to generate muscle tension during the performance of meaningful motor tasks. Equally problematic is the inflexibility of isokinetic devices – they do not lend themselves easily to testing of many different muscle groups, and few clinics can afford to have a suite of isokinetic machines specifically configured for every key muscle group.

Manual muscle testing

The reliability of manual muscle testing was discussed above, where it was noted that manual muscle testing provides an insensitive and only moderately reliable test of muscle strength. Though convenient, manual muscle testing is unlikely to be sufficiently sensitive and reliable to provide a satisfactory measure of the changes in strength of a magnitude that are often of interest clinically.

Functional tests

Functional measures of muscle strength are probably widely used in practice, but they have not often been described in the literature, and they have rarely been subject to experimental investigation. With a little bit of imagination, simple functional tasks such as stepping on to a block or standing up from a chair can easily be turned into a measure of strength. For example, a measure of the strength of lower limb muscle groups could be obtained by asking the person being tested to step up on blocks of increasing height (Fig. 6.6). The highest block on to which the person could step provides an indirect measure of the torque-generating capacity of muscles of the lower limb.

The types of muscle contraction utilized in these tests explicitly resemble those required for motor task performance, so they have a face validity – it is likely that these functional tests provide the best possible validity for this sort of inference. On the negative side, the reliability of these tests is not known. Reliability of functional tests probably varies with the functional task being tested. Also, functional tests demand that therapists are able to ensure that subjects do not utilize compensatory movement strategies which might enable successful task performance without generating large

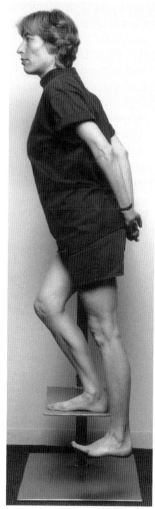

Figure 6.6 Functional exercises such as climbing stairs can be progressed by increasing the difficulty of the task, for example by increasing the height of the step.

forces with weak muscle groups. For example, when testing lower limb strength by testing the height of the step on to which subjects can stand, it is necessary to prevent subjects throwing their arms forward and pushing-off with the contralateral leg (this can be done by asking subjects to hold their hands behind their backs, keeping the contralateral knee extended and standing on the heel of the contralateral leg). Only then can the therapist be sure that the lower limb muscles of the test leg are being tested. Lastly, because these tests often test a number of muscle groups simultaneously they provide relatively little information about which muscle groups are weak, and sometimes this information is useful when structuring training.

MEASURING THE LENGTH OF MUSCLES

Measurement of muscle length really involves testing whether muscle–tendon units are short or inextensible. A number of clinical observations may be suggestive of muscle shortening, but it is often not possible to be certain that adaptive shortening of muscle (as distinct from other tissues which cross the joint) is responsible for a loss of passive joint range of motion. For example, it would be reasonable to suspect that soleus muscle shortening is responsible for a loss of dorsiflexion range of motion if the patient feels a stretch in the region of the soleus as the ankle is dorsiflexed, or if the tendon and belly of the soleus muscle become palpably very taut as the ankle is dorsiflexed to plantargrade with the knee flexed. When these conditions are met it is reasonable to hypothesize that the soleus muscle is short. However, even in these rather restrictive circumstances it is not possible definitively to implicate a short soleus muscle because it is still possible that the major limitation to joint range lies in other muscles or periarticular connective tissues.

In contrast, useful measures of the degree of shortening can be made on muscles which cross two or more mobile joints (see, for example, Harvey et al., 1994). These muscles can be stretched over one joint (e.g. the knee can be extended to lengthen gastrocnemius) so that the muscle becomes the sole or dominant restraint to movement at its other joint (i.e. with the knee extended, the gastrocnemius can become the major restraint to dorsiflexion). If the muscle does provide the dominant limitation to range of motion at the second joint, the test can logically be said to be a test of the muscle's length.

Note that, almost by definition, these tests can be performed in two ways. For example, the hamstring muscles' length can be tested either by measuring hip flexion with the knee extended or by measuring knee extension with the hip flexed (in this particular example the therapist would need to differentiate between the limitation provided by the hamstrings muscles and those due to neural

tension). In either case, the position of one joint must be standardized before the range of motion at the other joint can be measured. Thus, if hamstrings length is measured by flexing the hip and then measuring the amount of knee extension range, the hip must first be placed in a reproducible position (say, 90° of flexion), or else the final measure of knee extension range will not be reproducible.

In able-bodied people or people with only subtle muscle shortening, the logic of these tests does not necessarily hold up – it may not be possible to lengthen the muscle over one joint sufficiently to cause it to become the major limitation to range of motion at the second joint. Then the test is no more rigorous a test of muscle length than the tests of single joint muscles, discussed above. Fortunately it is possible to test whether the test does sufficiently lengthen the muscle of interest. This is done after measuring the length of the muscle, by releasing the stretch from the first joint (e.g. after measuring dorsiflexion with the knee extended as a measure of gastrocnemius shortening, flex the knee). If this causes the measured range to increase substantially (i.e. if there is then an increase in dorsiflexion range) the tester can be confident that the test did put sufficient stretch on the muscle to cause it to become the major limitation to the measured movement, and therefore that the measured range was a reasonable measure of the length of the muscle. This is an important part of the procedure for measuring muscle length, because the test is only valid if the muscle can be shown to be a major limitation to the movement tested.

The reliability of many commonly used procedures for measuring muscle length has received little attention in the experimental literature. However there is little reason to suspect that they should be any less reliable than other joint range-of-motion measures. Most joint range-of-motion measures have an acceptable to high level of reliability (for reviews, see Miller, 1985; Gadjosik and Bohannon, 1987). Any measure of joint range can be made more reliable by using a standardized procedure (Gadjosik and Bohannon, 1987), marking bony landmarks (Fish and Wingate, 1985), and (where practical and for passive measures) by standardizing the force applied by the therapist to the joint (Brand, 1985; Ada and Herbert, 1988).

Motor performance: evaluation and measurement

J. Carr and R. Shepherd

Lesions of the musculoskeletal system affect the sensorimotor apparatus, i.e. the effector part of the system through which we act to achieve our goals, and they therefore affect the way movements are performed. The effects can be far-reaching because of the natural coupling between body segments; i.e. if a lesion affects one segment or the link between two segments (a joint), then the movement of other segments along the linkage will also be affected. In this way, during walking, for example, a stiff ankle joint will affect not only movement at the ankle but will also affect motion at other joints, such as hip extension of that limb during stance phase.

The evaluation of human movement is made complex not only by the dynamics of the segmental linkage but also by the complexity of muscle activations, which is illustrated by the differing actions of monoarticular and multiarticular muscles and by the synergic relationships between muscle groups. Furthermore, muscle activation patterns (including postural adjustments) are specific to both task and the context in which the action is performed. The only way one can be certain that treatment directed toward local signs and symptoms (e.g. pain, joint stiffness or muscle weakness) is effective in improving the performance of a functional action is by measuring performance of that action in some way.

Evaluation of functional actions is increasingly being used both as a guide to intervention and as a measure of outcome. Individuals who experience musculoskeletal lesions, whether as a result of a sporting injury, a car accident, a back injury at work, a degenerative disease or surgery, attend the physiotherapist for relief of pain or stiffness as a means of improving the performance of actions critical to their daily lives. A major objective of physiotherapy for these individuals is, therefore,

to regain optimal performance of actions that have become dysfunctional.

Physiotherapy, however, has traditionally utilized methods for relieving pain, increasing joint range and strengthening muscles with the assumption that improved motor performance would naturally follow. Initial evaluation has been concentrated in assessments of relatively local phenomena such as range of painfree motion and strength of individual muscles. Tests of changes occurring during and at the conclusion of treatment have been similarly based.

We would argue that measuring performance of an action in its entirety is more relevant to functional ability than testing an isolated muscle or group of muscles as they act over one joint. Hence, the effect of intervention to decrease pain and stiffness is not only examined through measurement of specific local phenomena but also, in the context of the actions the individual wishes to carry out, through measurement of each action itself: for example, walking, stair climbing and descent, jogging, swimming, standing up and sitting down, reaching toward an object, grasping and manipulating different objects in order to carry out specific intentions.

Evaluation involves an analysis of the performance of any critical actions with which the individual is having difficulty because of the lesion. It is either based on observation, i.e. qualitative and subjective, or it involves some form of measurement, in which case it is quantitative and objective.

OBSERVATIONAL EVALUATION

Evaluation involves observing the individual performing the relevant action in order to compare performance against a biomechanical model. Only the kinematic features of an action, such as angular displacements at joints and linear displacements of body parts, are readily observable and for practical purposes it is these that can be matched against what would be expected for optimal (effective) performance. Velocity and force components underlying the kinematic pattern can only be inferred.

Simple visual observations lack reliability, accuracy and some validity, although for a therapist with an understanding of biomechanics, they can provide a guide for the development of a treatment or training programme. Nevertheless, Malouin (1995) has pointed out in a study of gait analyses, in which therapists' observational analyses of walking were compared with a biomechanical analysis, that there can be considerable discrepancy between the therapists' assessments of their own capabilities and their real ability. As a means of demonstrating a change in a patient's performance, objective and meaningful measures are required.

MEASUREMENT

A critical development in scientific rehabilitation practice has been the increasing development and use of valid and reliable measurement tools to provide the therapist, patient and health provider with accurate information. Such data provide an effective guide to treatment and training as well as quantitative methods of evaluating outcome.

Clinical practice includes the regular collecting of accurate and objective data about performance of actions most relevant to the individual's everyday life. These data drive the design and modification of the individual's training programme and, when outcome data from a number of different individuals are collected, they provide evidence that enables the ongoing development of evidence-based and best practice.

There are several methods of measuring motor performance. Some give information about the biomechanics of the entire action, others specific details of critical features of the action, such as how long it takes an individual to walk a certain distance. A selection of available tests for measuring aspects of major functional actions, which are reliable and valid, is described below. As with any

method of measurement, standardization of technique is necessary for a measure to be reliable.

The biomechanics of an action can be examined using a variety of tools. Smith (1990) describes many of the methods of kinematic, kinetic and muscle activation measures that have value in clinical measurement of motor performance. He illustrates how the equipment needed for measurement ranges from the simple and inexpensive (tape measure, stopwatch, camera) to the complex and expensive (electrogoniometers, accelerometers, forceplate, two- and three-dimensional imaging systems).

Gait, sit-to-stand and the ability to balance are motor functions whose performance is commonly measured in the clinic, by biomechanical methods where there are the necessary facilities, and by other valid and reliable tests.

Gait

Spatiotemporal variables of walking, such as stride length or width, can be measured using a stride analyser. They can also be measured (with somewhat less accuracy) by using non-permanent marking pens on the patient's heels, or by chalking the soles of the feet and having the patient walk on a darker surface. Time taken to walk a prescribed distance (e.g. 10 m) is measured with a stopwatch. Walking velocity is calculated as distance/time (m/s). To avoid the effects of acceleration and deceleration, the subject is timed only over the middle 10 m of a 14-m walkway. The 6- and 12-min walk tests, developed as tests of fitness, provide a measure of the distance which can be walked in a given time. Compared to biomechanical measures, these are somewhat indirect tests of locomotion yet they have been found to reflect improvement in performance (Wagenaar and Beck, 1992; Dean et al., 2000). If reliably performed, results of these tests constitute valid measures of change.

Although motion analysis utilizing videotaping of performance is often used to generate extensive and complex data about kinematic, and, if used with a forceplate, kinetic components, the use of videotape also enables quite simple measurements to be taken. A transparency placed over a still image on a videoscreen enables joint angles to be measured, and when measured frame by frame, angular velocity can be calculated. Van Vliet (1988) described the methodological details of this technique of deriving kinematic details of walking. Still photography (and a protractor) can also be used to measure joint angles and changes over time (Ada and Canning, 1990).

Sit-to-stand

This action can be measured using the sit-to-stand item of a functional scale, the Motor Assessment Scale (Carr et al., 1985). The Timed Up-and-Go Test was developed as a measure of balance. The patient stands up from a chair, walks 3 m (10 ft), turns around and returns to the chair (Podsialo and Richardson, 1991). Time taken to complete the test is measured with a stopwatch.

Balance

There are several methods of testing balance. Different tests, however, do not necessarily measure the same aspect of balance. The postural adjustments that comprise balance are specific to the action being performed and the environment. For balance in standing, some tests analyse the ability to stand still; others test the ability to move about within the limits of stability; others test the response to support surface perturbations. The Functional Reach Test measures the difference between arm's length and maximum reach forward (Duncan et al., 1990). It is a more dynamic test than those which measure the ability to stand still. Other functional tests are the Repetitive Reach Test (Goldie et al., 1990) and the Timed Up-and-Go Test. The Step Test (Hill et al., 1996) can be used to evaluate the ability to support and balance the body mass on one lower limb while stepping up and down on to a 7.5 cm block placed 5 cm in front of parallel feet. The number of steps is counted. Balance in sitting can be measured by the sitting balance item of the Motor Assessment Scale. Biomechanical tests utilize forceplate and high-speed camera.

Functional muscle strength

The amount of force generated by a muscle (or muscle group) is typically measured using a hand-held dynamometer or an isokinetic dynamometer. A more functional measure of the overall extensor force produced in a lower limb is the closed kinetic chain Lateral Step Test (Ross, 1997), which measures the number of step-ups which can be performed in a given period of time.

Self-assessments and self-efficacy scales

These provide patient input regarding the training programme together with factors such as perception of severity of symptoms and quality of life.

INTERPRETATION OF TEST RESULTS AND INTERVENTION

Increasing numbers of biomechanical and motor control studies are enabling the collection of normative data about common everyday, work-related and sporting actions. In addition, a growing number of studies of disabled individuals, utilizing biomechanical and other methods of measurement, help clarify the nature of the movement dysfunction associated with different types of lesion. Such information can enable the therapist to predict the likely dysfunction resulting from particular injuries or surgical interventions and, where possible, institute procedures to prevent unwanted adaptations such as muscle-length changes.

Studies of disabled motor performance include reports of walking and running patterns of individuals with lower limb amputations (Inman et al., 1981; Enoka et al., 1982; Winter and Sienko, 1988). Walking, stair ascent and descent and sit-to-stand have been studied in individuals following knee replacement surgery (Andriacchi et al., 1982; Weinstein et al., 1986; Jevsevar et al., 1993) and medial meniscectomy (Moffet et al., 1993), and in subjects with ACL-deficient knees (Andriacchi and Birac, 1993).

The measurement of motor performance, together with input from the patient, informs the therapist of the motor deficit and any adaptive motor behaviours the individual may be using, for example, to avoid pain or lessen the force produced over a joint. Using quantitative measures, a study of individuals discharged from rehabilitation after total hip replacement (THR) (Westwood, 1993) described both the biomechanical deficits and the adaptive motor behaviours during sit-to-stand. The fact that these individuals were taking little weight through the affected lower limb (measured with forceplate) and could only stand up using their arms to augment vertical propulsion suggests that discharge from rehabilitation without follow-up training was premature.

Other researchers have reported that many individuals following THR are discharged with residual muscle weakness and functional deficit (Kerslake et al., 1987; Harris and Sledge, 1990; Long et al., 1993; Shih et al., 1994; Drabsch et al., 1998). It is assumed that performance of functional activities will spontaneously improve once pain and stiffness at the hip have been reduced. Improvement may not, however, be so straightforward. The individual has usually spent many years developing adaptive motor patterns to enable some form of mobility to be maintained in the presence of severe symptoms and these habitual adaptations are likely to be maintained after surgery, irrespective of site.

Following lower limb surgery for long-standing joint dysfunction, the value of measuring performance of walking, sit-to-stand and balance lies in clearly identifying those individuals who need to continue with an exercise programme postdischarge. The same can be said following upper limb surgery, when the ability to reach, i.e. to place the hand in the appropriate part of the workplace for manipulative actions, has to be regained.

Several recent studies demonstrate the value of using measures of functional performance to provide a method of evaluating the relative outcomes of different rehabilitative strategies and the effects of training programmes. A study following THR and discharge (Drabsch et al., 1998) utilized a combination of measures. These included standardized observation, step and stride length measures using markers on subjects' heels, time taken to walk a standardized distance using a stopwatch and the amount of weight through affected limb during sit-to-stand with calibrated bathroom scales. These measures showed that subjects improved their performance of walking and sit-to-stand after a 6-week task-specific training programme that concentrated on the two actions of interest.

A randomized controlled trial of elderly individuals following hip fracture (Sherringon and Lord, 1997) used a selection of specific and functional motor performance measures to test the effects of a home-based exercise programme on strength, postural control and mobility. These measures included a measure of quadriceps strength, a version of the step test, a functional measure of lower limb strength, the Functional Reach Test for balance and stopwatch-measured time to walk a prescribed distance and cadence.

Baker and colleagues (1991) have reported the use of a footswitch system, myometer and goniometer in analysing the gait of subjects recovering from fractured neck of femur. The trained group, who had completed a period of gait training on a treadmill, was significantly superior to the control group in measures of double-support phase, stance/ swing ratio, strength of hip flexion and abduction and of knee extension. These findings provide a valuable measure of outcome, suggesting that treadmill training should become part of the rehabilitation programme of such individuals, with a high degree of probability that any individual with motor dysfunction following hip surgery may also benefit.

Despite successful remediation of symptoms such as pain and stiffness, the habituation of adaptive and usually relatively inefficient motor patterns may predispose the individual to recurring episodes of pain and stiffness and may provoke repeated injury. Provision of exercise programmes and periodic postdischarge measurement may, by ensuring that motor performance remains significantly improved, be one means of preventing reinjury or subsequent episodes of disability.

In conclusion, the aim of intervention is to enable the individual to improve functional performance. It is evident, therefore, that measurement of functional performance not only informs the development of evidence-based clinical practice but is also a critical part of the evaluation of dysfunction and of eventual outcome.

Muscle performance

K.M. Refshauge, C.G. Maher and J. Latimer

With expanding knowledge it has become apparent that muscle performance can be associated with dysfunction not only at the periphery, but also in the spine. For many years, the only aspect of muscle performance that was assessed in the spine was strength, and this was assessed quite poorly because of the complexity of the musculature, and the lack of availability of simple assessment tools. However, aspects of muscle performance other than strength are now commonly assessed for low back pain. These tests include: function of the stabilizing muscles around the spine, in particular of transversus abdominis and multifidus; endurance of the trunk extensor and sometimes the flexor muscles; and submaximal aerobic tests, particularly for chronic pain syndromes. For neck pain, endurance of the deep neck flexors may be tested. Some physiotherapists routinely examine muscle performance, while others examine specific tests when considered relevant.

LOW BACK PAIN

Specific stabilizing or motor control exercises

The use of specific spinal stabilization exercise is based upon research that has noted changes in the control and morphology of the deep spinal muscles, that are linked to the segmental control of the spine, in patients with spinal pain. The aim of specific exercise is therefore to re-establish the fine-tuned control of the deep spinal muscles prior to integration into high-demand tasks (Richardson et al., 1999). With the specific approach there is a requirement initially to retrain the control of the deep spinal muscles prior to commencing more functional exercise (Richardson et al., 1999). In order to teach patients to contract the deep muscles of the spine, therapists may use technical devices such as pressure monitors, electromyography and

ultrasound imaging (Richardson et al., 1999) to provide feedback to the patient. The premise of the specific approach is that simple functional exercise alone will not re-establish the control of the deep spinal muscles.

Although specific spinal stabilization exercise is widely promoted in physiotherapy texts (Twomey and Taylor, 1994; Richardson et al., 1999), its evidence base is currently small. For example there is no National Health and Medical Research Council level I evidence and only three clinical trials have directly evaluated treatment of chronic low back pain (O'Sullivan et al., 1997; Cairns et al., 2000; Goldby et al., 2001) The first trial (O'Sullivan et al., 1997; $n = 44$ subjects) concluded that individually supervised specific spinal stabilization exercise was more effective than standard medical care. However the trial subjects were restricted to those with symptomatic spondylolysis or spondylolisthesis, a group which represents a very small percentage of those with chronic low back pain, so it is unclear whether the specific spinal stabilization approach would benefit a wider population of patients with chronic low back pain. This issue has been addressed by two subsequent trials (Cairns et al., 2000; Goldby et al., 2001). Goldby's trial (Goldby et al., 2001) compared the effect of specific spinal stabilization exercise, manual therapy and a minimal-intervention placebo control in a group of 213 patients with non-specific chronic low back pain. The trial reported that the spinal stabilization rehabilitation programme was more effective at 12 months' follow-up in reducing disability and medication use and improving quality of life in patients with chronic low back pain than manual therapy or a minimal-intervention placebo control (Goldby et al., 2001). In contrast, Cairns and colleagues' (Cairns et al., 2000) trial of 97 subjects found that individually supervised specific spinal stabilization exercise provided no additional benefit to standard physiotherapy care at 6 months' (Cairns et al., 2000) or 12 months' follow-up (Cairns, 2002) for patients with chronic non-specific low back pain.

Readers are referred to Richardson et al. (1999) for further details about assessment, measurement and training.

Muscle endurance

The trunk extensor endurance test (Biering–Sorensen test)

The trunk extensor endurance test, as described by Biering-Sorensen (1984), has been shown to discriminate between patients with and without low back pain, and patients with a history of low back pain from patients who have never had low back pain. Poor performance in the test was found in a prospective study to be a risk factor for first-time occurrence of low back pain in the 12 months following testing for men but not for women (Biering-Sorensen, 1984; Luoto et al., 1995). Luoto et al. (1995) also found that if the holding time was less than 58 s, both men and women were three times more likely to develop low back pain in the next 12 months than subjects with a holding time in the normal range of 110–240 s. Most studies found that normal holding time is in the range of 150–190 s.

Test procedure   The patient lies prone with the upper body (from the upper border of the iliac crest) clear of the plinth. The buttocks and legs are firmly fixed to the plinth with three seat belts, one over the buttocks at the level of the greater trochanter, one over the popliteal fossa and one over the distal tibia close to the ankles. The arms are folded across the chest (see Fig. 6A10, in the Appendix). Prior to test commencement the upper part of the body is allowed to flex forward and rest on the stool.

The subject is asked to lift the upper trunk clear of the stool and maintain the trunk in neutral alignment for as long as possible. The examiner times how long the subject can maintain this position. The test is terminated when the subject: is unable to maintain the neutral posture, i.e. drops into forward flexion $> 10°$ and cannot correct position to regain neutral alignment; reaches tolerance

of symptoms; fatigues; or reaches a duration of 240 s. To measure whether the patient has dropped 10°, an inclinometer can be placed in the interscapular region (Latimer et al., 1999).

Reliability   A number of studies have examined the interrater reliability of painfree subjects and have reported reliabilities in the range 0.66–0.91. In contrast, Mayer et al. (1995) report a disappointing reliability of 0.20. Mayer et al.'s (1995) result was criticized by Delitto in an invited commentary on the paper, with the suggestion that Mayer et al. (1995) may have severely underestimated the reliability of the test. Latimer et al. (1999) suggested that one reason for the variability in reliability is that different researchers tested extensor muscle endurance using a variety of different trunk and limb positions. Using a strictly controlled protocol initially described by Biering-Sorensen (1984), Latimer et al. (1999) therefore conducted a reliability study in three groups of subjects: a group of asymptomatic subjects, a group currently suffering low back pain, and a group suffering previous episodes of low back pain. High reliability was obtained for the Biering-Sorensen test in subjects suffering current non-specific low back pain (NSLBP: $ICC_{1.1} = 0.88$, 95% CI $= 0.73–0.95$), in subjects suffering previous NSLBP ($ICC_{1.1} = 0.77$, 95% CI $= 0.52–0.90$) and in subjects asymptomatic for NSLBP ($ICC_{1.1} = 0.83$, 95% CI $= 0.62–0.93$). Therefore it appears that the Biering-Sorensen test provides reliable measures of holding time.

Validity   A number of studies have found that the Biering-Sorensen test discriminates between subjects with and without low back pain and discriminates those who have had a history of low back pain from those who have not. In a prospective study Biering-Sorensen (1984) found that low test performance was a risk indicator for first-time occurrence of low back pain in the follow-up year for men but not women. Similar results were found by Luoto et al. (1995), who found that both men and women were three times more likely to develop low back pain in the follow-up year if they had a holding time of less than 58 s compared to subjects with a good test result (holding time in the range 110–240 s. (Most studies that have evaluated normal subjects have reported a mean holding time in the range 150–190 s).

Factors other than endurance of the back extensor muscles, however, are known to contribute to the Biering-Sorensen holding time. Gender (Biering-Sorensen, 1984; Mannion et al., 1997; Kankaanpaa et al., 1998), body mass index (Kankaanpaa et al., 1998), age (Lattika et al., 1995) and motivation (Mayer et al., 1995) have all been shown to influence holding time. Interestingly, trunk extensor endurance did not correlate well with strength of the trunk extensor muscles (Holmstrom et al., 1992).

The trunk flexor endurance test (Ito test)

Endurance of the trunk flexor muscles is sometimes tested, although there is little evidence to support its use. The test as described by Ito et al. (1996) is a reliable test, although its ability to predict future episodes of low back pain has not been established.

Test procedure The patient lies supine with the arms folded across the chest and places the lower extremities in the position of 90° flexion of the hip and knee joints. The subject is asked to maintain maximal cervical spine flexion and to lift the head and shoulders clear of the bed while the pelvis remains stable on the plinth using gluteal contraction.

The patient is asked to maintain this position for as long as possible, not exceeding a 5-min time period. The examiner times in seconds how long the subject can maintain this position. The test is terminated when the subject is unable to maintain this posture, reaches the tolerance of symptoms or reaches the 5-min limit.

Reliability Ito et al. (1996) examined test–retest reliability of 90 subjects asymptomatic for low back pain and 100 subjects with chronic low back pain, the second test being performed 72 h after the first test. The test–retest correlations in healthy subjects were $r = 0.85$ in male subjects and 0.89 for female subjects. In subjects with chronic low back

pain, the correlations were $r = 0.91$ for men and $r = 0.85$ for women.

Validity The test has not been examined for validity.

Variations of the test Several variations of the test have been described (Kraus, 1970; McQuade et al., 1988; Moreland et al., 1997). The most common variations described by Moreland et al. (1997) include tests of static and dynamic abdominal endurance with reliabilities of ICC (2.1) = 0.51 and 0.59 respectively. The static test requires the subject to raise the head and shoulders from the initial crook lying position until the inferior angles of the scapulae clear the plinth and to maintain this position as long as possible (scored in seconds). The dynamic test requires the subject to curl the trunk from the crook lying position (with arms by the side) and either to reach 8 cm beyond the resting position of the hands (if aged >40 years) or 12 cm beyond the resting position of the hands (if aged <40 years). This test is scored in repetitions until fatigue.

Submaximal aerobic tests for cardiorespiratory endurance

In some patients, particularly those with subacute or chronic low back pain, return to function may be one of the treatment goals. Vigorous whole-body exercise programmes may be prescribed to facilitate return to function (Lindstrom et al., 1992a, b, 1995; Van Tulder et al., 1997). However, before undertaking such programmes, it may be necessary to determine the patient's cardiorespiratory endurance.

There are many ways to test cardiorespiratory endurance – cycle ergometry, 6-min walk tests and step tests. There are several protocols for these tests, all of which can be found in the *American College of Sports Medicine's Guidelines for Exercise Testing and Prescription* (Kenney, 1995). Kenney (1995) also discusses contraindications to testing, and provides ways to modify the tests for specific patient groups.

Appendix

C.G. Maher, K.M. Refshauge and J. Latimer

CLINICAL TESTS AND MEASURES

Lumbar spine range of movement measurements

Flexion of the lumbar spine (Fig. 6.A1)

Starting position of subject   Bare feet, feet hip-width apart, knees straight with weight borne evenly on the two legs, looking straight ahead, arms hanging at the sides relaxed. If this position is impossible for patients to adopt, they are asked to get as close to the position as possible. The subject's low back and upper buttocks should be exposed.

Procedure   The subject is instructed to bend forward and attempt to touch the floor with the fingertips. The therapist measures the distance between the subject's right long finger and the floor.

Common errors to avoid   Uncontrolled foot position, knee position or head position. Unclear or inconsistent instructions to patient as to whether to bend forward to onset of symptoms or to end of range. While these factors would logically seem to affect test performance, Gauvin et al. (1990) reported excellent reliability without the use of standardized instructions and patient positioning.

Variations of the test   The test is more commonly performed without the use of a stool because most subjects with low back pain are not able to reach the floor. In the case of a subject who is very flexible it may be necessary to position him or her on a stool for testing. Matyas and Bach (1985) reported a method that recorded results in terms of the measured distance between the tibial tuberosity and the fingertip and also noted the point in range where pain first came on (P1) and at its most extreme (P2) rather than range of motion *per se*.

Reliability   Evaluations of the various methods of the tests have consistently reported excellent intrarater and interrater reliability for patients and normal subjects (Matyas and Bach, 1985; Gauvin et al., 1990; Newton and Wadddell, 1991). For example, Newton and Waddell (1991) found that the intertester reliability for measuring 50 patients with low back pain and 10 normal subjects was excellent (ICC = 0.98).

Validity   The test has been criticized (Kippers and Parker, 1987) because it does not measure true lumbar flexion range of motion as it is also influenced by hip movement and a variety of associated structures. In contrast Matyas and Bach (1985) see the test's ability to be influenced by a number

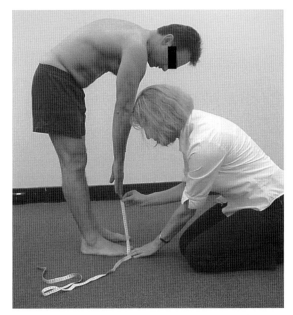

Figure 6.A1   Flexion of lumbar spine measured with tape measure fingertip to floor. The vertical distance from the tip of the middle finger to the floor is measured.

of structures as an advantage because a variety of structures may be responsible for the symptoms of patients presenting with low back pain.

Tests of themselves are not able to be evaluated for validity but rather it is the inferences made by an examiner based upon test results that can be evaluated for validity. If the results of the forward-bending test are used to make inferences about isolated lumbar flexion range, then this would be an invalid use of the test. If, however, the test is used to document a common impairment seen in patients with low back pain, and changes in forward-bending range are used as an index of resolution of this impairment, then the inference is probably acceptable. A paper by Rainville et al. (1994) that measured both isolated lumbar and total lumbo-pelvic range and disability in a group of chronic low back pain patients undergoing an intensive therapy programme provides an insight into this issue. The study found that total lumbopelvic range correlated more highly with disability scores at completion of the programme than did true lumbar flexion. Similarly, Waddell et al. (1992) noted that in chronic low back pain patients total lumbopelvic flexion range explained a greater proportion of variance of disability scores than did isolated lumbar flexion. Taken together, these two results suggest that global trunk movement may be more predictive of self-reported disability than its subcomponent of lumbar flexion.

Flexion of lumbar spine (Fig. 6.A2)

Description Measurement of lumbar flexion range of motion using a single inclinometer.

Starting position of subject Bare feet, feet hip-width apart, knees straight with the weight borne evenly on the two legs, looking straight ahead, arms hanging at the sides relaxed. If there is severe muscle spasm the patient is asked to get as close to the position as possible. The subject's low back and upper buttocks should be exposed.

Procedure Horizontal marks are made on the skin in the midline at S2 and T12–L1. The S2 spinous process is assumed to lie midway between the inferior aspects of the posterior superior iliac spines. T12–L1 is identified by counting up the spinous processes, checking that the iliac crests

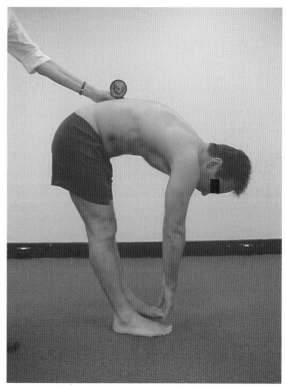

Figure 6.A2 Measurement of lumbar spine flexion range. End-of-range position with the third reading (T12–L1) being taken. After this reading is taken the inclinometer is moved to S2 and the final reading is taken.

approximate to the L4–L5 level. (Use standard Waddell skin markings.)

The inclinometer is first zeroed against a vertical surface. With the patient in the erect standing position, recordings are made at S2 and then at T12–L1. Holding the inclinometer on T12–L1, the patient is then asked to reach down with the fingertips of both hands as far as possible towards the toes, checking that the knees are kept straight. Keeping the patient fully flexed, the third recording is taken at T12–L1 and the fourth recording at S2.

Total flexion is obtained by subtracting the first reading at T12–L1 from the second reading at T12–L1. Pelvic flexion is obtained by subtracting the first reading at S2 from the second at S2. Lumbar flexion is obtained by subtracting pelvic flexion from total flexion.

Common errors to avoid Misreading the inclinometers.

Variations of the test Superior landmarks of T12, L1 or a point 15 cm above the the line joining the posterior superior iliac spine (PSIS) have also been used. A double inclinometer method has also been advocated; however the examiner has to position two inclinometers concurrently and read two angles concurrently and so the potential for error may be higher.

Some digital inclinometers have a memory function that records the angle at the upper and lower landmarks in the upright and flexed positions and so can calculate total flexion, lumbar flexion and pelvic flexion.

Reliability Waddell's protocol provides highly reliable (intertester) estimates of lumbar flexion (ICC = 0.87), pelvic flexion (ICC = 0.89) and total flexion (ICC = 0.94) for patients and normal subjects (Newton and Waddell, 1991; Waddell et al., 1992). Stude et al. (1994) report ICC values of 0.81–0.83 for measuring the lumbar flexion range of 28 asymptomatic subjects.

Validity There has been a preoccupation in the orthopaedic literature with measuring true or isolated lumbar flexion range rather than lumbopelvic range, which has been rejected as an invalid measure for patients with low back pain simply because it includes hip motion. This is an important issue because measuring true lumbar flexion takes more time, or the use of two inclin-ometers, and so more skill. This simplistic view however has been challenged by a paper (Rainville et al., 1994) that measured both isolated lumbar and total lumbopelvic range and disability in a group of chronic low back pain patients undergoing an intensive therapy programme. Interestingly, both measures of flexion were highly correlated at the beginning ($r = 0.88$) and end ($r = 0.84$) of the programme, suggesting that the two measures could be used interchangeably. More importantly, the more easily measured lumbopelvic range correlated more highly with disability scores at completion of the programme. Similarly, Waddell et al. (1992) noted that in chronic low back pain patients total lumbopelvic flexion range explained a greater proportion of variance of disability scores than did isolated lumbar flexion. Taken together these two results suggest that global trunk movement may

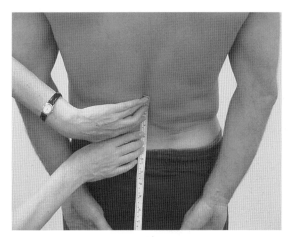

Figure 6.A3 Lumbar extension range of motion: modified-modified Schober method.

be more relevant to self-reported disability than its subcomponent of lumbar flexion.

Extension of lumbar spine (Fig. 6.A3)

Description Measurement of lumbar extension range of motion using a tape measure.

Starting position of subject Bare feet, feet hip-width apart, knees straight with the weight borne evenly on the two legs, looking straight ahead, arms hanging at the sides relaxed. If there is severe muscle spasm the patient is asked to get as close to the position as possible. The subject's low back and upper buttocks should be exposed.

Procedure The examiner places a mark along the midline of the spine horizontal to the PSIS and another on the spine 15 cm superior to the PSIS line. The tape measure is lined up against these marks and maintained firmly against the subject's skin with the examiner's fingers while the patient is then asked to bend backward. When the subject reaches full lumbar extension the new distance between the superior and inferior marks is measured to the nearest millimetre. The lumbar extension range is the difference between the original distance (15 cm) and the new distance.

Common errors to avoid Failure to maintain tape against skin surface, misreading the tape.

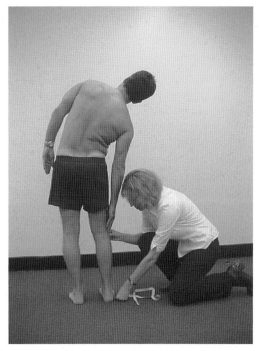

Figure 6.A4a   Lumbar lateral flexion range of movement, measured fingertip to floor.

Variations of the test   See above discussion of various methods. As with other procedures for measurement of spinal range, it would be possible to use this method to measure P1 and P2 if desired.

Reliability   Intertester reliability for the measurement of lumbar extension range of chronic low back pain patients has been shown to be very good, with an ICC value of 0.76. Intrarater reliability ranged between Pearson's $r = 0.70$ and 0.91 (Williams et al., 1993).

Validity   See section on validity at the beginning of this Appendix for a discussion of the issues related to measurement of lumbar range of movement.

Lateral flexion of lumbar spine (Fig. 6.A4)

Description   Measurement of lumbar lateral flexion range of motion using a tape measure.

Starting position of subject   Bare feet, feet hip-width apart, knees straight with the weight borne evenly on the two legs, looking straight ahead, arms hanging at the sides relaxed. If there is severe muscle spasm the patient is asked

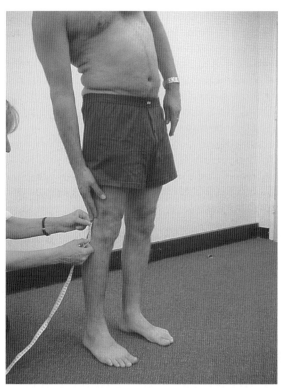

Figure 6.A4b   Lumbar lateral flexion range of movement – fingertip to head of fibula method.

to get as close to the position as possible. The subject's low back and upper buttocks should be exposed.

Procedure   The patient is instructed to lean over to the side as far as possible keeping the fingers in contact with the leg, making sure that the feet remain stationary and that the trunk does not rotate or flex. The distance from the middle finger to the floor (Fig. 6.4a) or to the head of the fibula (Fig. 6.4b) is then measured in centimetres.

Common errors to avoid   Allowing compensatory movements.

Reliability   Pile et al. (1991) report reliability values of 0.69–0.76 (unspecified statistic) using 10 patients and five observers for fingertip-to-floor method.

Validity   See the section on validity at the beginning of this Appendix for a discussion of the issues related to measurement of lumbar range of movement.

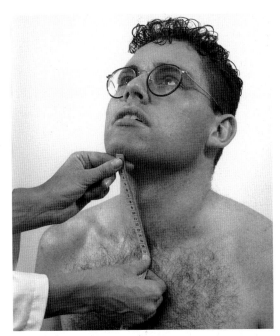

Figure 6.A5 Cervical spine extension measured between chin and sternal notch. Distance between chin and sternal notch is measured with a tape measure.

Cervical spine range of movement measurements

Extension and flexion of cervical spine (Fig. 6.A5)

Description Measurement of cervical spine extension and flexion using a tape measure.

Starting position of subject The patient's upper thorax and cervical spine should be exposed. The subject is positioned in a standardized seated position, i.e. sitting on a stool with no backrest, the lumbar lordosis maintained in neutral, arms comfortably at the sides, and the feet comfortably positioned on the floor, or positioned over the side of the treatment plinth. The subject should not slump or extend the legs as this can alter the position of the cervical spine, and therefore the starting position.

Procedure The examiner places a mark in the middle of the chin and another over the sternal notch. The tape measure is lined up against the chin with the examiner's fingers. The patient is then asked to look up at the ceiling (extension) or bend the chin towards the chest (flexion). When the subject reaches full cervical extension or flexion the distance between the marks over the chin and the sternal notch is measured to the nearest millimetre.

Common errors to avoid Failure to standardize patient starting position and failure to maintain neutral lordosis in the lumbar spine.

Variations of the test Range of motion can also be measured with a goniometer or a CROM device. The point in range where symptoms first commence (P1) and the behaviour of symptoms through range may be recorded. In irritable conditions a decision can generally be made to test only to P1 rather than to the end of range.

Rotation of cervical spine (Fig. 6.A6)

Description Measurement of cervical spine rotation using a tape measure.

Starting position of subject The patient's upper thorax and cervical spine should be exposed. The subject is positioned in a standardized seated position, i.e. sitting on a stool with no backrest, the lumbar lordosis maintained in neutral, arms comfortably at the sides and the feet comfortably positioned on the floor, or positioned over the side of the treatment plinth. The subject should not slump or extend the legs as this can alter the position of the cervical spine, and therefore the starting position.

Procedure The examiner places a mark in the middle of the chin and another over the acromion. The tape measure is lined up against the chin with the examiner's fingers while the patient is then asked to turn and look over the shoulder. When the subject reaches full cervical spine rotation the distance between the marks over the chin and the acromion is measured to the nearest millimetre.

Common errors to avoid Failure to standardize patient starting position, failure to maintain neutral lordosis in the lumbar spine and allowing deviations into side flexion or flexion/extension.

Variations of the test Range of motion can also be measured with a goniometer or a CROM device. The point in range where symptoms first

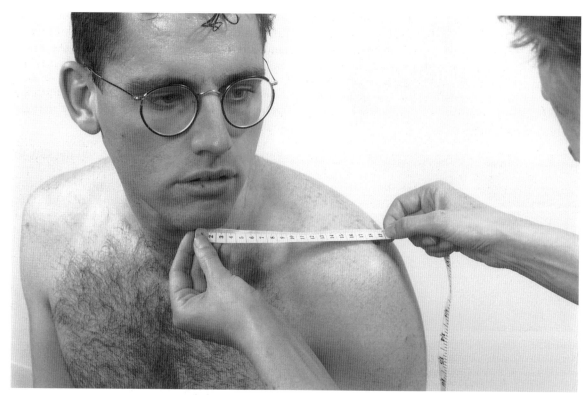

Figure 6.A6 Measurement of cervical spine rotation. Distance between chin and acromion is measured with a tape measure.

commence (P1) and the behaviour of symptoms through range may be recorded. In irritable conditions a decision can generally be made to test only to P1 rather than to the end of range.

Lateral flexion of cervical spine (Fig. 6.A7)

Description   Measurement of cervical spine lateral flexion using a tape measure.

Starting position of subject   The patient's upper thorax and cervical spine should be exposed. The subject is positioned in a standardized seated position, i.e. sitting on a stool with no backrest, the lumbar lordosis maintained in neutral, arms comfortably at the sides and the feet comfortably positioned on the floor, or positioned over the side of the treatment plinth. The subject should not slump or extend the legs as this can alter the position of the cervical spine, and therefore the starting position.

Procedure   The examiner places a mark at the lowest point of the ear lobe and another over the

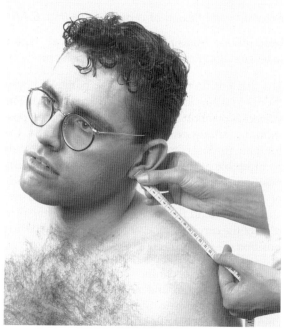

Figure 6.A7   Measurement of cervical spine lateral flexion. Distance between ear and acromion is measured with a tape measure.

acromion process. The tape measure is lined up against the ear lobe with the examiner's fingers while the patient is then asked to bend the ear towards the shoulder without turning the head. When the subject reaches full cervical spine lateral flexion the distance between the marks over the earlobe and the acromion process is measured to the nearest millimetre.

Common errors to avoid   Failure to standardize patient starting position, failure to maintain neutral lordosis in the lumbar spine and allowing deviations into rotation or flexion/extension.

Variations of the test   Range of motion can also be measured with a goniometer or a CROM device. The point in range where symptoms first commence (P1) and the behaviour of symptoms through range may be recorded. In irritable conditions a decision can generally be made to test only to P1 rather than to the end of range.

Reliability for all cervical spine range of motion measurements

Tape measure method   When measuring healthy young volunteers, intratester reliability is high for all cervical spine movements using the tape measure method. Pearson's r ranged between $r = 0.80$ for left rotation and $r = 0.95$ for flexion for an experienced therapist (Hsieh and Yeung, 1986), and between $r = 0.78$ for right rotation and 0.91 for right lateral flexion for an inexperienced therapist (Hsieh and Yeung, 1986).

CROM and goniometer   When measuring range of motion in 60 patients, intratester reliability and intertester reliability were found to be very high using both a CROM device and a goniometer. When using the CROM intratester reliability ranged between ICC = 0.84 for left lateral flexion and ICC = 0.95 for flexion (Youdas et al., 1991) and intertester reliability ranged between ICC = 0.73 for left lateral flexion and ICC = 0.92 for right rotation (Youdas et al., 1991).

Validity   In the same way that the tape measure method has been criticized for measurement of lumbar spine range of motion, this method does not measure true cervical spine range of motion because the measurement includes other joints and structures, e.g. the temporomandibular joint,

sometimes the shoulder and the thoracic spine and the anatomical variability of the chin and the ear lobe. In the same way as argued for the lumbar spine, there are advantages in such measurement methods because they account for the test's ability to be influenced by a number of structures that may be responsible for the symptoms of patients presenting with neck pain.

These tests cannot be evaluated for validity; instead it is the inferences made by an examiner based upon test results that can be evaluated for validity. If the results of the test are used to make inferences about isolated cervical flexion range then this would be an invalid use of the test. If, however, the test is used to document a common impairment seen in patients with neck pain, and changes in neck range are used as an index of resolution of this impairment then the inference is probably acceptable. It is also possible that global neck movement may be more predictive of self-reported disability than its subcomponent of cervical range of motion.

Measurement of tension tests

Straight leg raise test (Fig. 6.A8)

Description   Measurement of passive single SLR using an inclinometer.

Starting position of subject   The patient is positioned in the standard Waddell supine position, i.e. lying relaxed flat on the back, head lying on the couch without a pillow, arms at the sides with hips and knees as extended as possible without tension. The subject should not look up to watch what is happening.

Procedure   The foot is held with one hand, making sure that the hip is in neutral rotation. The inclinometer is positioned with the other hand on the tibial crest just below the tibial tubercle and set at zero. The leg is then raised passively by the examiner, whose other hand continues to hold the patient's knee fully extended. The leg is raised to the maximum tolerated SLR (not the onset of pain) and the maximum reading is recorded.

Common errors to avoid   Failure to standardize patient starting position, failure to maintain hip in neutral rotation and adduction, failure to control

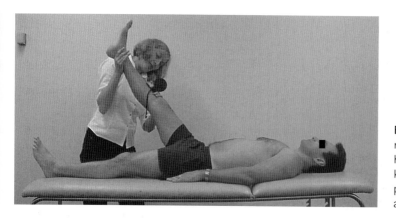

Figure 6.A8 Measurement of straight leg raise (SLR) using an inclinometer. The leg is held in neutral rotation. Extension of the knee is maintained by the examiner by pressure from the hand. A reading is taken at maximum tolerated SLR range.

knee extension and allowing patient to lift head or move trunk or limbs to watch test performance. Failure to zero inclinometer, misreading analogue inclinometer.

Variations of the test   The point in range where symptoms first commence (P1) and the behaviour of symptoms through range may be recorded. In irritable patients a decision can be generally made only to test to P1 rather than to the end of range. Sensitizing manoeuvres of ankle dorsiflexion, hip medial rotation, adduction or neck flexion may be added to the base test and the effect on symptoms noted; however the measurement then requires a second examiner to control patient position.

Reliability   The SLR has been found to have excellent intertester reliability in a number of studies (Matyas and Bach, 1985; Waddell et al., 1992; Chow et al., 1994; Boland and Adams, 2000). Matyas and Bach (1985) investigated the test–retest reliability of measuring SLR to P1 using a gravitational goniometer and obtained an r value of 0.96. Million et al (1982), cited in Matyas and Bach (1985), found a test–retest correlation of 0.97 for measurement of SLR in a patient population. This high reliability has been noted in acute and chronic low back pain patients, with analogue and digital inclinometers, and for testing to onset of symptoms or end of range.

Validity

Diagnostic validity   The SLR was originally described to differentiate hip from sciatic symptoms

and it is still used for this purpose today (see Boland and Adams, 2000, Ch. 6). However, Charnley's (1951) widely held view that a severely restricted SLR indicated the presence of a protruding disc has been challenged by several authors (Fahrni, 1966; Lerman and Drasnin, 1987). For example, some patients with SLR restricted to 35° or less have no disc pathology at surgery, but rather a nerve root adherent to the disc or intradural adhesions of specific nerve roots (Fahrni, 1966; McNab, 1971; see Boland and Adams, 2000, Ch. 6 for review). However, SLR has a sensitivity for detecting radiculopathy ranging from 0.88 to 1.00 (Kosteljanetz et al., 1988) and specificity ranging from 0.11 to 0.44 (Sprangfort, 1972; Kerr et al., 1988).

A crossed SLR has also been identified as a possible diagnostic indicator of disc pathology. A crossed SLR occurs when SLR performed on the asymptomatic leg reproduces symptoms in the symptomatic leg. A crossed SLR has a sensitivity of 0.42 and a specificity of 0.86 (Kosteljanetz et al., 1988).

Discriminative validity (see Boland and Adams, 2000, Ch. 6, for review)   During the performance of SLR many structures are moved and stressed, such as other lumbar spine structures, the SIJ, hip and hamstrings. In fact, SLR is also a test of hamstrings length, and putting hamstrings on maximal tension, as during SLR, would be expected to reproduce pain from a hamstrings lesion. This suggests relatively poor discriminative validity for SLR.

The response to sensitizing manoeuvres theoretically enhances the diagnostic capacity of the tests. If a sensitizing manoeuvre increases symptoms, it is generally believed that neuromeningeal

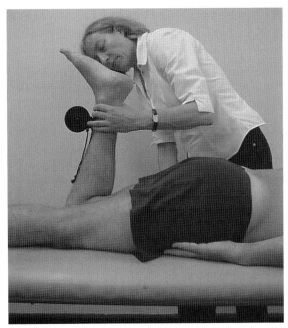

Figure 6.A9 Measurement of prone knee bend (PKB) using a tape measure. The hip is held in neutral extension. A reading is taken at maximal tolerated PKB range.

tissue is responsible for the symptoms, since other structures may not be further stressed. However, this belief is still being investigated (see Boland and Adams, 2000, Ch. 6).

Prone knee bend test (Fig. 6.A9)

Description   Measurement of passive PKB using a tape measure.

Starting position of subject   The subject is positioned in the standard prone position, i.e. lying relaxed flat on the stomach, arms at the side or comfortably raised into abduction and hips and knees in relaxed extension without tension. The subject should not look up to watch what is happening.

Procedure   The foot is held with one hand making sure that the hip is in neutral rotation. The tape measure is held in the same hand over the malleolus. The knee is then flexed passively by the examiner, whose other hand may be used to ensure that no spinal or hip extension occurs. The knee is flexed to the maximum tolerated PKB (not the onset of pain) and the distance from the malleolus to the bed is recorded.

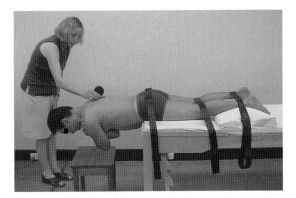

Figure 6.A10   Measurement of trunk extensor endurance using the Biering-Sorensen test. The patient maintains neutral trunk position with the arms folded across the chest for as long as possible. An inclinometer is positioned between the scapulae to ensure maintenance of the neutral trunk position. The test is terminated when the subject is unable to maintain the neutral posture (i.e. drops into forward flexion >10 degrees), reaches tolerance of symptoms or fatigue.

Common errors to avoid   Failure to standardize patient starting position, failure to maintain hip or lumbar spine in neutral extension and allowing the patient to lift head or move trunk or limbs to watch test performance.

Variations of the test   The point in range where symptoms first commence (P1) and the behaviour of symptoms through range may be recorded. In irritable patients a decision can be generally made only to test to P1 rather than to the end of range. Sensitizing manoeuvre of hip extension may be added to the standard test and the effect on symptoms noted; however the measurement then requires a second examiner to control patient position. An inclinometer, positioned over the anterior tibia or talus, can also be used to measure the range of knee flexion.

Reliability and validity   The PKB test has not been rigorously investigated. Therefore, reliability, sensitivity and discriminative or diagnostic validity are unknown.

Trunk extensor endurance – Biering-Sorensen test (Fig. 6.A10)

Description   Measurement of trunk extensor endurance.

Instruments required Stop watch, inclinometer, three belts (preferably wide) to strap patient to plinth, a plinth and a chair or stool slightly lower than the plinth.

Starting position of subject The subject lies prone with the upper part of the body (from the upper border of the iliac crest) clear of the plinth. The buttocks and legs are firmly fixed to the plinth by three seat belts, one over the buttocks at the level of the greater trochanter, one over the popliteal fossa and one over the distal tibia close to the ankles. The arms are folded across the chest. Prior to test commencement the upper part of the body is allowed to flex forward and rest on the stool.

Starting position of examiner The examiner stands to the side of the patient to observe trunk alignment and to assist the subject to rest back on stool at test termination.

Procedure The subject is asked to lift the upper trunk clear of the stool and maintain the trunk in neutral alignment for as long as possible. The examiner times how long the subject can maintain this position. The test is terminated when the subject is unable to maintain the neutral posture (i.e. drops into forward flexion $>10°$), reaches tolerance of symptoms or fatigue, or reaches duration of 240 s.

Common errors to avoid Failure to stabilize the buttocks and legs firmly, inconsistent positioning of the arms.

Variations of the test While not a part of the original protocol, an inclinometer can be placed on the trunk, in the interscapular region, to provide a more objective criterion for failure to maintain the neutral posture. A drop into flexion of $>10°$ that the subject is unable to correct is the criterion for test termination.

While Biering-Sorensen (1984) advocated stopping the test at 240 s this practice is illogical for a test of endurance and should be ignored.

Ito et al. (1996) measured trunk extensor endurance by positioning the subject in prone on the floor with a small pillow under the abdomen and then asked the subject to lift and hold the sternum off the floor. The test was shown to have high reliability with a Pearson correlation of 0.97 for male and 0.94 for female healthy subjects and 0.93 for male and 0.95 for female chronic low back pain patients, with a test–retest interval of 72 h.

REFERENCES

INTRODUCTION

Barrows, H.S. and Feltovich, P.J. (1987). The clinical reasoning process. *Med. Educ.*, **21**, 86–91.

Buckley, R.A. (1988). *The Modern Law of Negligence.* London: Butterworths.

Giesen, D. (1988). *International Medical Malpractice Law.* Dordrecht: Martinus Nijhoff.

Grieve, G.P. (1984). *Mobilisation of the Spine*, 4th edn. London: Churchill Livingstone.

Magee, D.J. (1987). *Orthopedic Physical Assessment.* London: W.B. Saunders.

Maher, C., Latimer, J. and Refshauge, K.M. (2001). *Atlas of Clinical Tests and Measures for Low Back Pain.* Sydney: Manipulative Physiotherapists Association of Australia.

Maitland, G.D. (1986). *Vertebral Manipulation*, 5th edn. London: Butterworth-Heinemann.

McCloskey, D.I. (1978). Kinesthetic sensibility. *Physiol. Rev.*, **58**, 763–820.

O'Sullivan, J. (1983). *Law for Nurses and Allied Health Professionals in Australia*, 3rd edn. Sydney: Law Book Company.

Richardson, C.A., Jull, G., Hodges, P. and Hides, J. (1999). *Therapeutic Exercises for Spinal Segmental Stabilization in Low Back Pain: Scientific Basis and Clinical Approach.* Sydney: Churchill Livingstone.

Siegler, M., Toulmin, S., Zimring, F.E. and Schaffner, K.F. (1987). *Medical Innovation and Bad Outcomes: Legal, Social, and Ethical Responses.* Ann Arbor, MI: Health Administration Press.

OBSERVATION

Braun, B. and Amundson, L. (1989). Quantitative assessment of head and shoulder posture. *Arch. Phys. Med. Rehabil.* **70**, 322–329.

Bullock, J.E., Jull, G.A. and Bullock, M.I. (1987). The relationship of low back pain to postural changes during pregnancy. *Aust. J. Physiother.*, **33**, 10–17.

Dieck, G., Kelsey, J., Goel, V., Pajnabi, M., Walter, S. and Laprade, M. (1985). An epidemiological study of the relationship between postural asymmetry in the teen years and subsequent back and neck pain. *Spine*, **10**, 872–877.

During, H., Goudfrooij, H., Keeson, W., Beedker, T.W. and Crowe, A. (1985). Towards standards for posture. *Spine*, **10**, 83–87.

Feldman, N., Refshauge, K.M., Goodsell, M. and Adams, R. (1994). The effect of chin retraction exercises on cervical and cervicothoracic posture in an asymptomatic population. In: *Proceedings of 4th International Physiotherapy Congress*, pp. 51–53. Bali: International Physiotherapy Association.

Franklin, M.E. and Conner-Kerr, T. (1998). An analysis of posture and back pain in the first and third trimesters of pregnancy. *J. Orthop. Sports Phys. Ther.*, **28**, 133–138.

Gerrard, B. (1989). The patello-femoral pain syndrome: a clinical trial of the McConnell programme. *Aust. J. Physiother.*, **35**, 71–80.

Griegel-Morris, P., Larson, K., Mueller-Klaus, K. and Oatis, C. (1992). Incidence of common postural abnormalities in the cervical, shoulder, and thoracic regions and their association with pain in two age groups of healthy subjects. *Phys. Ther.*, **72**, 425–430.

Grieve, G.P. (1986). Bony and soft-tissue anomalies of the vertebral column. In: *Modern Manual Therapy of the Vertebral Column*, ed. G. Grieve, pp. 3–20. London: Churchill Livingstone.

Harms-Ringdahl, K. and Ekholm, J. (1986). Intensity and character of pain and muscular activity levels elicited by maintained extreme flexion position of the lower-cervical-upper-thoracic spine. *Scand. J. Rehabil. Med.*, **18**, 117–126.

Hart, D.L. and Rose, S.J. (1986). Reliability of a noninvasive method for measuring the lumbar curve. *J. Orthop. Sports Phys. Ther.*, **8**, 180–184.

Levangie, P.K. (1999). The association between static pelvic asymmetry and low back pain. *Spine*, **24**, 1234–1242.

Magee, D.J. (1987). *Orthopedic Physical Assessment*. Philadelphia, PA: W.B. Saunders.

Magee, D.J. (1992). *Orthopedic Physical Assessment*, 2nd edn, pp. 120–122. Philadelphia, PA: W.B. Saunders.

McConnell, J. (1986). The management of chondromalacia patellae: a long term solution. *Aust. J. Physiother.*, **32**, 215–223.

McKenzie, R.A. (1981). *The Lumbar Spine – Mechanical Diagnosis and Therapy*, New Zealand: Spinal Publications.

Milne, J.S. and Lauder, I.J. (1974). Age effects in kyphosis and lordosis in adults. *Ann. Hum. Biol.*, **1**, 327–337.

Pope, M.H., Bevins, T., Wilder, D.G. and Frymoyer, J.W. (1985). The relationship between anthropometric, postural, muscular and mobility characteristics of males aged 18–55. *Spine*, **10**, 644–648.

Raine, S. and Twomey, L. (1994). Posture of the head, shoulders and thoracic spine in confortable erect standing. *Aust. J. Physiother.*, **40**, 25–32.

Refshauge, K.M., Goodsell, M. and Lee, M. (1994a). Consistency of natural cervical and cervicothoracic posture in standing. *Aust. J. Physiother.*, **40**, 235–240.

Refshauge, K.M., Goodsell, M. and Lee, M. (1994b). The relationship between surface contour and vertebral body measures of upper spine curvature. *Spine*, **19**, 2180–2185.

Refshauge, K.M., Bolst, L. and Goodsell, M. (1995). The relationship between cervicothoracic posture and pain. *J. Manual Manip. Ther.*, **3**, 21–24.

Soukka, A., Alaranta, H., Tallroth, K. and Heliovaara, M. (1991). Leg-length inequality in people of working age: the association between mild inequality and low-back pain is questionable. *Spine*, **16**, 429–431.

Twomey, L.T. (1992). A rationale for the treatment of back pain and joint pain by manual therapy. *Phys. Ther.*, **72**, 885–892.

Watson, D. and Trott, P. (1993). Cervical headache: an investigation of natural head posture and upper cervical flexor muscle performance. *Cephalalgia*, **13**, 272–284.

Williams, M.M., Hawley, J.A., McKenzie, R.A. and Wijmen, P.M. (1991). A comparison of the effects of two sitting postures on back and referred pain. *Spine*, **16**, 1185–1190.

TESTING OF ACTIVE MOVEMENTS

Beattie, P., Rothstein, J. and Lamb, R. (1987). Reliability of the attraction method for measuring lumbar spine backward bending. *Phys. Ther.*, **67**, 364–369.

Edwards, B. (1987). Clinical assessment: the use of combined movements in assessment and treatment. In: *Physical Therapy of the Low Back*, ed. L. Twomey and J. Taylor, pp. 175–198. New York: Churchill Livingstone.

Edwards, B. (1988). Combined movements of the cervical spine in examination and treatment. In: *Physical Therapy of the Cervical and Thoracic Spine*, ed. R.Grant, pp. 125–151. New York: Churchill Livingstone.

Garrett, T.R., Youdas, J.W. and Madson, T.J. (1993). Reliability of measuring forward head posture in a clinical setting. *J. Orthop. Sports Phys. Ther.*, **17**, 155–160.

Grieve, G.P. (1984). *Mobilisation of the Spine*. Edinburgh: Churchill Livingstone.

Hsieh, C. and Yeung, B. (1986). Active neck motion measurement with a tape measure. *J. Orthop. Sports Phys. Ther.*, **8**, 88–92.

Maitland, G.D. (1986). *Vertebral Manipulation*, 5th edn. London: Butterworth-Heinemann.

McKenzie, R.A. (1981). *The Lumbar Spine – Mechanical Diagnosis and Therapy*. Upper Hutt, New Zealand: Spinal Publications.

Perret, C., Poiraudeau, S., Fermanian, J., Colau, M.M., Benhamou, M.A. and Revel, M. (2001). Validity, reliability, and responsiveness of the fingertip-to-floor test. *Arch. Phys. Med. Rehabil*, **82**, 1566–1570.

Twomey, L.T. and Taylor, J. (1979). A description of two new instruments for measuring the ranges of sagittal and horizontal plane motions in the lumbar region. *Aust. J. Physiother.*, **25**, 201–204.

Youdas, J.W., Carey, J.R. and Garrett, T.R. (1991). Reliability of measurements of cervical spine range of motion – comparison of three methods. *Phys. Ther.*, **71**, 98–104.

TESTING ADEQUACY OF CEREBRAL BLOOD FLOW (VERTEBROBASILAR INSUFFICIENCY)

Abrahams, V.C. (1981). Sensory and motor specialization in some muscles of the neck. *Trends Neurosci.*, **January**, 24–27.

AJP Forum (2001). Pre-manipulative testing of the cervical spine. *Aust. J. Physiother.*, **47**, 163–167.

Bolton, P.S., Stick, P.E. and Lord, R.S.A. (1989). Failure of clinical tests to predict cerebral ischaemia before neck manipulation. *J. Manip. Physiol. Ther.*, **12**, 304–307.

Burton, A.C. (1965). *Physiology and Biophysics of the Circulation – An Introductory Text*, pp. 95–101. Chicago, IL: Year Book Medical.

Coman, W.B. (1986). Dizziness related to ENT conditions. In: *Modern Manual Therapy*, ed. G.P. Grieve, pp. 303–314. London: Churchill Livingstone.

de Jong, P.T.V.M., de Jong, J.M.B.V., Cohen, B. and Jongkees, L.B.W. (1977). Ataxia and nystagmus induced by injection of local anaesthetics in the neck. *Ann. Neurol.*, **1**, 240–246.

Drachman, D.A. (1998). A 69-year-old man with chronic dizziness. *J.A.M.A.*, **280**, 2111–2118.

Fisher, C.M., Karnes, W.E. and Kubik, C.S. (1961). Lateral medullary infarction: the pattern of vascular occlusion. *J. Neuropathol. Exp. Neurol.*, **20**, 323–379.

Frumkin, L. and Baloh, R.W. (1990). Wallenberg's syndrome following neck manipulation. *Neurology*, **40**, 611–615.

Fujita, N., Ueda, T., Yamanaka, T. et al. (1995). Clinical application of ultrasonic blood rheography in vertebral artery for vertigo. *Acta Oto-Laryngol. – Suppl.*, **519**, 178–183.

Goldberg, M.E., Eggers, H.M. and Couras, P. (1991). The ocular motor system. In: *Principles of Neural Science*, 3rd edn, ed. E.R. Kandel, J.H. Schwartz and T.M. Jessell, pp. 660–678. Connecticut: Prentice-Hall International.

Grant, R. (1988). *Dizziness Testing and Manipulation to the Cervical Spine*. New York: Churchill Livingstone.

Haldeman, S., Kohlbeck, F.J. and McGregor, M. (2002). Unpredictability of cerebrovascular ischemia associated with cervical spine manipulation therapy. *Spine*, **1**, 49–55.

Hardesty, W.H., Whitacre, W.B. and Toole, J.F. (1963). Studies on vertebral artery bloodflow in man. *Surg. Gynaecol. Obstet.*, **116**, 622–662.

Haynes, M.J. (1995). Cervical rotational effects on vertebral artery flow. *Chiropract. J. Aust.*, **25**, 73–76.

Haynes, M.J. (1996). Doppler studies comparing the effects of cervical rotation and lateral flexion on vertebral artery blood flow. *J. Manip. Physiol. Ther.*, **19**, 378–384.

Horn, S.W. (1983). 'The locked-in' syndrome following chiropractic manipulation of the cervical spine. *Ann. Emerg. Med.*, **12**, 648–650.

Hutchinson, M.S. (1989). An investigation of pre-manipulative dizziness testing. In: *Proceedings of 5th Biennial Conference of Manipulative Physiotherapists of Australia*, pp. 104–112. Sydney.

Kanshepolski, J., Danielson, H. and Flynn, R.E. (1972). Vertebral artery insufficiency and cerebellar infarct due to manipulation of the neck. *Bull. L.A. Neurol. Soc.*, **37**, 62–65.

Kelly, J.P. (1991). The sense of balance. In: *Principles of Neural Science*, ed. E.R. Kandell, J.H. Schwartz and T.M. Jessell, pp. 500–511. Connecticut: Prentice-Hall.

Loeb, C. and Meyer, J.S. (1965). *Strokes due to Vertebrobasilar Disease*. Springfield, IL: Charles C Thomas.

Lord, R.S.A. (1986). *Surgery of Occlusive Cerebrovascular Disease*. St Louis, MO: CV Mosby.

Lyness, S.S. and Wagman, A.D. (1974). Neurological deficit following cervical manipulation *Surg. Neurol.*, **2**, 121–123.

Magarey, M., Coughlan, B. and Rebbeck, T. (2000). Clinical guidelines for pre-manipulative procedures for the cervical spine. *Proceedings of the International Federation of Manipulative Therapists*, Perth, 88.

Maitland, G.D. (1986). *Vertebral Manipulation*. London: Butterworths.

Mann, T. and Refshauge, K.M. (2001). Complications from cervical spine manipulation without major arterial injury. Risk factors and implications for the pre-manipulative testing protocol. *Aust. J. Physiother.*, **47**, 255–266.

Mishkin, M.M. and Schreiber, M.N. (1974). Collateral circulation. In: *Radiology of the Skull and Brain: Angiography*, vol. 2, ed. T.H. Newton and D.G. Potts. St Louis, MO: CV Mosby.

Okawarra, S. and Nibbelink, D. (1974). Vertebral artery occlusion following hyperextension and rotation of the head. *Stroke*, **5**, 640–642

Olszewski, J., Zalewski, P., Machala, W. and Gaszynski, W. (1994). Applying of cervical torsion test by examination of Doppler's blood flow in vertebral arteries and basilar artery patients with degenerative cervical spine changes. *Otolaryngol. Pol.*, **48**, 549–555.

Patijn, J. (1991). Complications in manual medicine: a review of the literature. *J. Manual Med.*, **6**, 89–92.

Refshauge, K. (1994). Rotation: a valid premanipulative dizziness test? Does it predict safe manipulation? *J. Manip. Physiol. Ther.*, **17**, 15–19.

Refshauge, K.M., Parry, S., Shirley, D., Larsen, D., Rivett, D. and Boland, R. (2002). Professional responsibility in relation to cervical manipulation. *Aust. J. Physiother.*, **48**, 171–179.

Rivett, D.A., Sharples, K.J. and Milburn, P.D. (1999). Effect of premanipulative tests on vertebral artery and internal carotid artery blood flow: a pilot study. *J. Manip. Physiol. Ther.*, **22**, 368–375.

Rowell, L.B. (1986). *Human Circulation Regulation During Physical Stress*. New York: Oxford University Press.

Schellhas, K.P., Latchaw, R.E., Wendling, L.R. and Gold, L.H.A. (1980). Vertebrobasilar injuries following cervical manipulation. *J.A.M.A.*, **244**, 1450–1453.

Schmitt, H.P. (1991). Anatomical structure of the cervical spine with reference to pathology of manipulation complications. *J. Manual Med.*, **6**, 93–101.

Simon, N.M., Pollack, M.H., Tuby, K.S. and Stern, T.A. (1998). Dizziness and panic disorder: a review of the association between vestibular dysfunction and anxiety. *Ann. Clin. Psychiatry*, **10**, 75–80.

Sloane, P.D., Coeytaux, R.R., Beck, R.S. and Dallara, J. (2001). Dizziness: state of the science. *Ann. Intern. Med.*, **134**, 823–832.

Stevens, A. (1991). Functional Doppler sonography of the vertebral artery and some considerations about manual techniques. *J. Manual Med.*, **6**, 102–105.

Stopford, J.S.B. (1916). The arteries of the pons and medulla oblongata. Part II. *J. Anatomy*, **50**, 131–164.

Terrett, A.G. (1987). Vascular accidents from cervical spine manipulation: the mechanisms. *J. Aust. Chiropractors Assoc.*, **17**, 131–144.

Thiel, H.W. (1991). Gross morphology and pathoanatomy of the vertebral arteries. *J. Manip. Physiol. Ther.*, **14**, 133–141.

Thiel, H.W., Wallace, K., Donat, J. and Yong-Hing, K. (1994). Effect of vertebral arteryrious head and neck positions on vertebral artery blood flow. *Clin. Biomech.*, **9**, 105–110.

Tinetti, M.E., Williams, C.S. and Gill, T.M. (2000). Dizziness among older adults: a possible geriatric syndrome. *Ann. Intern. Med.*, **132**, 337–344.

Tissington Tatlow, W.F. and Bammer, H.G. (1957). Syndrome of vertebral artery compression. *Neurology*, **7**, 331–340.

Toole, J.F. and Tucker, S.H. (1960). Influence of head position upon cerebral circulation. *Arch. Neurol.*, **2**, 616–623.

Williams, P.R. and Warwick, R. (1980). *Gray's Anatomy*, 36th edn. London: Churchill Livingstone.

Zwiebel, W.J. (1986). *Introduction to Vascular Ultrasonography*, 2nd edn. New York: Harcourt Brace Jovanich.

TENSION TESTS

Beel, J.A., Groswald, D.E. and Luttges, M.W. (1984). Alterations in the mechanical properties of peripheral nerve following crush injury. *J. Biomech.*, **17**, 185–193.

Bell, A. (1987). The upper limb tension test-bilateral straight leg raising – a validating manouvre for the upper limb tension test. In: *Proceedings of the 5th Biennial Conference of the Manipulative Therapists Association of Australia*, ed. B.A. Dalziel and J.C. Snowshill, pp. 106–114. Melbourne, Australia: Manipulative Therapists Association of Australia.

Bogduk, N. and Twomey, L. (1991). *Clinical Anatomy of the Lumbar Spine*. London: Churchill Livingstone.

Bohannon, R., Gajdosik, R. and LeVeau, B. (1985). Contribution of pelvic and lower limb motion to increases in the angle of passive straight leg raising. *Phys. Ther.*, **65**, 474–476.

Boland, R.A. and Adams, R.D. (2000). Effects of ankle dorsiflexion on range and reliability of straight leg raising. *Aust. J. Physiother.*, **46**, 191–200.

Breig, A. (1978). *Adverse Mechanical Tension in the Central Nervous System: An Analysis of Cause and Effect by Functional Neurosurgery*. Stockholm: Almquist and Wiksell.

Breig, A. and Marions, O. (1963). Biomechanics of the lumbosacral nerve roots. *Acta Radiol.*, **1**, 1141–1160.

Breig, A. and Troup, J. (1979). Biomechanical considerations in the straight-leg-raising test. Cadaveric and clinical studies of the effects of medial hip rotation. *Spine*, **4**, 242–250.

Brudzinski, (1909). cited in O'Connell (1946). The clinical signs of meningeal irritation. *Brain*, **69**, 9–21.

Butler, D.S. (1991). *Mobilisation of the Nervous System*, pp. 127–146. Melbourne: Churchill Livingstone.

Charnley, J. (1951). Orthopaedic signs in the diagnosis of disc protrusion with special reference to the straight leg raising test. *Lancet*, **4**, 186–192.

Christodoulides, A.N. (1989). Ipsilateral sciatica on femoral nerve stretch test is pathognomonic of an L4/5 disc protrusion. *J. Bone Joint Surg. Ser. B*, **71**, 88–89.

Davidson, S. (1987). Prone knee bend – an investigation into the effect of cervical flexion and extension. In: *Proceedings of the 5th Biennial Conference of the Manipulative Therapists Association of Australia*, ed. B.A. Dalziel and J.C. Snowshill, pp. 235–246. Melbourne, Australia: Manipulative Therapists Association of Australia.

Dixon, J.K. and Keating, J.L. (2000). Variability in straight leg raise measurements: review. *Physiotherapy*, **86**, 361–370.

Dyck, P. (1976). The femoral nerve traction test with lumbar disc protrusions. *Surg. Neurol.*, **6**, 163–166.

Dyck, P. (1984). Lumbar nerve root: the enigmatic eponyms. *Spine*, **9**, 3–6.

Elvey, R. (1979). Brachial plexus tension tests and the pathoanatomical origin of arm pain. In: *Aspects of Manipulative Therapy.*, ed. R. Idczack, pp. 105–110. Melbourne: Lincoln Institute of Health Sciences.

Elvey, R. (1981). Brachial plexus tension tests and the pathoanatomical origin of arm pain. In: *Aspects of Manipulative Therapy*, ed. R. Idczack, pp. 116–122. Melbourne: Lincoln Institute of Health Sciences.

Elvey, R.L. (1983). The need to test the brachial plexus in painful shoulder and upper quadrant conditions. In: *Neck and Shoulder Symposium*, pp. 39–52. Sydney, Australia: Manipulative Therapists Association of Australia.

Elvey, R. (1986). Treatment of arm pain associated with abnormal brachial plexus tension. *Aust. J. Physiother.*, **32**, 225–230.

Estridge, M.N., Rouhe, S.A. and Johnson, N.G. (1982). The femoral stretching test. A valuable sign in diagnosing upper lumbar disc herniations. *J. Neurosurg.*, **57**, 813–817.

Fahrni, W. (1966). Observations on straight leg-raising with special reference to nerve root adhesions. *Can. J. Surg.*, **9**, 44–48.

Fidel, C., Martin, E., Dankaerts, W., Allison, G. and Hall, T. (1996). Cervical spine sensitizing maneuvers during the slump test. *J. Manual Manip. Ther.*, **4**, 16–21.

Fung, Y. (1981). *Biomechanics – Mechanical Properties of Living Tissues*. New York: Springer-Verlag.

Gajdosik, R.L., Rieck, M.A., Sullivan, D.K. and Wightman, S.E. (1993). Comparison of four clinical tests for assessing hamstring muscle length. *J. Orthop. Sports Phys. Ther.*, **18**, 614–618.

Gellman, H., Gelberman, R.H., Tan, A.M. and Botte, M.J. (1986). Carpal tunnel syndrome. An evaluation of the provocative diagnostic tests. *J. Bone Joint Surg.*, **68A**, 735–737.

Goddard, M. and Reid, J. (1965). Movements induced by straight leg raising in the lumbo-sacral roots, nerves and plexus, and in the intrapelvic section of the sciatic nerve. *J. Neurol., Neurosurg. Psychiatry*, **28**, 12–18.

Grant, R., Forrester, C. and Hides, J. (1995). Screen based keyboard operation: the adverse effects on the neural system. *Aust. J. Physiother.*, **41**, 99–107.

Grieve, G. (1984). *Mobilisation of the Spine*. London: Churchill Livingstone.

Hall, T., Zusman, M. and Elvey, R. (1998). Adverse mechanical tension in the nervous system? Analysis of straight leg raise. *Manual Ther.*, **3**, 140–146.

Herbert, R. (1988). The passive mechanical properties of muscle and their adaptations to altered patterns of use. *Aust. J. Physiother.*, **34**, 141–149.

Howe, J.F., Loeser, J.D. and Calvin, W.H. (1977). Mechanosensitivity of dorsal root ganglia and chronically injured axons: a physiological basis for the radicular pain of nerve root compression. *Pain*, **3**, 25–41.

Hsieh, C., Walker, J. and Gillis, K. (1983). Straight-leg-raising test. Comparison of three instruments. *Phys. Ther.*, **63**, 1429–1433.

Hudgins, W.R. (1979). The crossed straight leg raising test: a diagnostic sign of herniated disc. *J. Occup. Med.*, **21**, 407–408.

Johnson, E.K. and Chiarello, C.M. (1997). The slump test: the effects of head and lower extremity position on knee extension. *J. Orthop. Sports Phys. Ther.*, **26**, 310–317.

Kenneally, M. (1985). The upper limb tension test. In: *Proceedings of the 4th Biennial Conference of the Manipulative Therapists Association of Australia*, pp. 259–273. Brisbane, Australia: Manipulative Therapists Association of Australia.

Kleinrensink, G.J., Stoeckart, R., Mulder, P.G. et al. (2000). Upper limb tension tests as tools in the diagnosis of nerve and plexus lesions. Anatomical and biomechanical aspects. *Clin. Biomech.*, **15**, 9–14.

Kornberg, C. and Lew, P. (1989). The effect of stretching neural structures on grade one hamstring injuries. *J. Orthop. Sports Phys. Ther.*, **10**, 481–487.

Landers, J. (1987). The upper limb tension test. In: *Proceedings of the 5th Biennial Conference of the Manipulative Therapists Association of Australia*, pp. 1–12. Brisbane, Australia: Manipulative Therapists Association of Australia.

Lerman, V. and Drasnin, H. (1975). Adhesive lesions of the nerve root in the dural orifice as a cause of sciatica. *Surg. Neurol.*, **4**, 229–232.

Lew, P.C. and Briggs, C.A. (1997). Relationship between the cervical component of the slump test and change in hamstring muscle tension. *Manual Ther.*, **2**, 98–105.

Lewis, J., Ramot, R. and Green, A. (1998). Changes in mechanical tension in the median nerve: possible implications for the upper limb tension test. *Physiotherapy*, **84**, 254–261.

MacNab, I. (1971). Negative disc exploration. An analysis of the causes of nerve-root involvement in sixty-eight patients. *J. Bone Joint Surg.*, **53**, 891–903.

Maitland, G.D. (1978). Movement of pain sensitive structures in the vertebral canal in a group of physiotherapy students. In: *Proceedings of Inaugural Congress of the Manipulative Therapists Association of Australia*, pp. 37–52. Sydney, Australia: Manipulative Therapists Association of Australia.

Maitland, G.D. (1979). Negative disc exploration: positive canal signs. *Aust. J. Physiother.*, **25**, 129–133.

Maitland, G.D. (1985). The Slump Test: examination and treatment. *Aust. J. Physiother.*, **31**, 215–219.

Maitland, G.D. (1986). *Vertebral Manipulation*. London: Butterworths.

Philip, K., Lew, P. and Matyas, T. (1989). Inter-therapist reliability of the slump test. *Aust. J. Physiother.*, **35**, 89–94.

Quillen, W.S. and Rouillier, L.H. (1982). Initial management of acute ankle sprains with rapid pulsed pneumatic compression and cold. *J. Orthop. Sports Phys. Ther.*, **4**, 39–43.

Rubenach, H. (1985). The upper limb tension test – the effect of the position and movement of the contralateral arm. In: *Proceedings of the 4th Biennial Conference of the Manipulative Therapists Association of Australia*, pp. 274–283. Brisbane, Australia: Manipulative Therapists Association of Australia.

Scrimshaw, S.V. and Maher, C.G. (2001). Randomized controlled trial of neural mobilization after spinal surgery. *Spine*, **26**, 2647–2652.

Selvaratnam, P., Glasgow, E. and Matyas, T. (1989). Differential strain produced by the brachial plexus tension test on C5 to T1 nerve roots. In: *Proceedings of 6th Biennial Conference of the Manipulative Therapists Association of Australia*, ed. H.M. Jones, M.A. Jones and M.R. Milde, pp. 167–172. Adelaide, Australia: Manipulative Therapists Association of Australia.

Selvaratnam, P.J., Matyas, T.A. and Glasgow, E.F. (1994). Noninvasive discrimination of brachial plexus involvement in upper limb pain. *Spine*, **19**, 26–33.

Shacklock, M. (1995). Neurodynamics. *Physiotherapy*, **81**, 9–16.

Simionato, R., Stiller, K. and Butler, D. (1988). Neural tension signs in Guillan Barre syndrome: 2 case reports. *Aust. J. Physiother.*, **34**, 257–262.

Smyth, M.J. and Wright, V. (1958). Sciatica and the intervertebral disc. *J. Bone Joint Surg.*, **40A**, 1401–1418.

Sunderland, S. and Bradley, K. (1961a). Stress–strain phemomena in human peripheral nerve trunks. *Brain*, **84**, 102–119.

Sunderland, S. and Bradley, K. (1961b). Stress–strain phemomena in human spinal nerve roots. *Brain*, **84**, 120–127.

Tal-Akabi, A. and Rushton, A. (2000). An investigation to compare the effectiveness of carpal bone mobilisation and neurodynamic mobilisation as methods of treatment for carpal tunnel syndrome. *Manual Ther.*, **5**, 214–222.

Troup, J. (1981). Straight-leg-raising (SLR) and the qualifying tests for increased root tension: their predictive value after back and sciatic pain. *Spine*, **6**, 526–527.

Turl, S.E. and George, K.P. (1998). Adverse neural tension: a factor in repetitive hamstring strain? *J. Orthop. Sports Phys. Ther.*, **27**, 16–21.

Waddell, G. (1998). *The Back Pain Revolution*. Edinburgh: Churchill Livingstone.

Wasserman, S. (1918). Uber ein neues Schenkelnervneuritis nebst Bemerkungen aur diagnostik der Schenkelnerverkrankungen. *Dtsh Z Schft Nervenhk*, **63**, 140–143. Cited in Dyck, P. (1984). Lumbar nerve root: the enigmatic eponyms. *Spine*, **9**, 1983–1986.

Williams, P., Warwick, R., Dyson, M. and Bannister, L. (1989). *Gray's Anatomy*. Edinburgh: Churchill Livingstone.

Yaxley, G.A. and Jull, G.A. (1993). Adverse tension in the neural system. A preliminary study of tennis elbow. *Aust. J. Physiother.*, **39**, 15–22.

THE NEUROLOGICAL EXAMINATION

Appelberg, B., Hulliger, M., Johansson, H. and Sojka, P. (1983). Actions on gamma motor neurons by electrical stimulation of group I muscle afferents in the hind limb of the cat. *J. Physiol.*, **335**, 275–292.

Bannister, R. (ed.) (1992). *Brain and Bannister's Clinical Neurology*, 7th edn. Oxford: Oxford University Press.

Barr, M. (1974). *The Human Nervous System*. Maryland: Harper and Row.

Bickerstaff, E.R. (1980). *Neurological Examination in Clinical Practice*, 4th edn. Melbourne: Blackwell Scientific.

Bogduk, N. (1987). Innervation, pain patterns and mechanisms of pain production. In: *Clinics in Physical Therapy, Physical Therapy of the Low Back*, ed. L.T. Twomey and, J.R. Taylor. Melbourne: Churchill Livingstone.

Bohannon, R. (1986). Manual muscle test scores and dynamometer test scores of knee extension strength. *Arch. Phys. Med. Rehabil.*, **4**, 390–392.

Bohannon, R. and Gajdosik, R. (1987). Spinal nerve compression – some clinical implications. *Phys. Ther.*, **67**, 376–381.

Bouchier, I.A.D. and Morris, J.S. (1982). *Clinical Skills – A System of Clinical Examination*. London: W.B. Saunders.

Bowditch, M.G., Sanderson, P. and Livesey, J.P. (1996). The significance of an absent ankle reflex. *J. Bone Joint Surg.*, **78B**, 276–279.

Burke, D., Gracies, J.M., Mazevet, D. et al. (1992a). Convergence of descending and various peripheral inputs onto common propriospinal-like neurones in man. *J. Physiol.*, **449**, 655–671.

Burke, D., Gracies, J.M., Meunier, S. and Pierrot-Deseilligny, E. (1992b). Changes in presynaptic inhibition in man during voluntary contractions. *J. Physiol.*, **449**, 673–687.

Coscia, M., Leipzig, T. and Cooper, D. (1994). Acute cauda equina syndrome: diagnostic advantage of MRI. *Spine*, **19**, 475–478.

De Palma, A.F. and Rothman, R.H. (1970). *The Intervertebral Disc*. London: W.B. Saunders.

Foreman, S.M. and Croft, A.C. (1988). *Whiplash Injuries – The Cervical Acceleration/Deceleration Syndrome*. Sydney: Williams and Wilkins.

Gaines, J.M. and Talbot, L.A. (1999). Isokinetic strength testing in research and practice. *Biol. Res. Nurs.*, **1**, 57–64.

Gelberman, R., Szabo, R., Williamson, R. and Dimick, M. (1983). Sensibility testing in peripheral nerve compression syndromes. *J. Bone Joint Surg.*, **65-A**, 632–638.

Griffiths, D.M. (2002). The physiology of continence: idiopathic fecal constipation and soiling. *Semin. Pediat. Surg.*, **11**, 67–74.

Hagbath, K.-E., Wallin, G., Burke, D. and Lofstedt, L. (1975). Effects of Jendrassic manoeuvre on muscle spindle activity in man. *J. Neurol. Neurosurg. Psychiatry*, **38**, 1143–1153.

Helfet, A.J. and Gruebel, L. (1978). *Disorders of the Lumbar Spine*. Philadelphia: J.B. Lippincott.

Hoyland, J., Freemont, A.J. and Joyson, M.I.V. (1989). Intervertebral foramen venous obstruction. *Spine*, **14**, 553–567.

Janig, W. (1978). The autonomic nervous system. In: *Fundamentals of Neurophysiology*, ed. R.F. Schmidt. New York: Springer Verlag.

Kaiser, A.M. and Ortega, A.E. (2002). Anorectal anatomy: *Surg. Clin. North Am.*, **82**, 1125–1138.

Kandell, E.R., Schwartz, J.H. and Jessell, T.M. (1991). *Principles of Neural Science*, 3rd edn. Connecticut: Prentice-Hall International.

Knutsson, E., Skoglund, C.R. and Natchev, E. (1988). Changes in voluntary muscle strength, somatosensory transmission and skin temperature concomitant with pain relief during autotraction in patients with lumbar and sacral root lesions. *Pain*, **33**, 173–179.

Kortelainen, P., Puranen, J., Koivisto, E. and Lahde, S. (1985). Symptoms and signs of sciatica and their relation to the localization of the lumbar disc herniation. *Spine*, **10**, 88–92.

Lance, J.W. and McLeod, J.G. (1975). *A Physiological Approach to Clinical Neurology*, 2nd edn. London: Butterworths.

Lieberman, J., Corkill, G. and Taylor, R. (1983). Fatiguing weakness; an initial symptom in clinical compressive radiculopathy. *Surg. Neurol.*, **19**, 354–357.

Loeser, J.D. (1985). Pain due to nerve injury. *Spine*, **10**, 232–235.

Luhan, J. (1968). *Neurology, A Concise Clinical Textbook*. Baltimore: Williams and Wilkins.

Magee, D.J. (1987). *Orthopaedic Physical Assessment*. London: W.B. Saunders.

Maitland, G.D. (1986). *Vertebral Manipulation*, 5th edn. London: Butterworths.

McCall, I.W., Park, W.M. and O'Brien, J.P. (1979). Induced pain referral from posterior lumbar elements in normal subjects. *Spine*, **4**, 441–446.

McCulloch, J.A. and Waddell, G. (1980). Variations of the lumbosacral myotomes with bony segmental anomalies. *J. Bone Joint Surg.*, **62A**, 475–480.

McNab, I. (1972). The mechanism of spondylogenic pain. In: *Cervical Pain*, ed. C. Hirsch and Y. Zotterman. Oxford: Pergamon.

Mooney, V. and Robertson, J. (1976). The facet syndrome. *Clin. Orthop. Rel. Res.*, **115**, 149–156.

Neidre, A. and McNab, I. (1983). Anomalies of lumbar spine nerve roots. *Spine*, **8**, 294–299.

Olmarker, K., Rydevick, B. and Holm, S. (1989). Edema formation in spinal nerve roots induced by experimental, graded compression. *Spine*, **14**, 569–573.

Osol, A. (1972). *Blakiston's Gould Medical Dictionary*, 3rd edn. New York: McGraw-Hill.

Quinn, D. and Shannon, L. (2002). The colon and rectum. *Neonatal Network – J. Neonatal Nurs.*, **19**, 48–52.

Rydevick, B., Myer, R. and Powell, H. (1989). Pressure increases in the dorsal root ganglion following mechanical compression. Closed compartment syndrome in nerve roots. *Spine*, **14**, 574–576.

Shefchyk, S.J. (2002). Spinal cord neural organization controlling the urinary bladder and striated sphincter. *Prog. Brain Res.*, **137**, 71–82.

Skre, H. (1972). Neurological signs in a normal population. *Acta Neurol. Scand.*, **48**, 575–606.

Sunderland, S. (1978). *Nerve and Nerve Injuries*, 2nd edn. London: Churchill Livingstone.

Thorn, G.W. (1977). *Harrison's Principles of Internal Medicine*. Tokyo: McGraw-Hill Kogadusha.

Weiss, M.D., Garfin, S.R., Gelberman, R.H. et al. (1985). Lower extremity sensibility testing in patients with herniated lumbar intervertebral discs. *Spine*, **9**, 1219–1224.

Williams, P.R. and Warwick, R. (1980). *Gray's Anatomy*, 36th edn. London: Churchill Livingstone.

Young, A., Getty, J., Jackson, A. et al. (1983). Variations in the pattern of muscle innervation by the L5 and S1 nerve roots. *Spine*, **8**, 616–624.

Zimmerman, M. (1978). Regulatory functions of the nervous system as exemplified by the spinal motor system. In: *Fundamentals of Neurophysiology*, ed. R.F. Schmidt, pp. 205–211. New York: Springer-Verlag.

PASSIVE MOTION TESTS

Buch-Jaeger, N. and Foucher, G. (1994). Correlation of clinical signs with nerve conduction tests in the diagnosis of carpal tunnel syndrome. *J. Hand Surg.*, **19B**, 720–724.

Chiradejnant, A., Maher, C. and Latimer, J. (2002). Objective manual assessment of lumbar PA stiffness is now possible. *J. Manip. Physiol. Ther.* **26**, 34–39.

Cibulka, M., Delitto, A. and Koldehoff, R. (1988). Changes in innominate tilt after manipulation of the sacroiliac joint in patients with low back pain. An experimental study. *Phys. Ther.*, **68**, 1359–1363.

DiFabio, R. (1992). Efficacy of manual therapy. *Phys. Ther.*, **72**, 853–864.

Dreyfuss, P., Michaelsen, M., Pauza, K., McLarty, J. and Bogduk, N. (1996). The value of medical history and physical examination in diagnosing sacroiliac joint pain. *Spine*, **21**, 2594–2602.

Edmonston, S., Allison, G., Gregg, C., Purden, S., Svansson, G. and Watson, A. (1998). Effect of position on the posteroanterior stiffness of the lumbar spine. *Manual Ther.*, **3**, 21–26.

Fowler, P. and Lubliner, J. (1989). The predictive value of five clinical signs in the evaluation of meniscal pathology. *Arthroscopy*, **5**, 184–186.

Grieve, G. (1984). *Mobilisation of the Spine*, 4th edn. New York: Churchill Livingstone.

Harryman, D.T., Sidles, J.M., Clark, J.M., McQuade, K.J., Gibb, T.D. and Matsen, F.A. (1990). Translation of the humeral head on the glenoid with passive glenohumeral motion. *J. Bone Joint Surg.*, **72-A**, 1334–1343.

Jull, G., Bogduk, N. and Marsland, A. (1988). The accuracy of manual diagnosis for cervical zygapophysial joint pain syndromes. *Med. J. Aust.*, **148**, 233–236.

Kaltenborn, F. (1980). *Mobilization of the Extremity Joints*. Oslo: Olaf Noris Bokhandel Universitetsgaten.

Katz, J.W. and Fingeroth, R.J. (1986). The diagnostic accuracy of ruptures of the anterior cruciate ligament comparing the Lachman test, the anterior drawer sign, and the pivot shift test in acute and chronic knee injuries. *Am. J. Sports Med.*, **14**, 88–91.

Keating, J.C., Bergman, T.F., Jacobs, G.E., Finer, B.A. and Larson, K. (1990). Interexaminer reliability of eight evaluative dimensions of lumbar segmental abnormality. *J. Manip. Physiol. Ther.*, **13**, 463–470.

Koes, B., Bouter, L., Van Mameren, H., et al. (1993). A randomized clinical trial of manual therapy and physiotherapy for persistent back and neck complaints: subgroup analysis and relationship between outcome measures. *J. Manip. Physiol. Ther.*, **16**, 211–217.

Latimer, J., Goodsell, M., Lee, M., Maher, C., Wilkinson, B. and Moran, C. (1996a). Evaluation of a new device for measuring responses to posteroanterior forces in a patient population, part 1: reliability testing. *Phys. Ther.*, **76**, 158–165.

Latimer, J., Lee, M., Adams, R. and Moran, C. (1996b). An investigation of the relationship between low back pain and lumbar posteroanterior stiffness. *J. Manip. Physiol. Ther.*, **19**, 587–591.

Lee, R. and Evans, J. (1997). An in-vivo study of the intervertebral movements produced by posteroanterior mobilization. *Clin. Biomech.*, **12**, 400–408.

Lee, M. and Moseley, A. (1991). *Dynamics of the Human Body*, 2nd edn, pp. 153–156. Sydney: Zygal.

Lee, M., Kelly, D. and Steven, G. (1995). A model of spine, ribcage and pelvic responses to a specific lumbar manipulative force in relaxed subjects. *J. Biomech.*, **28**, 1403–1408.

Lee, M., Steven, G., Crosbie, J. and Higgs, J. (1996). Towards a theory of lumbar mobilisation – the relationship between applied force and movements of the spine. *Manual Ther.*, **2**, 67–75.

Liu, S.H., Henry, M.H. and Nuccion, S.L. (1996). A prospective evaluation of a new physical examination in predicting glenoid labral tears. *Am. J. Sports Med.*, **24**, 721–725.

MacConaill, M. and Basmajian, J. (1969). *Muscles and Movements: A Basis for Human Kinesiology*. Baltimore: Williams and Wilkins.

Maher, C. and Adams, R. (1994). Reliability of pain and stiffness assessments in clinical manual lumbar spine examination. *Phys. Ther.*, **74**, 801–811.

Maher, C. and Adams, R. (1996a). A comparison of pisiform and thumb grips in stiffness assessment. *Phys. Ther.*, **76**, 41–48.

Maher, C. and Adams, R. (1996b). Stiffness judgments are affected by visual occlusion. *J. Manip. Physiol. Ther.*, **19**, 250–256.

Maher, C. and Latimer, J. (1992). Pain or resistance – the manual therapists' dilemma. *Aust. J. Physiother.*, **38**, 257–260.

Maher, C.G., Latimer, J. and Adams, R. (1998). An investigation of the reliability and validity of posteroanterior spinal stiffness judgments made using a reference-based protocol. *Phys. Ther.*, **78**, 829–837.

Maher, C., Latimer, J. and Refshauge, K. (2001). *Atlas of Clinical Tests and Measures for Low Back Pain*. Melbourne: Australian Physiotherapy Association.

Maher, C., Latimer, J. and Starkey, I. (2002). An evaluation of Superthumb and the Kneeshaw device as manual therapy tools. *Aust. J. Physiother.*, **48**, 25–30.

Maitland, G. (1986). *Vertebral Manipulation.* London: Butterworths.

Matyas, T. and Bach, T. (1985). The reliability of selected techniques in clinical arthrometrics. *Aust. J. Physiother.*, **31**, 175–199.

McClure, P. and Flowers, K.R. (1992). Treatment of limited shoulder motion: a case study based upon biomechanical considerations. *Phys. Ther.*, **72**, 929–936.

Mior, S.A., McGregor, M. and Schut, B. (1990). The role of experience in clinical accuracy. *J. Manip. Physiol. Ther.*, **13**, 68–71.

Penning, L. (1992). Functional pathology of lumbar spinal stenosis. *Clin. Biomech.*, **7**, 3–17.

Phillips, D.R. and Twomey, L. (1996). A comparison of manual diagnosis with a diagnosis established by a uni-level lumbar spinal block procedure. *Manual Ther.*, **2**, 82–87.

Poppen, N. and Walker, P. (1976). Normal and abnormal motion of the shoulder. *J. Bone Joint Surg.*, **58**, 195–201.

Riddle, D. (1992). Measurement of accessory motion: critical issues and related concepts. *Phys. Ther.*, **72**, 865–874.

Shirley, D., Lee, M. and Ellis, E. (1999). The relationship between submaximal activity of the lumbar extensor muscles and lumbar posteroanterior stiffness. *Phys. Ther.*, **79**, 278–285.

Sidor, M.L., Zuckerman, J.D., Lyon, T., Koval, K., Cuomo, F. and Schoenberg, N. (1993). The Neer classification system for proximal humeral fractures. *J. Bone Joint Surg.*, **75A**, 1745–1750.

Siebenrock, K.A. and Gerber, C. (1993). The reproducibility of classification of fractures of the proximal end of the humerus. *J. Bone Joint Surg.*, **75A**, 1751–1755.

Squires, M., Latimer, J., Adams, R. and Maher, C. (2001). Indenter head area and testing frequency effects on posteroanterior lumbar stiffness and subjects' rated comfort. *Manual Ther.*, **6**, 41–47.

Stratford, P. and Binkley, J. (1995). A review of the McMurray test: definition, interpretation, and clinical usefulness. *J. Sports Phys. Ther.*, **22**, 116–120.

Sturesson, B., Selvile, G. and Uden, A. (1989). Movements of the sacroiliac joints. A roentgen stereophotogrammetric analysis. *Spine*, **14**, 162–165.

Waddell, G., Feder, G., McIntosh, A., Lewis, M. and Hutchison, A. (1996). *Low Back Pain Evidence Review.* London: Royal College of General Practitioners.

MUSCLE TESTING

Ada, L. and Herbert, R. (1988). Measurement of joint range of motion. *Aust. J. Physiother.*, **34**, 260–262.

Bohannon, R.W. (1990). Testing isometric limb muscle strength with dynamometers. *Crit. Rev. Phys. Rehab. Med.*, **2**, 75–86.

Brand, P.W. (1985). *Clinical Mechanics of the Hand.* St Louis: CV Mosby.

Corrigan, B. and Maitland, G.D. (1983). *Practical Orthopaedic Medicine.* London: Butterworths.

Daniels, L. and Worthingham, C. (1986). *Muscle Testing*, 5th edn. Philadelphia: WB Saunders.

Fish, D.R. and Wingate, L. (1985). Sources of goniometric error at the elbow. *Phys. Ther.*, **65**, 1666–1670.

Gadjosik, R.L. and Bohannon, R.W. (1987). Clinical measurement of range of motion. Review of goniometry emphasizing reliability and validity. *Phys. Ther.*, **67**, 1867–1872.

Gravel, D., Richards, C.L. and Filion, M. (1988). Influence of contractile tension development on dynamic strength measurements of the plantarflexors in man. *J. Biomech.*, **21**, 89–96.

Harvey, L., King, M. and Herbert, R.D. (1994). Test–retest reliability of a procedure for measuring extrinsic finger flexor muscle extensibility. *J. Hand Ther.*, **7**, 251–254.

Herzog, W. (1988). The relation between the resultant moments at a joint and the moments measured by an isokinetic dynamometer. *J. Biomech.*, **21**, 5–12.

Hortobagyi, T., Katch, F. and LaChance, P.F. (1989). Interrelationships among various measures of upper body strength assessed by different contraction modes. *Eur. J. Physiol.*, **58**, 749–755.

Kendall, F.P., McCreary, E.K and Provance, P.G. (1993). *Muscles. Testing and Function*, 4th edn. Baltimore: Williams and Wilkins.

Lamb, R.L. (1985). Manual muscle testing. In: *Measurement in Physical Therapy*, ed. J.M. Rothstein, pp. 47–55. New York: Churchill Livingstone.

Mayhew, T.P. and Rothstein, J.M. (1985). Measurement of muscle performance with instruments. In: *Measurement in Physical Therapy*, ed. J.M. Rothstein. pp. 57–102. New York: Churchill Livingstone.

McDonagh, M.J.N. and Davies, C.T.M. (1984). Adaptive response to mammalian skeletal muscle to exercise with high loads. *Eur. J. Appl. Physiol.*, **52**, 139–155.

Miller, P.J. (1985). Assessment of joint motion. In: *Measurement in Physical Therapy*, ed. J. M. Rothstein, pp. 120–127. New York: Churchill Livingstone.

Munsat, T.L. (1990). Clinical trials in neuromuscular disease. *Muscle Nerve* (suppl.), S3–S6.

Sapega, A.A., Nicholas, J.A., Sokolow, D. and Saraniti, A. (1982). The nature of torque "overshoot" in Cybex isokinetic dynamometry. *Med. Sci. Sports Exerc.*, **14**, 368–375.

Winter, D.A., Wells, R.P. and Orr, G.W. (1981). Errors in the use of isokinetic dynamometers. *Eur. J. Appl. Physiol.*, **46**, 397–408.

MOTOR PERFORMANCE: EVALUATION AND MEASUREMENT

Ada, L. and Canning, C. (1990). Anticipating and avoiding muscle shortening. In: *Key Issues in Neurological Physiotherapy*, eds. L. Ada and, C. Canning, pp. 219–236. Oxford: Butterworth-Heinemann.

Andriacchi, T.P., Galante, J.O. and Fermier, R.W. (1982). The influence of total knee-replacement design on walking and stair-climbing. *J. Bone Joint Surg.*, **64A**, 1328–1335.

Andriacchi, T.P. and Birac, D. (1993). Functional testing in the anterior cruciate ligament-deficient knee. *Clin. Orthop. Rel. Res.*, **288**, 40–47.

Baker, P.A., Evans, O.M. and Lee, C. (1991). Treadmill training following fractured neck-of-femur. *Arch. Phys. Med. Rehabil.*, **72**, 649–652.

Carr, J.H., Shepherd, R.B., Nordholm, L. and Lynne, D. (1985). Investigation of a new motor assessment scale for stroke patients. *Phys. Ther.*, **65**, 175–180.

Dean, C.M., Richards, C.L. and Malouin, F. (2000). Task-related circuit training improves performance of locomotor tasks in chronic stroke. A randomized controlled pilot trial. *Arch. Phys. Med. Rehabil.*, **81**, 409–417.

Drabsch, T., Lovenfosse, J., Fowler, V. et al. (1998). Effects of task-specific training on walking and sit-to-stand after total hip replacement. *Aust. J. Physiother.*, **44**, 193–198.

Duncan, P.W., Weiner, D.K., Chandler, J. et al. (1990). Functional reach: a new clinical measure of balance. *J. Gerontol.*, **45**, M192–197.

Enoka, R.M., Miller, D.I. and Burgess, E.M. (1982). Below-knee amputee running gait. *Amer. J. Phys. Med.*, **62**, 66–84.

Goldie, P.A., Matyas, T.A., Spencer, K.I. et al. (1990). Postural control in standing following stroke: test-retest reliability of some quantitative clinical test. *Phys. Ther.*, **70**, 234–243.

Harris, W.H. and Sledge, C.B. (1990). Total hip replacement. *N. Engl. J. Med.*, **323**, 725–731.

Hill, K., Bernhardt, J., McGann, A. et al. (1996). A new test of dynamic standing balance for stroke patients: reliability and comparison with healthy elderly. *Phys. Ther.*, **48**, 257–262.

Inman, V.T., Ralston, H.J. and Todd, F. (1981). *Human Walking*. Baltimore: Williams and Wilkins.

Jevsevar, D.S., Riley, P.O., Hodge, W.A. and Krebs, D.E. (1993). Knee kinematics and kinetics during locomotor activities of daily living in subjects with knee arthroplasty and in healthy control subjects. *Phys. Ther.*, **73**, (iv), 229–239.

Kerslake, J.M., Catton, L. and Ford, S.G. (1987). Functional activities following cementless isoelastic total hip replacement. *Proceedings of the Tenth International Congress of the World Confederation for Physical Therapy*, pp. 451–455, Sydney.

Long, W.T., Dorr, L.D., Healy, B. and Perry, J. (1993). Functional recovery of non cemented total hip arthroplasty. *Clin. Orthop. Rel. Res.*, **288**, 73–77.

Malouin, F. (1995). Observational gait analysis. In: *Gait Analysis: Theory and Application*, eds. R.L. Craik and C.A. Oatis, pp. 112–124, St Louis: Mosby.

Moffet, H., Richards, C., Malouin, F. and Bravo, G. (1993). Impact of knee extensor strength deficits on stair ascent performance in patients after medial meniscectomy. *Scand. J. Rehabil. Med.*, **25**, 63–71.

Podsialo, D. and Richardson, S. (1991). The timed 'Up & Go': a test of basic functional mobility for frail elderly persons. *J. Am. Gerontol. Soc.*, **39**, 142–148.

Ross, M. (1997). Test-retest reliability of the lateral step-up test in young adult healthy subjects. *J. Orthop. Sports Phys. Ther.*, **25**, 128–132.

Sherrington, C. and Lord, S.R. (1997). Home exercise to improve strength and walking velocity after hip fracture: A randomized controlled trial. *Arch. Phys. Med. Rehabil.*, **78**, 208–212.

Shih, C.H., Du, Y.K., Lin, Y.H. et al. (1994). Muscular recovery around the hip joint after total hip arthroplasty. *Clin. Orthop. Rel. Res.*, **302**, 115–120.

Smith, A. (1990). The measurement of human motor performance. In: *Key Issues in Neurological Physiotherapy*, eds. L. Ada and C. Canning. Oxford: Butterworth-Heinemann.

van Vliet, P. (1988). Kinematic analysis of videotape to measure walking following stroke: a case study. *Aust. J. Physiother.* **34**, 48–51.

Wagenaar, R.C. and Beck, W.J. (1992). Hemiplegic gait: a kinematic analysis using walking speed as a basis. *J. Biomech.*, **25**, 1007–1015.

Weinstein, J.N., Andriacchi, T.P. and Galante, J.O. (1986). Factors influencing walking and stair climbing following uncompartmental knee arthroplasty. *J. Arthroplasty*, **1**, 109–115.

Westwood, P. (1993). An investigation into the effects of task-specific training on the biomechanics of standing up in patients following total hip replacement. MAppSc Thesis, School of Physiotherapy, University of Sydney, Australia.

Winter, D.A. and Sienko, S.E. (1988). Biomechanics of below-knee amputee gait. *J. Biomech.*, **21**, 361–367.

MUSCLE PERFORMANCE

Biering-Sorensen, F. (1984). Physical measurements as risk indicators for low-back trouble over a one-year period. *Spine*, **9**, 106–119.

Cairns, M. (2002). Email correspondence, 8 February 2002.

Cairns, M., Foster, N. and Wright, C. (2000). A pragmatic randomised controlled trial of specific spinal stabilization exercises and conventional physiotherapy in the management of recurrent lumber spine pain and dysfunction. In: *Seventh Scientific Conference of the International Federation of Orthopaedic Manipulative Therapists* in conjunction with the 11th Biennial Conference of the Manipulative Physiotherapists Association of Australia, pp. 91–95, Perth.

Goldby, L., Moore, A., Doust, J., Trew, M. and Lewis, J. (2001). A randomised controlled trial investigating the efficacy of manual therapy, exercises to rehabilitate spinal stabilisation and an educational booklet in the conservative treatment of chronic low back disorder. In: *MACP/Kinetic Control 1st International Conference on Movement Dysfunction*, September 2001, Edinburgh, Scotland.

Holmstrom, E., Moritz, U. and Andersson, M. (1992). Trunk muscle strength and back muscle endurance in construction workers with and without low back disorders. *Scand. J. Rehabil. Med.*, **24**, 3–10.

Ito, T., Shirado, O., Suzuki, H. et al. (1996). Lumbar trunk muscle endurance testing: an inexpensive alternative to a machine for evaluation. *Arch. Phys. Med. Rehabil.*, **77**, 75–79.

Kankaanpaa, B., Laaksonen, D., Taimela, S., Kokko, S., Airaksinen, O. and Hanninen, O. (1998). Age, sex, and body mass index as determinants of back and hip extensor fatigue in the isometric Biering Sorensen back endurance test. *Arch. Phys. Med. Rehabil.*, **79**, 1069–1075.

Kenney, W. (1995). *ASCM's Guidelines for Exercise Testing and Prescription*, 5th edn. Baltimore: Williams and Wilkins.

Kraus, H. (1970). *Clinical Treatment of Back and Neck Pain*. New York: McGraw-Hill.

Latimer, J., Maher, C. and Refshauge, K.M. (1999). Reliability and validity of the Biering–Sorensen test in asymptomatic subjects and subjects reporting current or previous non specific low back pain. *Spine*, **24**, 2085–2090.

Lattika, P., Battie, M.C., Bideman, T. and Gibbons, L.E. (1995). Correlations of isokinetic and psychophysical back lift and static back extensor endurance tests in men. *Clin. Biomech.*, **10**, 325–330.

Lindstrom, I., Ohlund, C., Eek, C. et al. (1992a). The effect of graded activity on patients with subacute low back pain: a randomized prospective clinical study with an operant-conditioning behavioral approach. *Phys. Ther.*, **72**, 279–290.

Lindstrom, I., Ohlund, C., Eek, C., Wallin, L., Peterson, L.E. and Nachemson, A. (1992b). Mobility, strength, and fitness after a graded activity program for patients with subacute low back pain. A randomized prospective clinical study with a behavioral therapy approach. *Spine*, **17**, 641–652.

Lindstrom, I., Ohlund, C. and Nachemson, A. (1995). Physical performance, pain, pain behavior and subjective disability in patients with subacute low back pain. *Scand. J. Rehabil. Med.*, **27**, 153–160.

Luoto, S., Heliovaara, M., Hurri, H. and Alaranta, H. (1995). Static back endurance and the risk of low-back pain. *Clin. Biomech.*, **10**, 323–324.

Mannion, A.F., Connolly, B., Wood, K. and Dolan, P. (1997). The use of surface EMG power spectral analysis in the evaluation of back muscle function. *J. Rehabil. Res. Dev.*, **34**, 427–439.

Mayer, T., Gatchel, R., Betancur, J. and Bovasso, E. (1995). Trunk muscle endurance measurement: isometric contrasted to isokinetic testing in normal subjects. *Spine*, **20**, 920–927.

McQuade, K., Turner, J. and Buchner, D. (1988). Physical fitness and chronic low back pain: an analysis of the relationships among fitness, functional limitations and depression. *Clin. Orthop. Rel. Res.*, **233**, 198–204.

Moreland, J., Finch, E., Stratford, P., Balsor, B. and Gill, C. (1997). Intense reliability of six tests of trunk muscle function and endurance. *J. Orthop. Sports Phys. Ther.*, **26**, 200–208.

O'Sullivan, P., Twomey, L. and Allison, G. (1997). Evaluation of specific stabilizing exercise in the treatment of chronic low back pain with radiologic diagnosis of spondylolysis or spondylolisthesis. *Spine*, **22**, 2959–2967.

Richardson, C.A., Jull, G., Hodges, P. and Hides, J. (1999). *Therapeutic Exercise for Spinal Segmental Stabilization in Low Back Pain: Scientific Basis and Clinical Approach*. Sydney: Churchill Livingstone.

Twomey, L. and Taylor, J. (eds) (1994). *Physical Therapy of the Low Back*, 2nd edn. New York: Churchill Livingstone.

Van Tulder, M.W., Koes, B.W. and Bouter, L.M. (1997). Conservative treatment of acute and chronic nonspecific low back pain. A systematic review of randomized controlled trials of the most common interventions. *Spine*, **22**, 2128–2156.

CLINICAL TESTS AND MEASURES

Biering-Sorensen, F. (1984). Physical measurements as risk indicators for low-back trouble over a one-year period. *Spine*, **9**, 106–119.

Boland, R.A. and Adams, R.D. (2000). Effects of ankle dorsiflexion on range and reliability of straight leg raising. *Aust. J. Physiother.*, **46**, 191–200.

Charnley, J. (1951). Orthopaedic signs in the diagnosis of disc protrusion – with special reference to the straight-leg-raising test. *Lancet*, **4**, 186–192.

Chow, R., Adams, R. and Herbert, R. (1994). Straight leg raise test high reliability is not a motor memory artefact. *Aust. J. Physiother.*, **40**, 107–111.

Fahrni, W. (1966). Observations on straight leg-raising with special reference to nerve root adhesions. *Can. J. Surg.* **9**, 44–48.

Gauvin, M., Riddle, D. and Rothstein, J. (1990). Reliability of clinical measurements of forward bending using the modified fingertip-to-floor methods. *Phys. Ther.*, **70**, 443–447.

Hsieh, C.-Y. and Yeung, B.W. (1986). Active neck motion measurements with a tape measure. *J. Orthop. Sports Phys. Ther.*, **8**, 88–93.

Ito, T., Shirado, O., Suzuki, H. et al. (1996). Lumbar trunk muscle endurance testing: an inexpensive alternative to a machine for evaluation. *Arch. Phys. Med. Rehabil.*, **77**, 75–79.

Kerr, R., Cadoux-Hudson, T. and Adams, C. (1988). The value of accurate clinical assessment in the surgical management of the lumbar disc protrusion. *J. Neurol. Neurosurg. Psychiatry*, **51**, 169–173.

Kippers, V. and Parker, A. (1987). Toe-touch test a measure of its validity. *Phys. Ther.*, **67**, 1680–1684.

Kosteljanetz, M., Bang, F. and Schmidt-Olsen, S. (1988). The clinical significance of straight-leg raising (Lasegue's sign) in the diagnosis of prolapsed lumbar disc. Interobserver variation and correlation with surgical findings. *Spine*, **13**, 393–395.

Lerman, V. and Drasnin, H. (1987). Adhesive lesions of the nerve root in the dural orifice as a cause of sciatica. *Surg. Neurol.*, **4**, 229–232.

Matyas, T. and Bach, T. (1985). The reliability of selected techniques in clinical arthrometrics. *Aust. J. Physiother.*, **31**, 175–199.

McNab, I. (1971). Negative disc exploration – an analysis of the causes of nerve-root involvement in sixty-eight patients. *J. Bone Joint Surg.*, **53A**, 891–903.

Newton, M. and Waddell, G. (1991). Reliability and validity of clinical measurement of the lumbar spine in patients with chronic low back pain. *Physiotherapy*, **77**, 796–800.

Pile, K., Laurent, M., Salmond, C. et al. (1991). Clinical observation of ankylosing spondylitis: a study of observer variation in spinal measurements. *Br. J. Physiother.*, **30**, 11–13.

Rainville, J., Sobel, J. and Hartigan, C. (1994). Comparison of total lumbosacral flexion and true lumbar flexion measured by a dual inclinometer technique. *Spine*, **19**, 2698–2701.

Sprangfort, E. (1972). Lumbar disc herniation. A computer aided analysis of 2504 operations. *Acta Orthop. Scand.*, **42**, 459.

Stude, D., Goertz, C. and Gallinger, M. (1994). Inter- and intra-examiner reliability of a single, digital inclinometric range of motion measurement technique in the assessment of lumbar range of motion. *J. Manip. Physiol. Ther.*, **17**, 83–87.

Waddell, G., Somerville, D., Henderson, I. and Newton, M. (1992). Objective clinical evaluation of physical impairment in chronic low back pain. *Spine*, **17**, 617–628.

Williams, R., Binkley, J., Goldsmith, C. et al. (1993). Reliability of the modified-modified Schober and double inclinometer methods for measuring lumbar flexion and extension. *Phys. Ther.*, **73**, 26–37.

Youdas, J.W., Carey, J.R. and Garrett, T.R. (1991). Reliability of measurements of cervical spine range of motion – comparison of three methods. *Phys. Ther.*, **71**, 98–104.

P00FLMAQT

SANDWELL & WEST BIRMINGHAM NHS TR.

SANDWELL & WEST BIRMINGHA
SANDWELL DISTRICT HOSPITA
LYDON
WEST BROMWICH
WEST MIDLANDS
B71 4HJ

Bill To: 10930001

SANDWELL & WEST BIRMINGHA
FINANCE DEPT, BROOKFIELD
DUDLEY ROAD
BIRMINGHAM
WEST MIDLANDS
B18 7QH

Routing

Sorting
Y07A06X
Covering – ZXXXX
Despatch

0–7506–5356–6   1   F 7936617 1

Customer P/O No | Cust P/O List
68999 | 25.99 GBP

Fund:

Title: Musculoskeletal Physiotherapy : Its Clinical Science
Format: Paperback
Author: Refshauge, Kathy
Publisher: Butterworth Heinemann
Volume: 2004
Edition: 2nd Ed   Year: 2004

Order Specific Instructions

COUTTS LIBRARY SERVICES: UK 002556439 LGUK001R001 UKRWLG47

Chapter 7

Selection of treatment for musculoskeletal conditions

Edited by K.M. Refshauge

Selection and application of treatment

N. Bogduk and S. Mercer

Musculoskeletal physiotherapy embraces many conditions and circumstances. Physiotherapists may be involved in restoring or maintaining mobility in elderly patients, rehabilitating postoperative patients, or preventing or reversing joint contractures. These fields of endeavour are not at issue. They are not controversial, either because the interventions used and their results appear satisfactory, or because they have not yet been subject to scientific scrutiny.

Where issues can be raised is in the realm of regional musculoskeletal pain and the role of physical therapy for pain in general. For these conditions physiotherapists have at their disposal a variety of interventions. They may choose to use modalities such as heat, ice, ultrasound or shortwave diathermy; they may choose physical forces, in the form of traction or manual therapy; they may use exercises. Alternatively the interventions may not be physical. The physiotherapist may engage the patient in explanation, education and the management of psychosocial factors.

At the heart of professional practice is how to select a treatment for a given condition or for a given patient, particularly in the face of available and emerging evidence on how well these interventions work. The student is entitled to ask, and should ask, why am I being taught to do this? Established practitioners have cause to reflect on why they do what they do.

In basic terms, a physiotherapist might select a particular treatment out of habit or tradition, on the basis of sound clinicopathological correlations or on the basis of sensible principles. Each of these approaches has serious limitations that impact on the wisdom of what physiotherapists do.

HABIT AND TRADITION

The most arcane basis for selecting treatment is to retort: 'this is what I always do' or 'this was what I was taught to do'. It presupposes that what the therapist does or was taught to do does, in fact, work. This is not necessarily the case, and the emerging evidence base would suggest that it is most likely not the case.

Although they may have been believed, respected or even esteemed, teachers of the past were not necessarily correct. Although what was taught in the past may have been an honest and best distillation of what was known at the time, subsequent research has revealed that much traditional wisdom is at best questionable, and at worst, wrong. Persisting in that wisdom or perpetuating myths is not only intellectually moribund, it is a waste of resources. Not only the profession but also the public are poorly served by practitioners who continue to apply treatments that fundamentally do not work. Both are better served if those practitioners abandon ineffective practices and concentrate on what does work.

Students should be alert to the weaknesses of habit and tradition. Persons in authority, be they teachers, experts or gurus, may not be right. Students should learn to ask for evidence that a diagnostic technique is reliable and that it is valid. They should ask for evidence of efficacy for therapeutic techniques. Unless those data are forthcoming students will not know if what they are being taught is nothing more than something that the teacher imagined or made up. By the same token, established practitioners can ask if what they do is reliable, valid and efficacious.

Convention is often defended by reference to clinical experience. The implication is that someone who has been practising a particular therapy for a long time would know what is best. The telling argument in this context is that every craft group uses the same defence. Surgeons claim success; acupuncturists and naturopaths claim success; chiropractors as well as physiotherapists claim success. All defend their claims with 'clinical experience'. Yet they cannot all be right, for why then do so many patients continue to languish with musculoskeletal problems? The reason why convention is an intellectually flawed basis for therapy is that it is confounded by factors such as patient bias, recall bias, outcome measures, misperception and lack of controls.

Patient bias operates when a patient likes the therapist and for that reason is reluctant to disappoint him or her by reporting that the treatment did not work. Rather than confront or threaten the therapist's obvious dedication and kindness, the patient denies failure, fails to report it or tells a white lie by reporting modest success. As a result, the therapist, through no fault of his or her own, gains the impression that the therapy is not failing and therefore may, indeed, be quite good.

In pursuit of truth, patient bias is reduced, if not eliminated, by having independent observers evaluate the therapy. Since they lack any contractual relationship with an independent observer, patients are less inclined to fabricate a benevolent response when it is not due. Any study or any claim that lacks an independent observer can, therefore, be challenged in principle, for it is likely to be compromised by patient bias.

Recall bias operates when a therapist, in recounting experience, remembers only the 'good' cases.

Psychologically it is only natural for a therapist to suppress unpleasant memories of 'bad' experiences such as failures. Moreover, a therapist is likely to continue to see patients who are satisfied with their treatment and come back for more; dissatisfied patients simply do not return. Therefore, therapists' memories of their experience are dominated by the 'good' cases.

Recall bias is eliminated by studying all consecutive cases over a predetermined time frame. This eliminates intellectual cheating such as 'that case doesn't count because they did not come back to finish therapy'. The chances are that such patients did not finish therapy because they were dissatisfied with it. The effect of monitoring all consecutive patients is to dilute, but render more realistic, the reported or claimed percentage success rate.

Outcome measures is a vexatious issue. A success might be claimed by a therapist if the patient simply feels 'better'. A more cynical interpretation would be that 'better' does not count if the patient still has the problem and is continuing to seek therapy. Another consideration is the temporal stability of the outcome. A patient may feel totally relieved of symptoms upon rising from the plinth, but that does not count as a success if upon leaving the front door of the practice the patient suffers a total recurrence of the complaint.

There is no single or absolute outcome measure. All therapists are entitled to declare their own, but they must do so honestly. It is fair, legitimate and acceptable for therapists to declare that their intended or attained outcome was simply to make the patient feel better. That outcome, however, cannot be declared to constitute a 'cure'. The critical issue is that whatever success a therapy achieves should not be misrepresented or overplayed. In teaching a therapy a therapist should be obliged to declare clearly what outcome can honestly be expected. There is no justification for portraying a therapy as 'good' (because it makes the patient feel 'better') but implying that it will 'cure'. Nor should students be allowed to infer that a treatment will cure when in reality it will at best be only palliative.

Black-and-white outcome measures are easy to apply and interpret: 'the patient either has pain or has no pain'. Such outcome measures are severe, and many therapies are likely to fail if pitted against such demanding standards. Less demanding outcome measures, however, may be difficult to quantify and calibrate. For example, how big is a 25% reduction in pain? How worthwhile is a 25% loss? After all, the patient still has 75% of the pain.

It is important for any consumer of outcome data to be assured that the instruments used to measure outcome are appropriate. The size of interobserver errors should be known, lest their magnitude be greater than that of the purported therapeutic benefit. Natural variance must also be taken into account. Some patients improve more than others yet, at the same time, patients who do not undergo therapy will none the less show variations in the severity of their complaint. Random variations between or within patients should not be misinterpreted as being due to the therapy. For this reason, before any claim about the success of therapy can be sustained, it must be based on a sample size that takes into account natural variation. In formal statistical terms, the study must have the power to detect what it purports to show.

Misperception pertains to when a therapist noticing a genuine success ascribes that success erroneously to a particular therapy when in fact the success was due to some other factor. Of particular concern here are the covert or accidental psychotherapeutic dimensions of physiotherapy treatment. Patients may feel better not because of the exercise or manipulation but because the therapist appeared to care, spent time with them and tried to help. This effect has not been quantified in physiotherapy at large, but has attracted attention with respect to preventive measures for low back pain. It has been recognized that a public caring attitude achieves greater success than training in lifting techniques or a back school programme (Wood, 1987; Gundewall et al., 1993).

Related to misperception are *extrapolation* and *generalization*. Therapies useful for one region of the body may be erroneously extrapolated as useful for another homologous region. For example, although the neck and back are both regions of the vertebral column, therapies worthwhile for one are not necessarily equally efficacious for the other; the two regions differ sufficiently in anatomy, biomechanics and pathology for this caveat to apply. Similarly, therapies that might work for acute problems will not necessarily apply to chronic problems of the same body part. Acute back pain, for example, may have a different pathology from that of chronic back pain, and be responsive to different interventions. Or it may be that the biology (and psychology) of the same, original pathology evolves as the condition changes from acute to chronic, rendering it less responsive to therapy. Success with acute problems, therefore, does not constitute a basis for claiming or predicting success with chronic disorders.

Controls are ubiquitously the missing factor in clinical experience. Therapists in conventional practice are unlikely to be able to submit themselves or their patients to controlled studies. In institutional practice, the demand for services is usually too great to allow therapists either to double or to halve their workload in order to submit a cohort of age-matched and gender-matched patients to parallel sham therapy as a control. In private practice, ethical restrictions would apply to charging patients for control therapy, and therapists are unlikely to be able to afford to treat free of charge equal numbers of 'active' and 'control' patients. Controls, however, are crucial if illusions are to be eliminated.

Consider the claim 'my therapy has a 75% success rate' (Table 7.1). Are you impressed? Would you be inclined to adopt this treatment for your own patients? What if we now unveil a control (Table 7.2)? Are you still impressed? What if the control results are somewhat more modest (Table 7.3). Are you still convinced? How much difference should there be between the rows before you are 'sold' on the efficacy of the therapy?

When time is a factor in outcome, results may be displayed graphically in the form of survival curves (Fig. 7.1). These show the number of patients, or the proportion of patients, persisting with relief of symptoms over time. The superiority of a treatment over control is displayed by the difference between survival curves of the treated and control groups.

The formality of deciding statistically significant, and therefore convincing, differences between therapy and control lies in tests like chi-squared, the t-test and various rank tests (Sackett et al., 1985). In the case of graphic data, tests such as the Mantel–Haenszel procedure may be used (Kirkwood, 1988); these constitute a series of chi-squared tests looking for significance differences between the two curves along their entire length. Familiarity with these statistical tests is critical for consumers to be able to tell whether or not purported differences between therapy and control are significant. However, no truth is evident if the therapist fails to provide the second row in a two-by-two table or the second curve in a survival analysis.

Table 7.3 Hypothetical results of treatment of 100 patients and 100 matched controls

	Outcome	
	Success	Failure
Treatment	75	25
Control	65	35

Table 7.1 Hypothetical results of treatment of 100 patients

Outcome	
Success	Failure
75	25

Table 7.2 Hypothetical results of treatment of 100 patients and 100 matched controls

	Outcome	
	Success	Failure
Treatment	75	25
Control	75	25

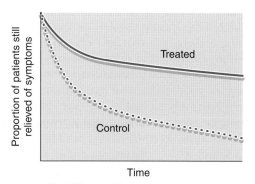

Figure 7.1 The difference in outcome over time between a hypothetical treatment and control, displayed graphically by survival curves.

CLINICOPATHOLOGICAL CORRELATION

The ideal approach to selecting treatment obtains when a particular constellation of clinical features correlates with a unique diagnosis for which there is a proven treatment. Under those conditions, all that is required of the practitioner is to be able to recognize the clinical features and to apply the established treatment. Unfortunately this ideal is not realized in musculoskeletal pain therapy.

Few painful musculoskeletal conditions can be diagnosed in pathoanatomical terms. Fractures can be diagnosed by X-ray. Rheumatoid arthritis can be diagnosed on the basis of classical clinical features and serological tests. Crystal arthropathies are diagnosed by laboratory examination of joint aspirates. Monoarthritis is diagnosed on the basis of focal joint effusion. Other conditions, however, defy such explicit and confident diagnosis.

Osteoarthritis is held to be a common basis for joint pain. Classically the diagnosis is applied to patients with the clinical features of a painful, stiff joint, with crepitus, supplemented by the radiological features of joint narrowing, subchondral sclerosis and osteophytes. However, doubts can be raised concerning the validity of these criteria. Radiographic findings of osteoarthritis are common in individuals with no symptoms (Lawrence et al., 1966; McAlindon, 1999), and not all painful joints exhibit the features of osteoarthritis. Accordingly, some authorities have questioned whether the pain of patients labelled as having osteoarthritis even stems from the incriminated joint, and whether osteoarthritis constitutes no more than another regional pain syndrome (Lane and Thompson, 1997; Croft, 1999).

Regional musculoskeletal pain syndromes are characterized essentially by pain in a particular region of the body. The pain is assumed to arise from one or other of the musculoskeletal structures in the region, but the actual source and cause defy detection.

Diagnosable conditions, such as tumours and infections, account for fewer than 1% of all cases of acute low back pain (Deyo and Diehl, 1988; Deyo et al., 1992) or acute neck pain (Heller et al., 1983; Johnson and Lucas, 1997). For the remainder of cases, although theories abound, there are no data in the literature on the actual sources, let alone causes, of acute low back pain, or of neck pain or thoracic spinal pain. Chronic low back pain may arise from the intervertebral discs (Schwarzer et al., 1994a, 1995a), the zygapophyseal joints (Schwarzer et al., 1994a, b, 1995b) or the sacroiliac joint (Schwarzer et al., 1995c; Maigne et al., 1996). Chronic neck pain may arise from the intervertebral discs (Grubb and Kelly, 2000) or zygapophyseal joints (Lord et al., 1996; Bogduk, 1999) but the diagnosis of these conditions requires invasive investigations. They cannot be diagnosed clinically.

The tools used for clinical diagnosis of spinal pain lack reliability, validity, or both. In the lumbar spine, tenderness is the only clinical sign for which interobserver reliability is reasonable, and is better between physiotherapists than between medical practitioners (Boline et al., 1993; Strender et al., 1997) but tenderness lacks any proven pathoanatomical validity. It is a reliable sign but does not implicate any particular underlying pathology. In the cervical spine, tenderness over the articular pillars is a reliable sign (Viikari-Juntura, 1987; Hubka and Phelan, 1994), but it lacks validity. It does not necessarily indicate that the pain stems from the underlying joint. Other clinical tests used to assess spinal pain abjectly lack reliability. For joint play, and passive intervertebral motion, interobserver agreement is fair to poor at best (de Boer et al., 1985; Mior et al., 1985; Nansel et al., 1989; Phillips and Twomey, 1996; Fjellner et al., 1999; Smedmark et al., 2000). Without reliability, these tests cannot be held to have any validity. Consequently, they cannot be used to make a specific diagnosis of spinal pain. Whereas some studies have found tests for sacroiliac joint pain to be reliable (Dreyfuss et al., 1996), others have found them to lack reliability (van der Wurff et al., 2000a). Nevertheless, the tests lack validity for pain stemming from the sacroiliac joint (Dreyfuss et al., 1996; van der Wurff et al., 2000b). McKenzie assessment for internal disc disruption is reliable and has some validity (Donelson et al., 1997), but the positive likelihood ratio is only 2 or less, which limits its diagnostic utility (Bogduk and Lord, 1997; Delaney and Hubka, 1999).

Classical teaching maintains that shoulder pain can be due to supraspinatus tendinitis, subacromial bursitis, rotator cuff tears, adhesive capsulitis or acromioclavicular osteoarthritis. The clinical diagnostic criteria for these classical conditions, however, lack content validity: they do not explicitly define each entity and distinguish it from others. For example, the signs of 'rotator cuff disease' include: no abnormality, generalized muscle atrophy, or atrophy localized to the infraspinatus or infraspinatus and supraspinatus; passive motion may be normal, mildly restricted or severely restricted; active motion may be normal, somewhat restricted or severely restricted; shoulder strength may be normal or there may be any level of reduction in strength (Cofield, 1993). Medical imaging is commonly used to confirm, if not establish, the diagnosis, but it too is confounded by the high prevalence of lesions in asymptomatic individuals (Needell et al., 1996). Formal studies have shown that expert rheumatologists fail to agree when asked to diagnose the same patient (Bamji et al., 1996). Expert physiotherapists have difficulty agreeing when asked simply to identify and distinguish between subacromial, glenohumeral and acromio-clavicular syndromes, without specifying classical pathology (de Winter et al., 1999). Classical tests for impingement syndrome lack validity (Calis et al., 2000), as do most tests for rotator cuff tears (Itoi et al., 1999; MacDonald et al., 2000; Naredo et al., 2002).

Other, common regional musculoskeletal pain syndromes include anterior knee pain, lateral epicondylalgia and various tendinopathies, such as biceps tendinitis and iliotibial band syndrome. The causes of anterior knee pain are in dispute, and remain fundamentally unknown. The various conditions implicating tendons are characterized by no more than pain and tenderness, but their pathology is unknown, as is the mechanism of the pain that they cause.

Essentially, therefore, only a descriptive diagnosis is possible for regional pain syndromes. Consequently, treatment cannot be selected and prescribed on the basis of a known and logical link between pathology and treatment. These conditions might only be treated symptomatically or empirically, i.e. the treatment is selected because it makes sense, or because it is known to work in practice even though a diagnosis is not possible.

SENSIBLE PRINCIPLES

If a therapist cannot select a treatment on the basis of an anatomicopathological diagnosis, he or she might at least be able to treat individual signs or symptoms. Weak muscles might be exercised to improve strength. Stiff joints might be mobilized to improve range of movement. Pain might be relieved by analgesic interventions. In selecting treatment on this basis, each of two principles applies: does the intervention have a sensible physiological basis; and does it actually work? In both respects, serious reservations can be raised concerning those treatments that are currently applied for musculoskeletal pain.

Physiological basis

A treatment can be attractive in principle if it is known to have a particular physiological effect. In that event, it might be used to treat patients for whom providing that effect is perceived as beneficial or advantageous. For some commonly used physiotherapy treatments there is reasonable evidence of a physiological basis, i.e. evidence of how the treatment works. For other interventions, evidence is lacking; there is only a purported physiological basis. In both instances, a further question is whether the use of the treatment in practice is consonant with its known or purported physiological basis.

The foremost effect of *cryotherapy* is vasoconstriction, which reduces blood flow and decreases metabolic activity (Stillwell, 1971; Basford, 1988). In principle, therefore, therapeutic cold has a place in the treatment of acute injuries to reduce swelling and minimize tissue damage. That, however, does not give it a place for chronic pain or when there is no evidence of tissue damage. In the cat, cooling blocks conduction along nerve fibres, particularly along small-diameter A fibres (Douglas and Malcolm, 1962). This most likely underlies the observation that in humans therapeutic cold produces a loss in perception first of light touch and cold, and later of pain and gross pressure (Fox, 1961). Therapeutic cold may, therefore, be applied as an analgesic.

Combining these observations offers the use of therapeutic cold a seemingly legitimate place in the treatment of acute injuries; the patient appreciates the temporary analgesia, and hopefully the reduction in swelling minimizes tissue damage. The rationale for the use of cold for chronic pain is more limited. There is no evidence that the analgesic effects of cold have any lasting influence on musculoskeletal pain. Analgesia occurs only so long as the cold is applied. Accordingly, cold might be used as an intermittent palliative measure, or applied by patients themselves as a first-aid measure; but it cannot be held to be a definitive means of treating the patient's pain.

Superficial heat, produced by hot packs, heat lamps or warm hydrotherapy, is portrayed as producing increased local temperature, increased local metabolic rate, arteriolar dilatation and increased capillary blood flow (Stillwell, 1971; Low, 1994; De Pace and Newton, 1996). These effects, however, occur in the skin, and there is no explicit evidence of analogous effects in deeper tissues. Concurrently, superficial heat appears to offer an analgesic effect (Grana, 1993), but the mechanism of this effect is not known. The use of superficial heat as an analgesic, therefore, is based on empirical observation, not on an established physiological precept. Claims that it constitutes a form of counterirritation may be attractive as an explanation, but have no greater status intellectually than that of a conjecture.

Therapeutic *ultrasound* is used for its deep heating and purported pain-relieving effects (Sweitzer, 1994). There is reasonable experimental evidence that ultrasound heats deep tissues and produces a variety of non-thermal effects such as cavitation, acoustic streaming and standing waves (Dyson, 1987; Miller, 1987; Kitchen and Partridge, 1990; Gann, 1991; Maxwell, 1992, Watson, 2000). Whether these effects are actually therapeutic in deep tissues, however, has not been clearly demonstrated and the evidence that ultrasound is analgetic is marginal at best.

Ultrasound is portrayed as being proinflammatory when applied to damaged tissues (Watson, 2000), i.e. enhancing fibroblast and endothelial cell activity, and the remodelling of scar. Much of the laboratory work underlying this contention, however, stems from *in vitro* studies (Young and Dyson, 1990a) and studies of cutaneous or superficial lesions (Dyson and Pond, 1973; Dyson and Suckling, 1978; Dyson and Niinikoski, 1982; Dyson and Luke, 1986; Young and Dyson, 1990b, 1990c). Whereas these studies may justify the use of ultrasound for wound healing and ulcers (Dyson and Suckling, 1978), their results are not indicative of what happens in deep, musculoskeletal tissues. Studies of the rat ankle have shown only that ultrasound causes a marginal increase in mast-cell degranulation (Fyfe and Chahl, 1984) and variable

increases or decreases in plasma extravasation that differ according to the frequency applied, the pulse ratio, the number of insonations and the duration after insonation (Fyfe and Chahl, 1985).

Other purported effects of ultrasound include increased blood flow, increased extensibility of collagenous tissues, decreased pain and decreased muscle spasm (Dyson, 1987; Kitchen and Partridge, 1990). However, blood flow does not necessarily increase (Imig et al., 1954). Earlier claims that ultrasound increases tendon extensibility (Gersten, 1955; Lehman et al., 1970) have not been borne out in subsequent studies (Stoller et al., 1983). Nor does it increase muscle strength (Black et al., 1984). Although ultrasound appears to increase the rate of repair of injured tendons (Jackson et al., 1991) it makes no difference to the strength or quality of repair (Turner et al., 1989).

There are few experimental data to show that ultrasound relieves pain. When applied to a nerve, ultrasound raises the pain threshold in the territory of that nerve (Lehman et al., 1958). This increase in threshold, however, is at best only of the order of 20% (Williams et al., 1987), and does not constitute evidence that ultrasound produces analgesia. The increase in threshold has been attributed to temporary blockade of conduction along C fibres (Lehman et al., 1970), but careful studies have shown that, whereas continuous ultrasound heats tissues and increases conduction velocities in nerves, pulsed ultrasound decreases conduction velocities but no more than placebo ultrasound (Kramer, 1984). The decreased conduction is due not to the ultrasound but to the cooling effects of the gel applied (Kramer, 1984). Nor is there any evidence that any change in pain perception substantially outlasts the period of application of ultrasound.

From first principles, therefore, ultrasound may have a role to promote healing of injured superficial tissues, but a beneficial effect on deep tissues has not been consistently demonstrated. In the absence of a definite physiological basis there is no reason to expect that ultrasound should relieve pain.

There is good evidence that *short-wave diathermy* heats deep tissues (Kitchen and Partridge, 1992), but inconsistent or weak evidence of any of its other purported effects. Heating tissues increases blood flow, but the increase is much less than what can be produced by gentle or moderate exercise

(Millard, 1961; Wyper and McNiven, 1976). In normal volunteers, short-wave diathermy raises the pain threshold in the region of application, but the effect dissipates within 30 min (Benson and Copp, 1974). Experimental studies on the rate of healing of wounds have yielded conflicting results (Kitchen and Partridge, 1992). In essence, there are few experimental data to support the purported therapeutic effects of short-wave diathermy. Its use, therefore, is sustained by habit and tradition, or the vain belief that it has a physiological rationale.

There is even less evidence for the purported effects of *interferential* therapy. This form of therapy has been promulgated by experts proclaiming presumed physiological effects, with few actual experimental data to substantiate those claims (Johnson, 1999; Watson, 2000). Critical to the rationale of interferential therapy is the ability to produce an amplitude modulated frequency, but a careful study has shown that this is immaterial to the effects that interferential has on motor or sensory nerves, or on pain perception; and that, in this regard, interferential offers no advantages over transcutaneous electrical nerve stimulation (Palmer et al., 1999).

There is no established biological basis for the therapeutic effects of *low-energy laser* therapy (Kitchen and Partridge, 1991; Beckerman et al., 1992). Some of the proposed, physiologic effects attributed to low-power laser energy are accelerated collagen synthesis, increased vascularization of healing tissues, a decrease in microorganisms and pain reduction (Synder-Mackler and Seitz, 1990), but none of these effects has been explicitly demonstrated. Studies on the superficial radial nerve have shown no effect of laser on conduction velocity (Greathouse et al., 1985; Kramer and Sandrin, 1993). Concepts such as *biostimulation* or *photoacceptance* do not constitute a valid explanation of the biological basis for laser therapy and do not provide a logical basis for the application of laser for conditions such as epicondylitis or radicular pain.

There is clear evidence that spinal *traction* separates vertebral bodies. However, in the lumbar spine much of the separation observed arises from flattening of the lumbar lordosis (Twomey, 1985). In the cervical spine 13.5 kg (30 lb) of traction achieves only fractions of a millimetre separation between vertebral bodies, amounting to 2 mm

total elongation anteriorly and 6 mm posteriorly between C2 and T1 (Colachis and Strohm, 1966). The purported benefit of this separation is, however, ambiguous.

When traction is used to treat radicular pain the implicit mechanism is decompression of the affected spinal nerve. However, separation of vertebrae increases the longitudinal dimension of the intervertebral foramina, but longitudinal compression of spinal nerves is an uncommon phenomenon. Most commonly, spinal nerves are affected in the sagittal dimension: anteriorly by disc herniations or osteophytes, or posteriorly by osteophytes of the zygapophyseal joints. Longitudinal separation does not relieve encroachment in the sagittal dimension. Moreover, upon the patient resuming the upright posture, any benefit of traction is immediately lost, as gravity restores the compression load on the spine. Indeed, it has been shown that, without rising, after simply resting on the traction table for 20 min, the effects of cervical traction are all but lost (Colachis and Strohm, 1966). Another conjecture is that traction reduces disc herniations. The available data, however, are limited and conflicting. In one small study, although traction did reduce disc herniations in two of three patients, the protrusions reappeared within 14 min of release of the force (Matthews, 1968).

In the absence of firm evidence for a mechanical effect of traction, some authorities have pursued alternative rationales, such as silencing ectopic impulse generators, and normalization of conduction in spinal nerves (Krause et al., 2000). These speculations, however, nevertheless presuppose that traction reverses compression of the spinal nerve, by separating the vertebral bodies. They also require that relatively brief traction somehow achieves lasting reversal of the pathophysiology that causes pain.

There is even less of a physiological rationale for traction when it is applied for spinal pain, as opposed to radicular pain. In the first instance, nerve root irritation causes pain in the limbs, not in the back or in the neck (Bogduk, 1997). The rationale for traction for spinal pain, therefore, cannot involve decompression of spinal nerves. Instead, it has been proposed that perhaps spinal pain might be relieved by 'increasing non-nociceptive input and recruitment of descending inhibition'

(Krause et al., 2000). While perhaps attractive as a conjecture, such a statement falls short of actually constituting evidence of how traction might relieve spinal pain. Another proposition is that traction serves to stretch spinal tissues (Krause et al., 2000), but in that event it is questionable whether elaborate and passive traction offers any advantage to simple stretching exercises that patients can undertake themselves. The proposition that traction reduces intervertebral disc pressures is confounded not only by the lack of experimental data that demonstrate this effect, but also by the lack of a cogent theory as to how raised disc pressure causes back pain and why that pain should stay relieved once the traction is released and the patient resumes an upright posture.

Corsets significantly reduce the range of flexion–extension and lateral bending of the trunk, but have no significant effect on axial rotation (van Poppel et al., 2000). Corsets have no significant effect on muscle activity or intra-abdominal pressure (Ciriello and Snook, 1995). The singular rationale for the use of corsets, therefore, is to reduce range of motion of the trunk. In contrast, soft collars have no effect on cervical mobility (Colachis et al., 1973). One can only deduce that collars have a behavioural effect in that they remind the patient not to move the neck.

Theories abound for the biological basis of *manipulative therapy*. The proposed mechanisms include restoration of vertebral movement by overcoming capsular, ligamentous or muscular shortening, or by breaking intra-articular adhesions; repositioning a subluxated vertebra, a zygapophyseal meniscoid or a disordered intervertebral disc; or altering the neural output of the affected segment or joint (Zusman, 1986; Geiringer et al., 1988). None of these mechanisms has been demonstrated in experimental animals, nor has their relationship to pain been established. They are but theories, and do not constitute a valid biological basis that justifies the application of manipulative therapy. Moreover, there is no evidence that a physiotherapist can tell in a given patient whether the pain is due to capsular stiffness, or subluxation, or a trapped meniscoid or a disordered disc. Therefore, there can be no legitimate match between operant pathology and purported mechanism of therapy. Manipulation cannot be portrayed as based on sound biological grounds; it is a therapy that rests only on convention and alleged empirical proof.

Mobilization is the gentle cousin of manipulation. Its attraction is that by intention and by experience it carries less risk of morbidity than manipulation. However, like manipulation it lacks any demonstrated biological mechanism. Clinically, mobilization involves moving a joint passively but slowly within its immediately available range of motion or slightly beyond the limit of that range. What this achieves biologically is unknown. On the one hand, mobilization may be perceived to stretch fibrous tissues in or around a joint. On the grounds that stretching fibrous tissue may cause it to creep, mobilization is sound in principle if the objective is to increase range of motion. It is contentious, however, that any gains achieved by this means are sustained. With respect to relief of pain, it has been postulated that mobilization promotes adaptation of capsular nerve endings, essentially decreasing their threshold for mechanical activation (Zusman, 1986). However, while attractive in theory, this mechanism of pain relief has not been expressly demonstrated. Like manipulation, mobilization cannot be justified on the basis of a sound, proven biological mechanism.

The classical role of *exercise* has been to strengthen the target muscle. That this can be achieved is not in doubt. Doubts arise, however, when exercise is prescribed to treat pain, for in that event there is no known relationship between increasing muscle strength and relief of pain. On the other hand, exercises might be used simply to encourage or increase mobility around a painful joint. In that event, the rationale is only a conjecture, for there is no experimental, physiological evidence upon which to believe that movement relieves pain.

A more sophisticated application of exercise requires training patients to coordinate their muscles differently, for example, to remember to cocontract their transversus abdominis and multifidus, in order to enhance the stability of the lumbar spine (Jull and Richardson, 1994; Richardson et al., 2000). With respect to rationale, the cardinal limitation to this model of intervention is that its physiological basis has not been elaborated. The supposed instability has not been defined. Nor has it been shown how the instability relates to the production of pain, and how it should be identified clinically. With respect to objective evidence, the model hinges on the perplexing demonstration that in certain patients with chronic low back pain the onset of activation of transversus abdominis is delayed during the performance of, for example, upper limb tasks (Hodges and Richardson, 1996). This delay has loosely been taken to imply impaired stability of the lumbar spine through lack of action of the transversus abdominis on the thoracolumbar fascia (Hodges and Richardson, 1996). What the model ignores is that, even at maximum contraction, the transversus abdominis contributes barely more than 5 Nm to the moments acting on the lumbar spine (Macintosh et al., 1987), which is no more than 2% of the moment required during lifting. The model, therefore, rests on the significance of a delayed onset of a less than trivial influence on the lumbar spine. In essence, this is a model with an ambiguous physiological basis. Nevertheless it has attracted adherents and has been tested clinically.

Evidence of efficacy

It is not mandatory for a treatment to have a known physiological basis. A treatment can be useful even if its mechanism of action is unknown, but provided that there is evidence that it does, in fact, work. When selecting a treatment for a particular condition or symptom, physiotherapists can, therefore, consult the available evidence from clinical trials of that treatment.

There have been no formal trials of cryotherapy or of superficial heat to show that these interventions relieve musculoskeletal pain. Their use remains based on reputation only.

Although ultrasound has been used for a variety of musculoskeletal conditions (McDiarmid and Burns, 1987), the early literature on its efficacy is descriptive or anecdotal. A systematic review of the literature found 'no convincing evidence confirming the efficacy of ultrasound' (Beckerman et al., 1993). Calls for physiotherapists to produce controlled trials to demonstrate the efficacy of ultrasound (Partridge, 1987; Kitchen and Partridge, 1990) have largely not been answered. Encouraging results in one early study of ultrasound for lateral elbow pain (Binder et al., 1985) have not been borne out by subsequent studies (Haker and

Lundeberg, 1991a) and systematic reviews (Labelle et al., 1992; Chandani et al., 1997).

When reviewed in 1992, there was scant evidence of the efficacy of short-wave diathermy for musculoskeletal pain (Kitchen and Partridge, 1992). For back pain its effects could not be distinguished from those of placebo treatment (Gibson et al., 1985). For neck pain statistically significant reduction of pain could be achieved, but required wearing a collar for 8 hours a day to deliver pulsed diathermy continuously, with no lasting effect greater than that of controls after ceasing therapy (Foley-Nolan et al., 1990, 1992). For the treatment of osteoarthritis of the knee by short-wave diathermy, a review found the literature to be of poor methodological quality, and the results to be equivocal (Marks et al., 1999). Although short-wave diathermy was superior to placebo tablets and to placebo injections in one study (Wright, 1964), in other controlled studies it was not superior to ice (Clarke et al., 1974), exercises alone (Chamberlain et al., 1982), cold short-wave diathermy, faradism or wax baths (Hamilton et al., 1959) or placebo short-wave diathermy (Klaber Moffett et al., 1996).

No controlled studies have yet demonstrated the efficacy of interferential therapy for musculoskeletal pain. One controlled study of the treatment of shoulder pain found no advantage and no difference in outcome when interferential and ultrasound, interferential or ultrasound, or dummy interferential, or dummy ultrasound was added to an exercise regimen (van der Heijden et al., 1999).

For laser therapy, positive and negative results have been reported for a variety of disorders of joints, tendons and muscles; but overall, the literature is poor (Beckerman et al., 1992). A systematic review found that the better-quality studies suggest that laser does have a therapeutic effect greater than that of placebo (Beckerman et al., 1992), but subsequent studies have negated that view (Haker and Lundeberg, 1991b; Vasseljen et al., 1992; Krasheninnikoff et al., 1994). Although laser may appear to improve pain during treatment, it provides no lasting benefit greater than placebo (Haker and Lundeberg, 1991b; Vasseljen et al., 1992). For low back pain, laser treatment is slightly better than placebo during therapy, but any differences all but evaporate by 1 month after ceasing treatment (Basford et al., 1999).

Although one trial of lumbar traction for back pain found it to be superior to rest (Larsson et al., 1980) and another found it to be better than hot packs and rest (Lidstrom and Zachrisson, 1970), others have found it to be no better than sham traction (Matthews and Hickling, 1975; Pal et al., 1986; Beurskens et al., 1997) and no better than other interventions or no intervention (Coxhead et al., 1981). For sciatica, traction is not better than isometric exercises (Weber et al., 1984), bedrest (Moret et al., 1998), or 10 kg of autotraction (Weber, 1973). Studies of cervical traction have found it to be no better than placebo (British Association of Physical Medicine, 1966; Tan and Nordin, 1992) or no better than isometric exercises (Goldie and Landquist, 1970). Another study, comparing cervical traction with instruction only, found significant improvements in some ranges of movement as a result of traction, but no significant improvement in pain (Zylbergold and Piper, 1985).

For the treatment of low back pain with corsets, a systematic review (Koes and van den Hoogen, 1994) was somewhat encouraging in its conclusions. It reported that: 'the efficacy of orthoses for treating low-back pain remains controversial, although there are some promising results in the literature'. Closer examination of that literature reveals that, of three trials that included patients with acute low back pain, two found negative results. The one positive study reported that patients who wore orthoses improved more than patients treated with advice, in terms of speed of recovery, the number of patients improved and the ability to work normally.

There are no data that explicitly show any therapeutic benefit of collars for neck pain. Rather, collars have often been used as part of the control treatment in studies of other interventions. By implication they are inferior to other interventions, and are regarded as offering no greater benefit than placebo (Huston, 1988; Harms-Ringdahl and Nachemson, 2000).

The efficacy of manual therapy (manipulation or mobilization) is a vexatious and contentious issue: vexatious because of the generally poor quality of published studies and the often limited duration of follow-up; contentious because proponents of manual therapy readily and rapidly find flaws in any study that threatens to discredit their practice. A discussion of all the issues involved would merit a complete chapter in its own right. For present purposes, readers are directed to the conclusions of the most comprehensive, systematic review published to date (van Tulder et al., 1997). They are that: 'There is limited evidence that manipulation is more effective than a placebo treatment for acute low back pain. There is no evidence that manipulation is more effective than (other) physiotherapeutic applications (massage, shortwave diathermy, exercises) or drug therapy (analgesics, NSAIDs) for acute low back pain, because of the contradictory results.' For chronic low back pain, the review is somewhat more generous: 'there is strong evidence that manipulation is more effective than a placebo treatment for chronic low back pain. There is moderate evidence that manipulation is more effective for chronic low back pain than usual care by the general practitioner, bed-rest, analgesics, and massage.'

A close inspection of the original literature reveals that these conclusions may be overly generous. Manual therapy has not been shown to be more effective than placebo for the relief of pain; and those studies with positive results had only short-term follow-up, whereas those with longer follow-up typically had negative results (Bogduk and McGuirk, 2002). Quantitative estimates suggest that manual therapy is little more than 16% better than comparison treatments (Shekelle et al., 1992).

For manual therapy for neck pain, the evidence of efficacy is less compelling. A systematic review pooled all available studies and calculated an effect size of 16% (Aker et al., 1996). This, however, was the effect evident between 1 and 4 weeks after treatment. Few studies have reported longer-term follow-up. The one study that did found that, at 2 years, 56% of those patients who received mobilization as part of a package of tailored physiotherapy were painfree (McKinney, 1989), but 54% of patients who were prescribed rest were also painfree, as were 77% of patients who received home exercises. Although not recognized in the systematic review, that same study showed that the short-term results of mobilization were not better than a simple home exercise package

(McKinney et al., 1989). Similarly, although another study (Brodin, 1984, 1985) reported that manual therapy was more effective than physiotherapy, it also showed that manual therapy was not better than being prescribed salicylates and placed on a waiting list.

The data on the efficacy of exercises offer mixed conclusions. For acute low back pain, a systematic review found that: 'there is strong evidence that exercise therapy is not more effective than other conservative treatments, including no intervention' (van Tulder et al., 1997). For chronic back pain, the same review found that 'there is strong evidence that exercise therapy is effective for chronic low back pain,' but 'there is no evidence in favour of one of the exercises due to the contradictory results' (van Tulder et al., 1997). For neck pain, a comparable body of data is lacking. No studies have vindicated any utility of exercises for chronic neck pain. With respect to acute neck pain, one study has shown that home exercises are at least as effective as tailored physiotherapy in the short term, and more effective in the long term (McKinney, 1989; McKinney et al., 1989); another has shown that active exercises are more effective than rest, collar and gradual mobilization (Rosenfeld et al., 2000). For acute shoulder pain, exercises are not more effective than injection therapy (Winters et al., 1997), although the long-term results are no worse than those of injection (Winters et al., 1999); For chronic impingement syndrome, exercises are superior to placebo therapy, and are as effective as arthroscopic surgery, both in the short term (Brox et al., 1993) and at follow-up 2½ years later (Brox et al., 1999). However, about one in four patients treated by exercise ultimately turn to surgery (Brox et al., 1999).

Specific stabilizing exercises have been shown to be more effective than usual care for patients with spondylosis or spondylolisthesis (O'Sullivan et al., 1997). They improve pain and function by a factor of 50%, and the effects are enduring. It is not evident from this study, however, whether the therapeutic benefit is due to a biomechanically specific stabilizing effect on the lumbar spine, or the intensity of intervention and attention during the 10-week treatment programme is the operant factor.

IMPLICATIONS

Of the traditional interventions available to the physiotherapist:

- Cold and superficial heat are not definitive forms of treatment, but are palliative measures that patients can apply for themselves.
- Ultrasound lacks a firm physiological basis for the treatment of musculoskeletal pain, and controlled clinical trials indicate that it lacks efficacy.
- There is no evidence of a physiological basis for short-wave diathermy, and controlled clinical trials indicate that it is not more effective than simpler, less passive measures, or placebo.
- There is no proven physiological basis for interferential therapy, and what little information there is from controlled clinical trials indicates that it does not work.
- Low-energy laser therapy lacks a physiological rationale, and clinical trials at best show that any pain relief obtained is limited in magnitude and in duration.
- Traction lacks a cogent rationale, and clinical trials fail to substantiate its reputed efficacy.
- No evidence vindicates the efficacy of corsets and collars beyond that of a placebo.

Physiotherapists, therefore, would be hard-pressed to justify selecting these interventions as a form of treatment. Yet, it may be that some physiotherapists believe that these interventions do work in their hands, despite what the research says. In that event, however, surely they are duty-bound to provide new data that refute the available data, for there is no reason, *a priori*, to believe that one therapist's personal experience constitutes better evidence than that issuing from an objective, scientific assessment of the intervention. On the contrary, because of the influences of observer bias, recall bias and lack of follow-up, it is far more likely that personal experience is flawed.

Manual therapy and exercise remain reasonable options in the physiotherapy armamentarium, but with reservations. Manipulation and mobilization are superior to some interventions for back pain but not superior to others; their attributable effect is small. Of all conservative measures, intensive exercise seems to be the best option for chronic low back pain, but even there it is not a panacea. Home exercises seem to be the most effective intervention for acute neck pain. Exercises seem worthwhile for chronic shoulder pain.

When the evidence underpinning musculoskeletal physiotherapy is reviewed it is evident that much of what was taught and practised in the past either lacks a valid rationale or lacks evidence of efficacy, or both. This calls for a paradigm shift. Upon investigating practices of the past, physiotherapists have the option to desist in perpetrating those that do not work, while maintaining those interventions that do work. But in addition, they have the option to contribute to the development and evaluation of new and emerging interventions, and to embrace those shown to be of greater benefit than past practices.

Amongst the emerging paradigms is a lessening emphasis on passive interventions for acute musculoskeletal pain, with greater emphasis on psychosocial issues. Passive interventions are not curative, and many are a profligate waste of time and resources. They perpetuate the illusion that the physiotherapist can and will cure the problem with a physical intervention. Yet, strong evidence indicates that the more worthwhile interventions involve explanation, reassurance, and simple encouragement and assistance to remain active (Maher et al., 1999). For subacute back pain and for acute neck pain after whiplash, minimal passive yet maximal active and cognitive intervention has proved as effective as any other intervention (Borchgrevink et al., 1998; Indahl et al., 1995, 1998; Hagen et al., 2000). For chronic neck pain, cognitive multimodal therapy, although still not proven, promises to be more effective than traditional physical interventions (Vendrig et al., 2000). Within this milieu, some physiotherapists have urged a greater, and overtly psychological, involvement of their fellows in the management of patients (Watson, 1999).

These developments, however, have occurred largely if not exclusively in the treatment of spinal pain. Whether a new paradigm is applicable and effective for other musculoskeletal conditions has yet to be seen. But whatever the new developments may be, the same two operant questions remain for evaluating and selecting treatment:

1. Is there any reason why this treatment should or might work?
2. Is there any evidence that, in fact, it does work?

Positive answers to these questions will secure a cogent, responsible and accountable basis for musculoskeletal physiotherapy.

Using evidence in clinical practice

M. Elkins, A. Moseley, C. Sherrington, R. Herbert and C.G. Maher

Physiotherapists have a professional and ethical obligation to offer optimal treatment to their patients. This is challenging, however, because optimal treatment is changing continuously.

This section describes how physiotherapists can use research evidence, particularly evidence from randomized trials and systematic reviews of randomized trials, to assess the effectiveness of therapeutic interventions. It describes design features that confer validity to randomized trials and systematic reviews, and it presents methods for assessing the quality of randomized controlled trials and systematic reviews, assessing the size of treatment effects and applying the results to local clinical practice. The initial steps of the process of using evidence in patient care are then illustrated using a clinical example.

RANDOMIZED CONTROLLED TRIALS

Clinical trials test the effect of interventions on patients. One type of clinical trial is a controlled trial, in which the participants are divided into groups. The intervention of interest is applied to those allocated to the treatment group, while those allocated to the control group do not receive the intervention of interest. The following arrangements are types of controlled trials.

Treatment group receives	Control group receives
Treatment A	No treatment
or Treatment A + standard treatment	Standard treatment only
or Treatment A	Treatment B
or Treatment A	Sham treatment

At the end of the trial, outcomes of subjects in each group are measured. The average difference in outcomes between groups is used as an estimate of the size of the treatment effect.

Although the use of a control group protects against some sources of bias, it does not prevent all possible sources of bias. For example, bias will arise in controlled trials if treatment and control groups are not comparable (i.e. if the groups would have had different outcomes even if they were treated in the same way). This source of bias ('allocation bias') can be greatly reduced if the trial is randomized, because randomization ensures that the groups are comparable. In randomized trials, subjects are randomly allocated to treatment or control group. Randomization minimizes allocation bias, so the randomized controlled trial is considered to provide the least biased test of the effects of an intervention (Chalmers et al., 1983).

SYSTEMATIC REVIEWS

Often more than one trial of a particular intervention has been performed and published. When

this is the case, the findings of several trials of a particular intervention can be put together in a literature review. These reviews are intended to assist clinicians by surveying all relevant studies and summarizing the information in them. In the field of health, most reviews assess the effects of interventions for the treatment and/or prevention of conditions or symptoms. Others assess the accuracy of diagnostic tests (Dixon and Keating, 2000; Solomon et al., 2001), or the prevalence or prognosis of a particular condition (Loney and Stratford, 1999; Cote et al., 2001).

Some reviews of the literature examine a broad topic, leave the method of gathering the literature undefined, and do not appraise the quality of the included trials. All of these features can bias the conclusions of the review (Oxman and Guyatt, 1993). Systematic reviews are reviews designed to minimize these sources of bias (Petticrew, 2001).

In systematic reviews, there is an explicit description of the sequence of steps to be followed in the conduct of the review. This means there is a description of a comprehensive search strategy used to locate studies for possible inclusion in the review, the criteria used to determine whether a study is included in the review, the quality of the included trials and the methods of synthesizing trial findings. Such methods minimize bias and maximize transparency, so good-quality systematic reviews are often considered the best single source of information of the effects of treatment (National Health and Medical Research Council, 1999).

EVIDENCE–BASED PRACTICE

The model of evidence-based practice proposed by Sackett and colleagues (2000) provides a practical framework for using research evidence to guide clinical practice. The five steps are:

1. Convert the need for information into an answerable question.
2. Search for evidence to answer the question.
3. Critically appraise the evidence identified.
4. Integrate the appraisal with clinical expertise and the patient's circumstances.

5. Evaluate the effectiveness of the treatment, and efficacy at steps 1–4.

We will cover the first four steps in this chapter.

Step 1: Formulate an answerable question

An answerable question asks for specific information that is directly relevant to management of a patient or group of patients. It should contain the following elements: (1) the problem; (2) a proposed intervention; (3) the outcome you are hoping to affect; and (4) any alternative intervention (Richardson et al., 1995). An example is: among people with (1) acute ankle inversion sprains, does (2) the addition of passive accessory joint mobilization lead to (3) faster recovery of full painfree dorsiflexion, when compared to (4) standard treatment alone? These elements guide which terms you will use when searching for evidence.

Step 2: Search for evidence

To answer our question, we will use electronic resources available through the internet to search for randomized controlled trials and systematic reviews. Our initial search will use the Physiotherapy Evidence Database (PEDro). PEDro is freely available and specifically indexes systematic reviews and randomized controlled trials in physiotherapy (http://www.pedro.fhs.usyd.edu.au/; Sherrington et al., 2000). We will then check if any other reviews and trials are available, but not indexed on PEDro, using subscription databases of Medline, EMBASE and CINAHL (Booth and Madge 1998).

Step 3: Critically appraise the evidence

Unfortunately, not all randomized controlled trials and systematic reviews are of uniformly high quality. Trials and reviews of lower quality are likely to produce results that are systematically biased (Oxman and Guyatt, 1993). A series of screening questions can be used to identify quickly higher-quality reviews and trials. Sackett and colleagues (2000) suggest that readers should ask several questions to evaluate the validity of trials and reviews. These are described below and are discussed

more fully elsewhere (Sackett et al., 2000; Maher et al., 2003).

Screening questions for randomized controlled trials

1. Were subjects randomly allocated to groups?
2. Was there blinding of subjects and assessors?
3. Was there adequate follow-up?

Were subjects randomly allocated to groups?

Ideally, the allocation of subjects to treatment and control groups should be random. When a trial is published, the randomization procedure should be explained in detail. Random allocation can be achieved, for example, using a computer-generated list of random numbers or (perhaps less satisfactorily) by tossing a coin. However, not every trial that is described as randomized has used a truly random procedure. Other procedures, such as allocation by hospital record number or by alternation, are sometimes called random but would be better considered as quasi-randomized. Quasi-random allocation can produce comparable groups in the same way randomization does, but it is more easily corrupted (Schulz, 1995).

True randomization eliminates allocation bias (Chalmers et al., 1983). Trials without random allocation are potentially biased and should not generally be used as a source of information on which to base clinical decisions.

As well as being random, the allocation sequence should also be concealed. This means that the investigator enrolling patients in the trial cannot know to which group the next subject to be enrolled will be allocated. Awareness of the allocation sequence could influence the investigator's decision to enrol someone in the trial. This could corrupt the randomization process and bias which subjects are enrolled into each group. Concealment prevents this type of mechanism from introducing a systematic bias. In practice, trials with inadequate or unclear concealment of allocation typically report a treatment effect that is almost 30% greater than those with concealed allocation (Egger et al., 2002). Concealed allocation can be achieved using consecutively numbered, sealed opaque envelopes that contain the group allocation and are opened only after the subject is recruited to the trial, or by telephoning an investigator off-site after the subject is recruited to the trial.

Was there blinding of subjects and assessors?

Blinding of subjects means that subjects cannot tell whether they have received the experimental or control intervention. Without blinding, subjects in the treatment group may tend to report better outcomes than they really experienced because they perceive that this is what is expected of them (Wickstrom and Bendix, 2000). Blinding of subjects minimizes this source of bias.

Blinding of subjects may be achieved by administering a 'sham' intervention to the control group. A true sham intervention cannot be distinguished from the treatment group intervention and has no therapeutic effects. To avoid corruption of subject blinding, it is helpful also to blind care providers, so that they do not inadvertently unblind the subject. It is often not possible to provide a true sham in physiotherapy trials. In this situation, an intervention that is as similar as possible to the treatment group intervention, still with no therapeutic effect, may be the best alternative.

If the outcome assessor is aware to which group a subject has been allocated, this may bias measurement of outcomes. Assessor blinding eliminates this source of bias. For objective measures, blinding of assessors can be achieved by having an independent assessor, who is unaware of allocations, to take the measurements. For subjective measures, blinding assessors requires blinding of subjects.

Double-blinding involves blinding of both subjects and assessors. Trials that are not double-blinded tend to exaggerate the effects of treatment. They typically report a treatment effect that is almost 15% greater than double-blinded trials (Egger et al., 2002).

Was there adequate follow-up?

In most physiotherapy trials, outcome measures are not obtained from some subjects who enter the trial. Collectively, this is known as 'loss to follow-up'. Subjects may be lost to follow-up for various reasons, including that they lose interest in the trial, emigrate, return to work, become ill, and so on.

Loss to follow-up is another potential source of bias. This bias can be systematic if the loss to follow-up is associated with outcome. For example, if subjects with poorer outcomes are more commonly lost to follow-up, the remaining subjects will indicate a spuriously good outcome. If the treatment and control groups differ in their pattern of loss to follow-up, estimates of the treatment effect will also be biased. Because follow-up data are not available, it is difficult to know if subjects lost to follow-up have good or poor outcomes. The larger the loss to follow-up, the greater the potential for bias. Because the number of subjects lost to follow-up usually increases over time, a trial may have valid conclusions about the short-term effects of therapy but the long-term results may be biased.

Most experts would agree that losses to follow-up of greater than 20% create potential for serious bias. However, complete follow-up is not absolutely necessary for the results of the trial to be used in clinical decision-making. As a rule of thumb we might choose to treat the findings of the study with some suspicion if loss to follow-up is greater than 15%. Alternatively, hypothetical results can be calculated by assuming all those who were lost to follow-up had either a good outcome or a bad outcome. If the two hypothetical results are not very different from each other, then you can assume that no serious bias was created by the loss to follow-up.

In most studies there are some protocol violations. For example, subjects may not receive the allocated intervention, outcome measurements may not be taken at the scheduled time or subjects may be too ill for the measurements to be taken. The least biased way to deal with protocol violations is called 'analysis by intention to treat' (Hollis and Campbell, 1999). This approach involves collecting data from all subjects regardless of protocol violations and then analysing the data as if the protocol violations had not occurred. For example, data from subjects who did not receive the intervention as intended for their allocation group are analysed as though the treatment had been received. Although this approach may seem counterintuitive, it avoids the unnecessary biases introduced by other strategies for dealing with protocol violations. The concept of analysis by intention to treat was introduced relatively recently, so many trials in physiotherapy have not adopted it or do not explicitly state that they did so (Moseley et al., 2002).

Screening questions for systematic reviews

1. Was an adequate search strategy described?
2. Was the quality of individual trials taken into account when synthesizing the trials' findings?
3. Was the method used to draw conclusions appropriate?

Was an adequate search strategy described?

In a literature review, the method used to search for relevant studies can produce bias. For example, reviewers may include only their own trials, or only trials that support a particular viewpoint. This is likely to make the included studies unrepresentative of all trials in the area. Because systematic reviews seek to use methods which minimize bias, they should conduct a thorough and transparent search for reports of relevant studies.

The search strategy also needs to be as extensive as possible. This is because studies with the most positive findings are likely to be published in the most accessible journals. Unless the search goes beyond the leading journals, an unrepresentatively optimistic subset of trials tends to be reviewed (Stern and Simes, 1997). At the very least, reviewers should search several key databases, using a sensitive search strategy formulated prior to conducting the review. An example of a description of such a search strategy developed by the Cochrane Collaboration Back Review Group is provided by Gross and colleagues (2002).

Was the quality of individual trials taken into account when synthesizing the trials' findings?

Trials of low quality are potentially biased so systematic reviews should not use them to draw conclusions about the effects of therapy. There is general agreement that trials that are not randomized should be excluded. Beyond this, the best method for assessing trial quality in systematic reviews is still unclear (Juni et al., 1999). Many reviewers report the quality of the randomized trials using checklists or scales (for reviews of checklists and scales, see Moher et al., 1995; Verhagen et al., 2001). Some then only synthesize results

from those studies attaining a certain score. These approaches appear sensible but have not been empirically validated. As a general rule, systematic reviews which have used an explicit and sensible procedure for considering trial quality should be regarded as acceptable.

Was the method used to draw conclusions appropriate?

One of the advantages of systematic reviews is that they can combine the results of several trials to produce a summary result. Several methods are available.

One method is to count the number of studies indicating a beneficial effect of the intervention and the number which do not. This 'vote-counting' method is not recommended for several reasons. First, the relative size and methodological quality of the studies are ignored, as each receives equal weighting (Jones, 1995). Also this method provides no information on the size of the treatment effect. Vote counting is very insensitive to true effects, and will often tend to lead to the conclusion of 'no evidence of effect' even if the intervention is effective. Finally, the result may be influenced by how the reviewer chooses to deal with studies with non-significant results (Antman et al., 1992).

A related method is the 'levels of evidence' approach which considers the methodological quality of trials in the pooling process and provides a qualitative descriptor of the evidence for a therapy, for example, 'no evidence', 'limited evidence', 'strong evidence', etc. Unfortunately this system retains most of the flaws of vote-counting methods. Additionally there are a number of different systems for pooling levels of evidence and the systems often produce different conclusions from the same set of trials (Ferreira et al., 2002).

These potential biases are avoided in the statistical method for synthesizing the results of several trials, known as meta-analysis. Meta-analysis involves weighting the treatment effects from individual studies according to their precision (which depends on sample size), and statistically combining them to produce a pooled estimate of the size of the treatment effect (Hedges and Olkin, 1980; Cooper and Hedges, 1994; Egger et al., 2001). Meta-analysis is not always possible. Individual trials may not be sufficiently similar or the necessary data may not be given in the individual trial reports. However, when meta-analysis is possible it provides the best method currently available for obtaining estimates of the size of treatment effects in systematic reviews.

An understanding of the clinical use of the intervention is required to decide whether meta-analysis has been used appropriately. Consider the characteristics of the subjects, how the interventions were applied, the study design and the trial outcomes. If, from a clinical perspective, these factors differ marginally between the combined studies, this supports the use of meta-analysis. The appropriateness of meta-analysis can be further examined statistically by assessing whether the results of studies are similar for a given outcome (i.e. statistical homogeneity). If they differ substantially, meta-analysis may not be appropriate. A simple indicator of this is whether the confidence intervals for estimates of treatment effects from each study overlap. If not, differences between estimates of treatment effects are probably not just due to chance, in which case pooled estimates from meta-analyses may be difficult to interpret (Walker et al., 1988).

Further appraisal of evidence – is the treatment effect clinically worthwhile?

The last components of the evidence that should be appraised are the size of the treatment effect and its relevance to the patient. These are relevant whether the result comes from an individual trial or from a systematic review. If a treatment is to be useful it must do more good than harm. Well-designed research evidence can indicate if a treatment is useful by assessing how much good (or harm) the treatment can do (Herbert 2000a, b). One way to judge the amount of good a treatment can do is to examine the size of the treatment effect.

Unfortunately, many randomized controlled trials and systematic reviews focus on statistical significance instead of emphasizing the size of treatment effects. Statistical significance is conventionally reported using *P*-values, which convey no information about the size of the treatment effect, only an estimate of whether the result could have arisen by chance. Statistical significance does not guarantee that the size of a treatment's effect will be big

enough to make it clinically useful. Conversely, treatment effects can be of great clinical significance yet statistically non-significant, especially in studies with small sample sizes.

A group's outcome may be reported in various ways, depending on how the outcome is measured. Some outcome measures are continuous. This means the outcome can take on any of many values for a single subject. Examples of continuous outcomes are walking speed, time to recovery of full painfree range or visual analogue scale measures of pain. In these cases, it is useful to consider typical outcomes, such as the mean (or sometimes median) outcome. Thus, when outcomes are continuous, the best estimate of the size of the treatment effect is usually the difference between group means (or medians).

A group's outcome needs to be reported in a different way if the outcome measure is dichotomous. Dichotomous outcomes do not take on a range of values. They are events that either happen or do not. Some dichotomous outcomes are recovered/did not recover, recurred/did not recur and returned to work/did not return to work. When outcomes are dichotomous, the proportion of subjects to whom the event occurs should be reported. For example, in the trial of specific stabilizing exercise by Hides and colleagues (2001), six of the 20 subjects in the exercise group reported a recurrence of low back pain during the follow-up year compared to 16 out of 19 in the control group. Thus the risk of recurrence was 30% (6/20) in the exercise group and 84% (16/19) in the control group.

The changes that occur within a group do not provide an estimate of the size of treatment effects because the outcomes of people in that group are determined partly by treatment but also by a range of other factors including natural recovery, statistical regression, placebo effects, Hawthorne effects and so on (Campbell and Stanley, 1963; Cook and Campbell, 1979). Estimates of the size of treatment effects can only be provided by contrasts between groups. The difference in outcome of groups that do and do not receive treatment provides a measure of the effect of treatment.

When outcomes are measured on a continuous scale the (average) effects of therapy are best measured by the difference between group means. For example, in the trial of physiotherapy aimed at restoring muscle function in subjects with shoulder pain by Ginn and colleagues (1997), one outcome measured on a continuous scale was the range of painfree shoulder abduction. Among the subjects in the treatment group, painfree abduction increased by a mean of 22°, while among those in the control group it decreased by a mean of 5°. Thus the best estimate of the treatment effect for this outcome measure is an improvement at 1 month of 27°. (The authors also calculated a 95% confidence interval around this estimate, which was 6.7 to 49.4° improvement. This means the 'true' average effect probably lies between these extremes.) Sometimes the effect is divided by (a pooled estimate of) the standard deviation. This is called, amongst other things, the 'effect size' or 'standardized mean effect'.

When the outcome is measured on a dichotomous scale we need to contrast the risk of that outcome occurring in the two groups. The simplest way to do this is to take the difference in the risk, known as the 'absolute risk reduction'. In the study by Hides and colleagues (2001) the absolute risk reduction is 84% minus 30%, or 54%. The number needed to treat (in this case the number of subjects needed to be treated with exercises rather than control to prevent one recurrence of low back pain) is calculated by dividing 100 by the absolute risk reduction. Thus the Hides study shows that one recurrence of back pain is prevented for approximately every two subjects treated.

We stated earlier that if a treatment is to be useful it must do more good than harm. 'Harm' from treatment can include inconvenience, anxiety, discomfort and cost of treatment. The harm of a programme of stabilizing exercise might include the inconvenience associated with attending for several sessions of therapy and performing exercise. If the exercise produces any adverse effects, we should consider how frequent and how serious they are. The harm of a treatment can be calculated in the same way as benefit. For example, in the trial by Hoving et al. (2002), 11 of 60 subjects (18%) in the manual therapy group reported increased neck pain for greater than 2 days compared to only three of 64 in the medical care group (5%). The absolute risk increase is 13% and the number needed to harm is 8. Serious adverse responses to manual therapy (such as stroke or death) occur

infrequently (Ernst, 2002), so it is difficult to obtain accurate estimates of the frequency of such events. Clearly it would be helpful for patients and physiotherapists to be able to estimate the risk of serious adverse events accurately.

Because the absolute risk reduction or the difference between group means only estimate the treatment effect, there is uncertainty about the true treatment effect. The degree of uncertainty can be represented with a confidence interval (Sim and Reid, 1999; Altman et al., 2000). Roughly speaking, a 95% confidence interval gives a range within which we can be 95% certain the true average treatment effect lies (see Herbert 2000a, b, for an overview and for details on how to extract confidence intervals about estimates of the size of treatment effects from reports of clinical trials). If a trial has few subjects, the confidence interval will cover a wide range, which means that the treatment effect has not been estimated with precision. Wide confidence intervals often include effect sizes that are so small as to not be clinically worthwhile and effect sizes that are large and clinically important. This prevents any firm conclusion about the usefulness of the intervention. Meta-analysis can be useful in this situation. When the results of several small trials are combined, the pooled result usually provides a more precise estimate of the size of treatment effects (i.e. the pooled estimate has narrower confidence intervals) than any provided by each small study.

Step 4: Integrate the appraisal with clinical expertise and the patient's circumstances

The physiotherapist has a responsibility not only to obtain the best evidence, but also to use evidence to assist patients to make informed decisions about whether treatment is likely to be worthwhile. If the patient makes an informed estimate that the benefit is likely to outweigh the harm, the therapy is generally indicated.

These decisions are influenced by individual patients' values and preferences, so they can be complex. Some patients consider it very inconvenient to make several visits to the physiotherapist and to follow a programme of exercise. Other patients may enjoy the outing or the exercise, or both. Some patients would not regard, for example, a temporary increase in neck pain as a serious adverse effect and many would probably proceed with manual therapy treatment despite some risk of a temporary increase in neck pain. This same risk may be interpreted as unacceptable by someone with mild symptoms, with a good prognosis for spontaneous recovery or where the likely beneficial treatment effect cannot be predicted with much certainty.

It may be reasonable mentally to 'adjust' estimates of the size of treatment effects when applying the findings of a trial to a patient who might be expected to respond particularly well to therapy, or when the treatment to be administered differs substantially from that described in the study. For example, if a particular intervention was found to lead to a large improvement in symptoms when offered daily, and in your clinical setting the intervention can only be offered every second day, it may be reasonable to expect a less positive response in your setting than in the trial.

A clinical example

The practical application of the first four steps of the evidence-based practice framework will now be illustrated using a clinical case.

> ### Case
>
> A 60-year-old woman presents with osteoarthritis of the right knee. She has had medial joint pain for the last 6 months and X-rays reveal slight narrowing of the medial joint space. Her knee pain is increased by walking and stair climbing, so she has been trying to walk as little as possible and avoids stairs completely. This has meant that she no longer goes shopping or to work as a volunteer at the local school. Your initial assessment reveals a walking capacity (i.e. distance covered in a 6-min walk test) of 350 m, with a visual analogue scale pain rating of 6/10 when descending stairs.

Step 1: Define an answerable question

Several answerable questions could be generated in relation to this case. Let us consider one related

to the use of land-based exercise:

In a person with (1: problem) osteoarthritis of the knee, does (2: intervention) exercise decrease (3: outcome) pain and disability, compared to (4: alternative intervention) rest?

Step 2: Search for evidence

Using selected terms from our answerable question, we can create a specific search strategy which will help pinpoint the most relevant evidence. The best approach is to use search terms that will be satisfied by all relevant studies, but by relatively few irrelevant studies. This involves thinking about terms that relate closely, but uniquely, to the search question. Consider, for example, the following search strategy applied on PEDro:

> In the 'Abstract & Title' field, enter the terms 'osteoarthritis' and 'exercise', in the 'Body Part' field, select 'lower leg or knee', and combine with 'AND'.

This approach makes the PEDro database find all trials and systematic reviews that contain both the words osteoarthritis and exercise in their titles or abstracts and which have been coded as relevant to the lower leg or knee. The search (conducted December 2002) produced 24 records: seven systematic reviews and 17 randomized controlled trials. Scanning the titles, six of the systematic reviews were relevant to our question. Fourteen trials were relevant to our question, none of which had been published since the most recent systematic review. No other relevant trials or reviews were identified using searches in Medline, EMBASE and CINAHL.

In general, systematic reviews are preferred over individual trials as sources of evidence about treatment effects. The topic of the most recent systematic review was 'therapeutic exercise for people with osteoarthritis of the hip or knee' (Fransen et al., 2002). Having found some relevant evidence, the next step is to apply the screening questions for systematic reviews to appraise its methodological quality.

Step 3: Critically appraise the evidence

Fransen et al. (2002): Was an adequate search strategy described? An extensive search strategy was described by the authors. Five major electronic databases were searched: Medline, CINAHL, the Cochrane Controlled Trials Register, the Cochrane Musculoskeletal Group Trials Register and PEDro.

The search terms used in the review were similar to those we had chosen: 'osteoarthritis', 'knee', 'hip', and 'exercise or exercise therapy'. Because some databases were not limited to physiotherapy research, the terms 'physical therapy or physiotherapy' and 'rehabilitation' were also used.

The search was then extended by reviewing the reference lists of the retrieved articles for further relevant trials. This process, sometimes known as 'snowballing', has been shown to improve the results of the overall search (Helmer et al., 2001). Only English-language articles were reviewed due to limited resources for translation. In addition to making the review less extensive, this strategy introduces the possibility of language bias. Language bias arises because there are some systematic differences between trials published in English and those published in other languages (Moher et al., 1996; Juni et al., 2002). Omitting trials published in languages other than English can alter the magnitude or direction of the overall treatment effect determined by the review (Gregoire et al., 1995). The effect of language bias is difficult to predict, so it is preferable if reviews consider all relevant reports and exclude trials only on the basis of quality (Juni et al., 2002).

The published versions of clinical trials do not always describe the methods used in an exhaustive and unambiguous way. This creates the potential for uncertainty or disagreement among reviewers about the eligibility of a study for inclusion in the review. Fransen and colleagues (2002) used two strategies in their review to ensure the data collected were as complete and correct as possible. First, two reviewers independently screened retrieved clinical studies for inclusion, extracted data from all included studies and scored methodological quality. If the two reviewers disagreed, the third reviewer, blinded to the first two authors' decisions, adjudicated. Second, authors were contacted if the data could not be extrapolated in the desired form from the published article. Contacting authors may further improve the quality of the systematic review by allowing access to unpublished data which can allow further analysis (e.g. subgroup analysis).

The strategies used by Fransen and colleagues (2002) to search the literature were such that we can be reasonably confident the authors obtained most published trials relevant to their question. This should increase our confidence in the findings of the review.

Fransen et al. (2002): Was the quality of individual trials taken into account when synthesizing the trials' findings?
Fransen and colleagues (2002) assessed and reported the methodological quality of the studies included. This allows readers of the review to make their own decisions about the overall quality of studies in the review, as well as individual studies. The quality of the included studies was assessed using a quality scale (Jadad et al., 1986). The three concepts examined by this scale match those addressed by our screening questions for clinical trials: randomization, double-blinding and follow-up.

Fransen et al. (2002): Was any synthesis of data appropriate?
Meta-analysis was used to draw conclusions about the effects of exercise on each of the prespecified outcomes.

The clinical judgement of the authors was applied when considering the suitability of studies to be combined. For example, the pain outcome measure for one study was not included as the subjects were required to take daily analgesic medication, which may spuriously diminish the analgesic effect attributable to the exercise regimen. Homogeneity of the results being combined was examined statistically as well. In most cases there was insignificant heterogeneity among the studies, indicating that the small differences between different estimates of the effect of the exercise could be due to chance.

The appropriate use of meta-analysis in this review should increase confidence in the findings of the review.

Fransen et al. (2002): Summary
Overall, the systematic review by Fransen and colleagues (2002) appears to be a good-quality review, so the evidence it contains would be suitable to use to answer our question. It is also the most recent

review retrieved by our search. It should therefore report an equal or greater number of trials than older reviews. But there are other reasons to expect more recent reviews to provide better evidence. The number of reviews in physiotherapy with explicit systematic methods being published is increasing exponentially (Moseley et al., 2002), and they appear to be replacing qualitative or narrative reviews (Khan et al., 1996). Also, recently several bodies have issued guidelines for the conduct and reporting of systematic reviews (Moher et al., 1999; Clarke and Oxman, 2000). These changes support the notion that older systematic reviews would be expected to be of lower quality. Let us look at the oldest systematic review retrieved by our search.

La Mantia and Marks (1995): Was an adequate search strategy described?

The topic of this systematic review was 'the efficacy of aerobic exercises for treating osteoarthritis of the knee' (La Mantia and Marks, 1995). The methods section indicates that the search strategy was less extensive than that used by Fransen et al. (2002). The two electronic databases searched, Medline and CINAHL, were only searched for the years 1985–1994 and 1980–1994, respectively. Good-quality randomized trials of interventions that could be used by physiotherapists were published as early as 1931 (Doull et al., 1931: this trial scored 6/10, which is better than the mean score of trials on PEDro published in 2000 or 2001 (mean = 5.7; Moseley et al., 2002)), so there does not appear to be any advantage in restricting searches of electronic databases to more recent years. The search terms were similar: 'arthritis or osteoarthritis' and 'exercise, exercise therapy, or aerobic exercises'. The searching was extended using 'a manual search' and by consulting experts in this clinical field. These methods have been shown to improve the quality of the resulting systematic review (McManus et al., 1998).

Although not conducted by either of these reviews, searches can be further improved by contacting manufacturers for any equipment or therapeutic devices used as part of the intervention and asking them if they know about any ongoing or unpublished trials (Helmer et al., 2001). Eysenbach and colleagues (2001) have also identified general internet searches as being effective in retrieving unpublished and particularly ongoing trials.

La Mantia and Marks (1995) did not report the total number of citations retrieved by the search nor the reasons for excluding the trials they do not discuss. All of these trials may have been seriously flawed, or irrelevant items captured in the search and therefore suitable for exclusion. Without the reasons for exclusion, the reader is unable to interpret whether reviewer bias could have influenced the selection of trials reviewed.

The exclusion of trials only reported as abstracts rather than full papers is a restriction Fransen et al. (2002) imposed which La Mantia and Marks (1995) did not. Excluding trials published only as abstracts may appear advantageous because it is more convenient and the extent of reporting in the included trials will be more comprehensive. However, on average, published trials show a 10% greater treatment effect than unpublished trials (Egger et al., 2002). This may be because journals prefer to publish trials which indicate a treatment should be used. Regardless of the reason, this 'publication bias' can influence the results of the systematic review. The exclusion of unpublished trials is therefore not recommended.

La Mantia and Marks (1995): Was the quality of individual trials taken into account when synthesizing the trials' findings?

La Mantia and Marks (1995) did not formally assess the methodological quality of the studies included. Instead, the results section takes a narrative approach. Although only three trials are the focus of their review, the results are not always consistent between the trials. Without comparable statements with regard to quality, it is difficult for the reader to interpret which trials should be given the most importance when weighing their relative merits. A potentially less biased and more interpretable approach would be to use meta-analysis, as used by Fransen et al. (2002).

La Mantia and Marks (1995): Was any synthesis of data appropriate?

Although formal vote counting was not presented in their results, La Mantia and Marks (1995) do review which of their three included trials indicates a beneficial treatment effect for each outcome. The subsequent conclusions include broad statements such as 'the overall beneficial effects of aerobic exercise seem overwhelming' and they state they gained 'an overall favourable impression' of the effects of the intervention.

Step 4: Integrate the appraisal with clinical expertise and the patient's circumstances

The review by Fransen and colleagues (2002) is more recent and used a more extensive search strategy when compared to the La Mantia and Marks (1995) review. Fransen and colleagues also specified reasons for exclusions, rated the quality of the included trials and used meta-analysis to synthesize overall results on key outcomes. These are all important factors in ensuring that a systematic review represents the best evidence available. Therefore the Fransen review provides a better source of evidence than the La Mantia review.

The primary finding of the Fransen et al. (2002) review was that exercise improved self-reported measures of pain over a non-exercise or sham exercise control. The overall mean effect size was reported as a standardized mean difference of 0.46, with a 95% confidence interval of 0.35–0.57. (The standardized mean difference is the size of the effect divided by a pooled estimate of the standard deviation.) This effect size is considered moderate. For the outcome measure of self-reported physical function, exercise was again more beneficial than control, with a mean effect size of 0.33 and a 95% confidence interval of 0.23–0.42. This effect size is considered small. These measures reflect the magnitude of changes from baseline at the completion of the exercise intervention, over and above any change experienced by the control groups.

To assess the relevance of the review to our patient we can compare the disease severity experienced by our patient with that experienced by patients included in the review. The discussion section of the review notes that many of the larger trials included in the review had mostly participants with early or mild symptomatic disease. This appears similar to our patient's situation.

To assist us to draw clinical conclusions from the Fransen et al. (2002) review we can convert the standardized effect size found by the review back to common clinical units of measurement (Oxman

et al., 2003). The review found an average reduction in pain of 46% (with a 95% CI of 35–57%) if a patient was to carry out a land-based exercise programme for 1–3 months, compared with no exercise. This translates to an average improvement from the 6/10 pain our patient has on descending stairs of 2.8 points with a 95% CI of 2.1–3.4. In other words, the new visual analogue scale score will be around 3/10. This seems to be a clinically important difference which would warrant the possible perceived inconvenience of exercising. After further assessment of our patient we might decide to adjust the average expected effect up or down. For example, if she also had another medical condition which limited her ability to exercise, we might expect a smaller effect. We could then assist her in deciding whether she wants to undertake an exercise programme by providing information about likely benefits.

The review reports studies with exercise programmes of various durations, from 1 to 3 months, so we cannot draw firm conclusions about the optimal length of the programme we should prescribe. Similarly, the duration of exercise sessions investigated in the review ranged from 30 to 90 min.

The other main outcome measure of the review is self-reported physical function. While these data can provide a rough indication of the likely effects on walking capacity, they cannot be directly translated to predict likely improvement on walking distance. We could look at the other trials retrieved in our PEDro search to see if any use walking capacity as an outcome measure to assist us in predicting effect of exercise on this variable.

Now that we have decided that exercise has a role to play in the treatment of this patient we need to decide the type of exercise we will suggest. The Fransen et al. (2002) review included a range of different land-based exercise interventions (e.g. range of motion, resistance, walking), some of which were conducted individually and some in groups. The authors state that they were unable to draw firm conclusions about the mode of delivery and type of exercise due to the few studies which investigated these questions.

Let us now look at the only trial included in the review (also identified on our PEDro search) which compared resistance and aerobic exercise (Ettinger et al., 1997). We will first appraise this source of evidence with our three screening questions for trials.

Ettinger et al. (1997): Were subjects randomly allocated to groups?

The randomization procedure is described in detail in the methods section. A random order of allocation was computer-generated and stored off-site. The centres recruiting subjects were only sent the next allocation at the time of enrolment of each new subject, after baseline data collection. Thus, the allocation also meets the criterion of concealment.

Ettinger et al. (1997): Was there blinding of subjects and assessors?

Neither the subjects nor the assessors were blinded to the treatment group allocation. Assessor blinding is nearly always possible, but subject blinding is fairly rare in trials of physiotherapy. This is probably because of the difficulty in providing a sham intervention which is indistinguishable from the treatment of interest. As a result, the size of the treatment effect reported in unblinded trials tends to be slightly inflated (Egger et al., 2002).

Ettinger et al. (1997): Was there adequate follow-up?

Of the 439 participants randomized, 364 returned for the final data collection visit at 18 months. This represents a 17% loss to follow-up, which is just over our suggested limit of 15%. In most trials where posttreatment outcomes are measured repeatedly over time, loss to follow-up varies from one measurement point to the next. The 3- and 9-month posttreatment measurement points had loss to follow-up of 11% and 19%, respectively. The results from the 3-month posttreatment measurement point therefore satisfy this criterion and presumably would be less influenced by bias from loss to follow-up than the 9- and 18-month measurements.

Ettinger and colleagues (1997) used an intention-to-treat analysis, reporting that subjects were 'analysed according to the initial randomized assignments' in the statistical analysis section.

Ettinger et al. (1997): Summary

As this study employed concealed random allocation and had adequate follow-up, but did not have blind outcome assessment, a reasonable assessment might be that this study probably provides good evidence

with which to answer our question, though there is a small potential for bias.

The study by Ettinger and colleagues (1997) found that the aerobic exercise group were an average of only 0.07 points better on a six-point pain intensity scale than the resistance exercise group, with a 95% confidence interval of −0.08 to 0.22 points. Because the confidence interval spans zero, the difference seen between the groups could be due to chance. Regardless of the source of this difference, however, it is unlikely to be of clinical relevance due to its small magnitude.

Ettinger and colleagues (1997) measured disability using a self-reported physical disability questionnaire. Twenty-three activities of daily living were scored on a Likert scale from 1 (usually done with no difficulty) to 5 (unable to do). A composite disability score was created by averaging the scores on all 23 items. The aerobic group were an average of 0.02 points better on their composite score than the resistance exercise group, with a 95% confidence interval of −0.09 to 0.13. Again, this result is of such small magnitude that any difference in treatment effect between aerobic and resistance exercise is unlikely to be of any clinical significance.

EXERCISE PRESCRIPTION AND THE CLINICAL EXAMPLE

Based on the Fransen et al. (2002) review, we can say that the research evidence shows benefits from land-based exercise on pain and functional limitation associated with knee osteoarthritis. So we can be confident that land-based exercise is likely moderately to reduce the pain experienced on stair descent by patients like our patient.

However we can be less sure of the most effective type of exercise for her. The study by Ettinger and colleagues (1997) showed little difference between aerobic and resistance exercise. We did not find other studies which could help us answer this question. To be sure that there are equal benefits from the two types of exercise among people with knee osteoarthritis we would probably need more studies to be conducted. It may be helpful to conduct searches about exercise for similar patient groups, for example, older people with mobility limitation but no diagnosis of osteoarthritis. We could get some indication of likely effects in people with osteoarthritis from these studies.

Other factors which we can use to decide on the type of exercise to prescribe include clinical skills (e.g. further assessment, identification of limiting factors for different forms of exercise), patient preference (she may be unwilling to carry out an aerobic exercise programme but keen on the idea of strength training), service availability (a group exercise programme for people with osteoarthritis may be running in a local hall) and basic science (an understanding of the theoretical benefits of various forms of exercise may be helpful).

CONCLUSION

In this section we have described how evidence, in the form of high-quality clinical research, can be used to assist clinical decision-making. The process involves asking clear questions, finding the best evidence, critically appraising the evidence and applying it to the individual patient. These are the first four steps in the process of evidence-based practice. The body of evidence will change and improve with time, so we need to incorporate this process into clinical practice continuously. The information retrieved with this process can assist physiotherapists and their patients to make the best possible decisions about management of health problems.

REFERENCES

SELECTION AND APPLICATION OF TREATMENT

Aker, P.D., Gross, A.R., Goldsmith, C.H. and Peloso, P. (1996). Conservative management of mechanical neck pain: systematic overview and meta-analysis. *Br. Med. J.*, **313**, 1291–1296.

Bamji, A.N., Erhadt, C.C., Price, T.R. and Williams, P.L. (1996). The painful shoulder: can consultants agree? *Br. J. Rheumatol.*, **35**, 1172–1174.

Basford, J.R. (1988). Physical agents and biofeedback. In: *Rehabilitation Medicine. Principles and Practice*, ed. J.A. DeLisa, pp. 257–275. Philadelphia: J.B. Lippincott.

Basford, J.R., Sheffield, C.G. and Harmsen, W.S. (1999). Laser therapy: a randomized, controlled trial of the effects of low-intensity Nd:YAG laser irradiation on musculoskeletal back pain. *Arch. Phys. Med. Rehabil.*, **80**, 647–652.

Beckerman, H., de Bie, R.A., Bouter, L.M., de Cuyper, H.J. and Oosterdorp, R.A.B. (1992). The efficacy of laser therapy for musculoskeletal and skin disorders: a criteria-based meta-analysis of randomised clinical trials. *Phys. Ther.*, **72**, 483–491.

Beckerman, H., Bouter, L.M., van der Heijden, G.J.M.G., Bie, R.A. and Koes, B.W. (1993). Efficacy of physiotherapy for musculoskeletal disorders: what can we learn from research? *Br. J. Gen. Pract.*, **43**, 73–77.

Benson, T.B. and Copp, E.P. (1974). The effect of therapeutic forms of heat and ice on the pain threshold of the normal shoulder. *Rheumatol. Rehabil.*, **13**, 101–104.

Beurskens, A.J., de Vet, H.C., Koke, A.J. et al. (1997). Efficacy of traction for nonspecific low back pain. 12-week and 60 month results of a randomized clinical trial. *Spine*, **22**, 2756–2762.

Binder, A., Hodge, G., Greenwood, A.M., Hazelman, B.L. and Page Thomas D.P. (1985). Is therapeutic ultrasound effective in treating soft tissue lesions? *Br. Med. J.*, **290**, 512–514.

Black, K.D., Halverson, J.L., Majerus K.A. and Soldberg G.L. (1984). Alterations in ankle dorsiflexion torque as a result of continuous ultrasound to the anterior tibial compartment. *Phys. Ther.*, **64**, 910–913.

Bogduk, N. (1997). *Clinical Anatomy of the Lumbar Spine and Sacrum*, 3rd edn, pp. 187–213. Edinburgh: Churchill Livingstone.

Bogduk, N. (1999). The neck. *Bailliere's Clin. Rheumatol.*, **13**, 261–285.

Bogduk, N. and Lord, S.M. (1997). Commentary on: A prospective study of centralization of lumbar and referred pain: a predictor of symptomatic discs and anular competence. *Pain Med. J. Club J.*, **3**, 246–248.

Bogduk, N. and McGuirk, B. (2002). *Medical Management of Acute and Chronic Low Back Pain. An Evidence-Based Approach*. Amsterdam: Elsevier.

Boline, P.D., Haas, M., Meyer, J.J., Kassak, K., Nelson, C. and Keating, J.C. (1993). Interexaminer reliability of eight evaluative dimensions of lumbar segmental abnormality: Part II. *J. Manip. Physiol. Ther.*, **16**, 363–374.

Borchgrevink, G.E., Kaasa, A., McDonagh, D., Stiles, T.C., Haraldseth, O. and Lereim, I. (1998). Acute treatment of whiplash neck sprain injuries. *Spine*, **23**, 25–31.

British Association of Physical Medicine (1966). Pain in the neck and arm: a multicentre trial of the effects of physiotherapy. *Br. Med. J.*, **1**, 243–258.

Brodin, H. (1984). Cervical pain and mobilization. *Int. J. Rehabil. Res.*, **7**, 190–191.

Brodin, H. (1985). Cervical pain and mobilization. *Manual Med.*, **2**, 18–22.

Brox, I., Staff, P.H., Ljunggren, A.E. and Brevik, J.I. (1993). Arthroscopic surgery compared with supervised exercises in patients with rotator cuff disease (stage II impingement syndrome). *Br. Med. J.*, **307**, 899–903.

Brox, J.I., Gjengedal, E., Uppheim, G. et al. (1999). Arthroscopic surgery versus supervised exercises in patients with rotator cuff disease (stage II impingement syndrome). *J. Shoulder Elbow Surg.*, **8**, 102–111.

Calis, M., Akgun, K., Birtane, M., Karacan, I., Calis, H. and Tuzun, F. (2000). Diagnostic values of clinical diagnostic tests in subacromial impingement syndrome. *Ann. Rheum. Dis.*, **59**, 44–47.

Chamberlain, M.A., Care, G. and Harfield, B. (1982). Physiotherapy in osteoarthritis of the knees. A controlled trial of hospital versus home exercises. *Int. J. Rehabil. Med.*, **4**, 101–106.

Chandani, A., Waldron, D., Teng, S.S. and Glasziou, P. (1997). A systematic review of treatments for "tennis elbow". *Aust. Musculoskel. Med.*, **2**, 21–26.

Ciriello, V.M. and Snook, S.H. (1995). The effect of back belts on lumbar muscle fatigue. *Spine*, **20**, 1271–1278.

Clarke, G.R., Willis, L.A., Stenner, L. and Nichils, P.J.R. (1974). Evaluation of physiotherapy in the treatment of osteo-arthrosis of the knee. *Rheumatol. Rehabil.*, **13**, 190–197.

Cofield, R.H. (1993). Physical examination of the shoulder: effectiveness in assessing shoulder stability. In: *The Shoulder: A Balance of Mobility and Stability*, ed. F.A. Matsen, F.H. Fu and R.J. Hawkins, pp. 331–343. Rosemont, IL: American Academy of Orthopaedic Surgeons.

Colachis, S.C. and Strohm, B.R. (1966). Effect of duration of intermittent cervical traction on vertebral separation. *Arch. Phys. Med. Rehabil.*, **47**, 353–359.

Colachis, S.C., Strohm, B.R. and Ganter, E.L. (1973). Cervical spine motion in normal women: radiographic study of the effect of cervical collars. *Arch. Phys. Med. Rehabil.*, **54**, 161–169.

Coxhead, C.E., Inskip, H., Meade, T.W., North, W.R.S. and Troup, J.D.G. (1981). Multicentre trial of physiotherapy in the management of sciatic symptoms. *Lancet*, **1**, 1065–1068.

Croft, P. (1999). Diagnosing regional pain: the view from primary care. *Bailliere's Clin. Rheumatol.*, **13**, 231–242.

de Boer, K.F., Harman, R., Tuttle, C.D. and Wallace, H. (1985). Reliability study of detection of somatic dysfunctions in the cervical spine. *J. Manip. Physiol. Ther.*, **8**, 9–16.

Delaney, P.M. and Hubka, M.J. (1999). The diagnostic utility of McKenzie clinical assessment for lower back pain. *J. Manip. Physiol. Ther.*, **22**, 628–630.

De Pace, D.M. and Newton, R. (1996). Anatomic and functional aspects of pain: evaluation and management with thermal agents. In: *Thermal Agents in Rehabilitation*, ed. S.L. Michlovitz, pp. 320–358. Philadelphia: F.A. Davis.

de Winter, A.F., Jans, M.P., Scholten, R.J.P.M., Deville, W., van Schaardenburg, D. and Bouter, L. (1999). Diagnostic classification of shoulder disorders: interobserver agreement and determinants of disagreement. *Ann. Rheum. Dis.*, **58**, 272–277.

Deyo, R.A. and Diehl, A.K. (1988). Cancer as a cause of back pain: frequency, clinical presentation and diagnostic strategies. *J. Gen. Intern. Med.*, **3**, 230–238.

Deyo, R.A., Rainville, J. and Kent, D.L. (1992). What can the history and physical examination tell us about low back pain? *J.A.M.A.*, **268**, 760–765.

Donelson, R., Aprill, C., Medcalf, R. and Grant, W. (1997). A prospective study of centralization of lumbar and referred pain. *Spine*, **33**, 1115–1122.

Douglas, W.W. and Malcolm, J.L. (1962). The effect of localized cooling on conduction in cat nerves. *J. Physiol.*, **130**, 53–71.

Dreyfuss, P., Michaelsen, M., Pauza, K., McLarty, J. and Bogduk, N. (1996). The value of history and physical examination in diagnosing sacroiliac joint pain. *Spine*, **21**, 2594–2602.

Dyson, M. (1987). Mechanisms involved in therapeutic ultrasound. *Physiotherapy*, **73**, 116–120.

Dyson, M. and Pond, J.B. (1973). Biological effects of therapeutic ultrasound. *Rheumatol. Rehabil.*, **12**, 209–213.

Dyson, M. and Suckling, J. (1978). Stimulation of tissue repair by ultrasound: a survey of the mechanisms involved. *Physiotherapy*, **64**, 105–108.

Dyson, M. and Niinikoski, J. (1982). Stimulation of tissue repair by ultrasound. *Infect. Surg.*, **September**, 37–44.

Dyson, M. and Luke, D.A. (1986). Induction of mast cell degranulation in skin by ultrasound. *Institute of Electrical and Electronic Engineers Transactions in Ultrasonics, Ferroelectrics and Frequency Control*, **33**, 194–201.

Fjellner, A., Bexander, C., Faleij, R. and Strender L.E. (1999). Interexaminer reliability in physical examination of the cervical spine. *J. Manip. Physiol. Ther.*, **22**, 511–516.

Foley-Nolan, D., Barry, C., Coughlan, R.J., O'Connor, P. and Roden, D. (1990). Pulsed high frequency (27 MHz) electromagnetic therapy for persistent neck pain. *Orthopaedics*, **13**, 445–451.

Foley-Nolan, D., Moore, K., Codd, M., Barry, C., O'Connor, P. and Coughlan, R.J. (1992). Low energy high frequency pulsed electromagnetic therapy for acute whiplash injuries. *Scand. J. Rehabil. Med.*, **24**, 51–59.

Fox, R.H. (1961). Local cooling in man. *Br. Med. Bull.*, **17**, 14–18.

Fyfe, M.C. and Chahl L.A. (1984). Mast cell degranulation and increased vascular permeability induced by "therapeutic" ultrasound in the rat ankle joint. *Br. J. Exp. Pathol.*, **65**, 671–676.

Fyfe, M.C. and Chahl L.A. (1985). The effect of single or repeated applications of "therapeutic" ultrasound on plasma extravasation during silver nitrate induced inflammation of the rat hindpaw ankle joint *in vivo*. *Ultrasound Med. Biol.*, **11**, 273–283.

Gann, N. (1991). Ultrasound: current concepts. *Clin. Manage.*, **11**, 64–69.

Gersten, J.W. (1955). Effect of ultrasound on tendon extensibility. *Am. J. Phys. Med.*, **34**, 362–369.

Geiringer, S.R., Kincaid, C.B. and Rechtien, J.J. (1988). Traction, manipulation, and massage. In: *Rehabilitation Medicine. Principles and Practice*, ed. J.A. DeLisa, pp. 276–294. Philadelphia: J.B. Lippincott.

Gibson, T., Grahame, R., Harkness, J., Woo, P., Belgrave, P. and Hills, R. (1985). Controlled comparison of shortwave diathermy treatment with osteopathic treatment in non-specific low-back pain. *Lancet*, **i**, 1258–1261.

Goldie, I. and Landquist, A., (1970). Evaluation of the effects of different forms of physiotherapy in cervical pain. *Scand. J. Rehabil. Med.*, **2–3**, 117.

Grana, W.A. (1993). Physical agents in musculoskeletal problems: heat and cold therapy modalities. In: *Instructional Course Lectures*, ed. J.D. Heckman, pp. 439–442. Park Ridge: American Academy of Orthopaedic Surgeons.

Greathouse, D.G., Currier, D.P. and Gilmore, R.L. (1985). Effects of clinical infrared laser on superficial radial nerve conduction. *Phys. Ther.*, **65**, 1184–1187.

Grubb, S.A. and Kelly, C.K. (2000). Cervical discography: clinical implications from 12 years of experience. *Spine*, **25**, 1382–1389.

Gundewall, B., Lijquist, M. and Hansson, T. (1993). Primary prevention of back symptoms and absence from work. A prospective randomized study among hospital employees. *Spine*, **18**, 587–594.

Hagen, E.M., Eriksen, H.R. and Ursin, H. (2000). Does early intervention with a light mobilization program reduce long-term sick leave for low back pain? *Spine*, **25**, 1973–1976.

Haker, E. and Lundeberg, T. (1991a). Pulsed ultrasound treatment in lateral epicondylalgia. *Scand. J. Rehabil. Med.*, **23**, 115–118.

Haker, E. and Lundeberg, T. (1991b). Is low-energy laser treatment effective in lateral epicondylalgia? *J. Pain Symptom Manage.*, **6**, 241–246.

Hamilton, D.E., Bywaters, E.G.L. and Please, N.W. (1959). A controlled trial of various forms of physiotherapy in arthritis. *Br. Med. J.*, **2**, 542–545.

Harms-Ringdahl, K. and Nachemson, A. (2000). Acute and subacute neck pain: non-surgical treatment. In: *Neck and Back Pain: The Scientific Evidence of Causes, Diagnosis, and Treatment*, ed. A. Nachemson and E. Jonsson, pp. 327–338. Philadelphia: Lippincott, Williams & Wilkins.

Heller, C.A., Stanley, P., Lewis-Jones, B. and Heller, R.F. (1983). Value of X ray examinations of the cervical spine. *Br. Med. J.*, **287**, 1276–1278.

Hodges, P.W. and Richardson, C. (1996). Inefficient muscular stabilization of the lumbar spine associated with low back pain. A motor control evaluation of transversus abdominis. *Spine*, **21**, 2640–2650.

Hubka, M.J. and Phelan, S.P. (1994). Interexaminer reliability of palpation for cervical spine tenderness. *J. Manip. Physiol. Ther.*, **17**, 591–595.

Huston, G.J. (1988). Collars and corsets. *Br. Med. J.*, **296**, 276.

Imig, C.J., Randall, B.F. and Hines, H.M. (1954). Effect of ultrasonic energy on blood flow. *Am. J. Phys. Med.*, **53**, 100–102.

Indahl, A., Velund, L. and Reikeraas, O. (1995). Good prognosis for low back pain when left untampered: a randomised clinical trial. *Spine*, **20**, 473–477.

Indahl, A., Haldorsen, E.H., Holm, S., Reikeras, O. and Ursin, H. (1998). Five-year follow-up study of a controlled clinical trial using light mobilisation and an informative approach to low back pain. *Spine*, **23**, 2625–2630.

Itoi, E., Kido, T., Sano, A., Urayama, M. and Sato, K. (1999). Which is more useful, the "full can test" or the "empty can test", in detecting the torn supraspinatus tendon? *Am. J. Sports Med.*, **27**, 65–68.

Jackson, B.A., Schwane, J.A. and Starcher, B.C. (1991). Effect of ultrasound therapy on repair of Achilles tendon injuries in rats. *Med. Sci. Sports Exerc.*, **23**, 171–176.

Johnson, M.I. (1999). The mystique of interferential currents when used to manage pain. *Physiotherapy*, **85**, 294–297.

Johnson, M.J. and Lucas, G.L. (1997). Value of cervical spine radiographs as a screening tool. *Clin. Orthop.*, **340**, 102–108.

Jull, G.A. and Richardson, C.A. (1994). Rehabilitation and active stabilization of the lumbar spine. In: *Physical Therapy of the Low Back*, 2nd edn, ed. L.T. Twomey and J.R. Taylor, pp. 251–273. New York: Churchill Livingstone.

Kirkwood, B.R. (1988). *Essentials of Medical Statistics*, p. 121. Oxford: Blackwell.

Kitchen, S.S. and Partridge C.J. (1990). A review of therapeutic ultrasound. *Physiotherapy*, **76**, 593–600.

Kitchen, S.S. and Partridge, C.J. (1991). A review of low-level laser therapy. *Physiotherapy*, **77**, 161–168.

Kitchen, S. and Partridge, C. (1992). Review of shortwave diathermy continuous and pulsed patterns. *Physiotherapy*, **78**, 243–252.

Klaber Moffett, J.A., Richardson, P.H., Frost, H. and Osborn, A. (1996). A placebo-controlled double-blind trial to evaluate the effectiveness of pulsed short wave therapy for osteo-arthritic hip and knee pain. *Pain*, **67**, 121–127.

Koes, B.W. and van den Hoogen, H.M.M. (1994). Efficacy of bed rest and orthoses of low-back pain. A review of randomized clinical trials. *Eur. J. Phys. Med. Rehabil.*, **4**, 86–93.

Kramer, J.F. (1984). Ultrasound: evaluation of its mechanical and thermal effects. *Arch. Phys. Med. Rehabil.*, **65**, 223–227.

Kramer, J.F. and Sandrin, M. (1993). Effect of low-power laser and white light on sensory conduction rate of the superficial radial nerve. *Physiother. Can.*, **45**, 165–170.

Krasheninnikoff, M., Ellitsgaard, N., Rogvi-Hansen, B. et al. (1994). No effect of low power laser in lateral epicondylitis. *Scand. J. Rheumatol.*, **23**, 260–263.

Krause, M., Refshauge, K.M., Dessen, M. and Boland, R. (2000). Lumbar spine traction: evaluation of effects and recommended application for treatment. *Manual Ther.*, **5**, 72–81.

Labelle, H., Guibert, R., Joncas, J., Newman, N., Fallaha, M. and Rivard, C.H. (1992). Lack of scientific evidence for the treatment of lateral epicondylitis of the elbow. An attempted meta-analysis. *J. Bone Joint Surg.*, **74B**, 646–651.

Lane, N.E. and Thompson, J.M. (1997). Management of osteoarthritis in the primary care setting: an evidence-based approach to treatment. *Am. J. Med.*, **103**, 25S–30S.

Larsson, U., Choler, U., Lidstrom, A. et al. (1980). Auto-traction for treatment of lumbago-sciatica. *Acta Orthop. Scand.*, **51**, 791–798.

Lawrence, J.S., Bremner, J.M. and Bier, F. (1966). Osteo-arthrosis. Prevalence in the population and relationship between symptoms and x-ray changes. *Ann. Rheum. Dis.*, **25**, 1–24.

Lehman, J.F., Brunner, G.D. and Stow, R.W. (1958). Pain threshold measurements after therapeutic application of ultrasound microwaves and infrared. *Arch. Phys. Med.*, **39**, 560–565.

Lehman, J.F., Masock, A.J., Warren, C.G. and Koblanski, J.N. (1970). Effects of therapeutic temperatures on tendon extensibility. *Arch. Phys. Med.*, **51**, 481–487.

Lidstrom, A. and Zachrisson, M. (1970). Physical therapy on low back pain and sciatica. *Scand. J. Rehabil. Med.*, **2**, 37–42.

Lord, S., Barnsley, L., Wallis, B.J. and Bogduk, N. (1996). Chronic cervical zygapophysial joint pain after whiplash: a placebo-controlled prevalence study. *Spine*, **21**, 1737–1745.

Low, J. (1994). Electrotherapeutic modalities. In: *Pain Management in Physical Therapy*, 2nd edn, ed. P.E. Wells, V. Framplton and D. Bowsher, pp. 140–176. Oxford: Butterworth-Heinemann.

MacDonald, P.B., Clark, P. and Sutherland, K. (2000). An analysis of the diagnostic accuracy of the Hawkins and Neer subacromial impingement signs. *J. Shoulder Elbow Surg.*, **9**, 299–301.

Macintosh, J.E., Bogduk, N. and Gracovetsky, S. (1987). The biomechanics of the thoracolumbar fascia. *Clin. Biomech.*, **2**, 78–83.

Maher, C., Latimer, J. and Refshauge, K. (1999). Prescription of activity for low back pain: what works? *Aust. J. Physiother.*, **45**, 121–132.

Maigne, J.Y., Aivaliklis, A. and Pfefer, F. (1996). Results of sacroiliac joint double block and value of sacroiliac pain provocation tests in 54 patients with low-back pain. *Spine*, **21**, 1889–1892.

Marks, R., Ghassemi, M., Duarte, R. and Van Nguyen, J.P. (1999). A review of the literature on shortwave diathermy as applied to osteo-arthritis of the knee. *Physiotherapy*, **85**, 304–316.

Matthews, J.A. (1968). Dynamic discography: a study of lumbar traction. *Ann. Phys. Med.*, **9**, 275–279.

Matthews, J.A. and Hickling, J. (1975) Lumbar traction: a double-blind controlled study for sciatica. *Rheumatol. Rehabil.*, **14**, 222–225.

Maxwell, J. (1992). Therapeutic ultrasound: its effects on the cellular and molecular mechanisms of inflammation and repair. *Physiotherapy*, **78**, 421–426.

McAlindon, T.E. (1999). The knee. *Bailliere's Clin. Rheumatol.*, **13**, 329–344.

McDiarmid, T. and Burns P.N. (1987). Clinical applications of therapeutic ultrasound. *Physiotherapy*, **73**, 155–162.

McKinney, L.A. (1989). Early mobilisation and outcomes in acute sprains of the neck. *Br. Med. J.*, **299**, 1006–1008.

McKinney, L.A., Dornan, J.O. and Ryan, M. (1989). The role of physiotherapy in the management of acute neck sprains following road-traffic accidents. *Arch. Emerg. Med.*, **6**, 27–33.

Millard, J.B. (1961). Effect of high frequency currents and infrared rays on the circulation of the lower limb in man. *Ann. Phys. Med.*, **6**, 45–65.

Miller, D.L. (1987). A review of the ultrasonic bioeffects of microsonation, gas body activation and related cavitation-like phenomena. *Ultrasound Med. Biol.*, **13**, 443–470.

Mior, S.A., King, R.S., McGregor, M. and Bernard, M. (1985). Intra and interexaminer reliability of motion palpation in the cervical spine. *J. Can. Chiro. Ass.*, **29**, 195–198.

Moret, N.C., van der Stap, M., Hagmeijer, R., Molenaar, A. and Koes, B.W. (1998). Design and feasibility of a randomized clinical trial to evaluate the effect of vertical traction in patients with a lumbar radicular syndrome. *Manual Ther.*, **3**, 203–211.

Nansel, D.D., Peneff, A.L., Jansen, R.D. and Cooperstein, R. (1989). Interexaminer concordance in detecting joint-play asymmetries in the cervical spines of otherwise asymptomatic subjects. *J. Manip. Physiol. Ther.*, **12**, 428–433.

Naredo, E., Aguado, P., De Miguel, E. et al. (2002). Painful shoulder: comparison of physical examination and ultrasound findings. *Ann. Rheum. Dis.*, **61**, 132–136.

Needell, S.D., Zlatkin, M.B., Sher, J.S., Murphy, B.J. and Uribe, J.W. (1996). MR imaging of the rotator cuff: peritendinous and bone abnormalities in an asymptomatic population. *Am. J. Roentgenol.*, **166**, 863–867.

O'Sullivan, P.B., Twomey, L.T. and Allison, G.T. (1997). Evaluation of specific stabilizing exercise in the treatment of chronic low back pain with radiologic diagnosis of spondylolysis or spondylolisthesis. *Spine*, **22**, 2959–2967.

Pal, B., Mangion, P., Hossain, M.A. and Diffey, B.L. (1986). A controlled trial of continuous lumbar traction in the treatment of back pain and sciatica. *Br. J. Rheumatol.*, **25**, 181–183.

Palmer, S.T., Martin, D.J., Steedman, W.M. and Ravey, J. (1999). Alteration of interferential current and transcutaneous electrical nerve stimulation frequency: effects on nerve excitation. *Arch. Phys. Med. Rehabil.*, **90**, 1065–1071.

Partridge, C. (1987). Evaluation of the efficacy of ultrasound. *Physiotherapy*, **83**, 166–168.

Phillips, D.R. and Twomey, L.T. (1996). A comparison of manual diagnosis with a diagnosis established by a uni-level lumbar spinal block procedure. *Manual Ther.*, **2**, 82–87.

Richardson, C.A., Jull, G.A. and Hides, J.A. (2000). A new clinical model of the muscle dysfunction linked to the disturbance of spinal stability: implications for treatment of low back pain. In: *Physical Therapy of the Low Back*, 3rd edn, ed. L.T. Twomey and J.R. Taylor, pp. 249–267. New York: Churchill Livingstone.

Rosenfeld, M., Gunnersson, R. and Borenstein, P. (2000). Early intervention in whiplash-associated disorders. *Spine*, **25**, 1782–1787.

Sackett, D.L., Haynes, R.B. and Tugwell, P. (1985). *Clinical Epidemiology. A Basic Science for Clinical Medicine*. Boston: Little, Brown.

Schwarzer, A.C., Aprill, C.N., Derby, R., Fortin, J., Kine, G. and Bogduk, N. (1994a). The relative contributions of the disc and zygapophyseal joint in chronic low back pain. *Spine*, **19**, 801–806.

Schwarzer, A.C., Aprill, C.N., Derby, R., Fortin, J., Kine, G. and Bogduk, N. (1994b). Clinical features of patients with pain stemming from the lumbar zygapophysial joints. Is the lumbar facet syndrome a clinical entity? *Spine*, **19**, 1132–1137.

Schwarzer, A.C., Aprill, C.N., Derby, R., Fortin, J., Kine, G., and Bogduk, N. (1995a). The prevalence and clinical features of internal disc disruption in patients with chronic low back pain. *Spine*, **20**, 1878–1883.

Schwarzer, A.C., Wang, S., Bogduk N., McNaught, P.J., and Laurent, R. (1995b). Prevalence and clinical features of lumbar zygapophysial joint pain: a study in an Australian population with chronic low back pain. *Ann. Rheum. Dis.*, **54**, 100–106.

Schwarzer, A.C., Aprill, C.N. and Bogduk, N. (1995c). The sacroiliac joint in chronic low back pain. *Spine*, **20**, 31–37.

Shekelle, P.G., Adams, A.H., Chassin, M.R., Hurwitz, E.L. and Brook, R.H. (1992). Spinal manipulation for low-back pain. *Ann. Intern. Med.*, **117**, 590–598.

Smedmark, V., Wallin, M. and Arvidsson, I. (2000). Inter-examiner reliability in assessing passive intervertebral motion of the cervical spine. *Manual Ther.*, **5**, 97–101.

Stillwell, G.K. (1971). Therapeutic heat and cold. In: *Handbook of Physical Medicine and Rehabilitation*, 2nd edn, ed. F.H. Krusen, pp. 259–272. Philadelphia: W.B. Saunders.

Stoller, D.W., Markholf, K.L., Zager S.A. and Shoemaker, S.C. (1983). The effects of exercise, ice and ultrasonography on torsional laxity of the knee joint. *Clin. Orthop.*, **174**, 172–180.

Strender, L.E., Sjoblom, A., Sundell, K., Ludwig, R. and Taube, A. (1997). Interexaminer reliability in physical examination of patients with low back pain. *Spine*, **22**, 814–820.

Sweitzer, R.W. (1994). Ultrasound. In: *Physical Agents. A Comprehensive Text for Physical Therapists*, ed. B. Hecox, T.A. Mehretab and J. Weisberg, Ch. 13, pp. 91–114. Norwalk, CT: Appleton and Lange.

Synder-Mackler, L. and Seitz, L. (1990). Therapeutic uses of light in rehabilitation. In: *Thermal Agents in Rehabilitation*, 2nd edn, ed. S.L. Michlovitz, Ch. 9, pp. 200–218. Philadelphia: F.A. Davis.

Tan, J.C. and Nordin, M. (1992). Role of physical therapy in the treatment of cervical disk disease. *Orthop. Clin. North Am.*, **23**, 435–449.

Turner, S.M., Powell, E.S. and Ng, C.S.S. (1989). The effect of ultrasound on the healing of repaired cockerel tendon: is collagen crosslinkage a factor? *J. Hand Surg.*, **14B**, 428–433.

Twomey, L. (1985). Sustained lumbar traction. An experimental study of long spine segments. *Spine*, **10**, 146–149.

van der Heijden, G.J.M.G., Leffers, P., Wolters, P.J.M.X. et al. (1999). No effect of bipolar interferential electrotherapy and pulsed ultrasound for soft tissue shoulder disorders: a randomised controlled trial. *Ann. Rheum. Dis.*, **58**, 530–540.

van der Wurff, P., Hagmeijer, R.H.M. and Meyne, W. (2000a). Clinical tests of the sacroiliac joint. A systematic methodological review. Part I: reliability. *Manual Ther.*, **5**, 30–36.

van der Wurff, P., Meyne, W. and Hagmeijer, R.H.M. (2000b). Clinical tests of the sacroiliac joint. A systematic methodological review. Part 2: validity. *Manual Ther.*, **5**, 89–96.

van Poppel, M.N.M., de Looze, M.P., Koes, B.W., Smid, T. and Bouter, L. (2000). Mechanisms of action of lumbar supports: a systematic review. *Spine*, **25**, 2103–2113.

van Tulder, M.W., Koes, B.W. and Bouter, L.M. (1997). Conservative treatment of acute and chronic non-specific low back pain: a systematic review of randomised controlled trials of the most common interventions. *Spine*, **22**, 2128–2156.

Vasseljen, O., Hoeg, N., Kjeldstad, B., Johnsson, A. and Larsen, S. (1992). Low level laser versus placebo in the treatment of tennis elbow. *Scand. J. Rehabil. Med.*, **24**, 37–42.

Vendrig, A.A., van Akkerveeken, P.F. and McWhorter, K.R. (2000). Results of a multimodal treatment program for patients with chronic symptoms after a whiplash injury of the neck. *Spine*, **25**, 238–244.

Viikari-Juntura, E. (1987). Interexaminer reliability of observations in physical examinations of the neck. *Phys. Ther.*, **67**, 1526–1532.

Watson, P.J. (1999). Psychosocial assessment. The emergence of a new fashion, or a new tool in physiotherapy for musculoskeletal pain? *Physiotherapy*, **85**, 530–535.

Watson, T. (2000). The role of electrotherapy in contemporary physiotherapy practice. *Manual Ther.*, **5**, 132–141.

Weber, H. (1973). Traction therapy in sciatica due to disc prolapse. *J. Oslo City Hosp.*, **23**, 167–176.

Weber, H., Ljunggren, E. and Walker, L. (1984). Traction therapy in patients with herniated lumbar intervertebral discs. *J. Oslo City Hosp.*, **34**, 61–70.

Williams, A.R., McHale, J., Bowditch, M., Miller, D.L. and Reed, B. (1987). Effects of MHz ultrasound on electrical pain threshold perception in humans. *Ultrasound Med. Biol.*, **13**, 249–258.

Winters, J.C., Sobel, J.S., Groenier, K.H., Arendzen, H.J. and Meyboom-de-Jong, B. (1997). Comparison of physiotherapy, manipulation, and corticosteroid injection for treating shoulder complaints in general practice: randomised, single blind study. *Br. Med. J.*, **314**, 1320–1325.

Winters, J.C., Jorritsma, W., Groenier, H., Sobel, S.J., Meyboom-de-Jong, B. and Arendzen, H.J. (1999). Treatment of shoulder complaints in general practice: long-term results of a randomised, single blind study comparing physiotherapy, manipulation, and corticosteroid injection. *Br. Med. J.*, **318**, 1395–1396.

Wood, D.J. (1987). Design and evaluation of a back injury prevention program within a geriatric hospital. *Spine*, **12**, 77–82.

Wright, V. (1964). Treatment of osteoarthritis of the knees. *Ann. Rheum. Dis.*, **23**, 389–391.

Wyper, D.J. and McNiven, D.R. (1976). Effects of some physiotherapeutic agents on skeletal muscle blood flow. *Physiotherapy*, **63**, 83–85.

Young, S.R. and Dyson, M. (1990a). Macrophage responsiveness to therapeutic ultrasound. *Ultrasound Med. Biol.*, **16**, 809–816.

Young, S.R. and Dyson, M. (1990b). The effect of therapeutic ultrasound on angiogenesis. *Ultrasound Med. Biol.*, **16**, 261–269.

Young, S.R. and Dyson, M. (1990c). Effect of therapeutic ultrasound on the healing of full-thickness excised skin lesions. *Ultrasonics*, **28**, 175–180.

Zusman, M. (1986) Spinal manipulative therapy: review of some proposed mechanisms, and a new hypothesis. *Aust. J. Physiother.*, **32**, 89–99.

Zylbergold, R.S. and Piper, M.C. (1985) Cervical spine disorders: a comparison of three types of traction. *Spine*, **10**, 867–871.

USING EVIDENCE IN CLINICAL PRACTICE

Altman, D.G., Machin, D., Bryant, T.N. and Gardner, M.J. (eds) (2000). *Statistics with Confidence*, 2nd edn. London: British Medical Journal Books.

Antman, E.M., Lau, J., Kupelnick, B., Mosteller, F. and Chalmers, T.C. (1992). A comparison of results of meta-analyses of randomized control trials and recommendations of clinical experts. Treatments for myocardial infarction. *J.A.M.A.*, **268**, 240–248.

Booth, A. and Madge, B. (1998). Finding the evidence. In: *Evidence-based Healthcare: A Practical Guide for Therapists*, ed. T. Bury and J. Mead, pp. 107–135. Oxford: Butterworth-Heinemann.

Campbell, D.T. and Stanley, J.C. (1963). *Experimental and Quasi-Experimental Designs for Research*. Chicago, IL: Rand McNally College.

Chalmers, T., Celano, P., Sacks, H. and Smith, H. (1983). Bias in treatment assignment in controlled clinical trials. *N. Engl. J. Med.*, **309**, 1358–1361.

Clarke, M. and Oxman, A.D. (eds) (2000). *Cochrane Reviewers' Handbook 4.1* (updated June 2000). Review Manager (RevMan) (computer program). Version 4.1. Oxford, England: Cochrane Collaboration.

Cook, T. and Campbell, D. (1979). *Quasi-Experimentation: Design and Analysis Issues for Field Settings*. Chicago, IL: Rand McNally.

Cooper, H.M. and Hedges, L.V. (eds) (1994). *The Handbook of Research Synthesis*. New York: Russell Sage Foundation.

Cote, P., Cassidy, D., Carroll, L., Frank, J. and Bombardier, C. (2001). A systematic review of the prognosis of acute whiplash and a new conceptual framework to synthesise the literature. *Spine*, 26, E445–E458.

Dixon, J.K. and Keating, J.L. (2000). Variability in straight leg raise measurements: review. *Physiotherapy*, **86**, 361–370.

Doull, J.A., Hardy, M., Clark, J.H. and Herman, N.B. (1931). The effect of irradiation with ultra-violet light on the frequency of attacks of upper respiratory disease (common colds). *Am. J. Hyg.*, **13**, 460–477.

Egger, M., Davey Smith, G. and Altman, D.G. (eds) (2001). *Systematic Reviews in Health Care. Meta-analysis in Context*. London: British Medical Journal Books.

Egger, M., Ebrahim, S. and Smith, G.D. (2002). Where now for meta-analysis? *Int. J. Epidemiol.*, **31**, 1–5.

Ernst, E. (2002). Manipulation of the cervical spine: a systematic review of case reports of serious adverse events, 1995–2001. *Med. J. Aust.*, **15**, 376–380.

Ettinger, W.H. Jr., Burns, R., Messier, S.P. et al. (1997). A randomized trial comparing aerobic exercise and resistance exercise with a health education program in older adults with knee osteoarthritis. The Fitness Arthritis and Seniors Trial (FAST). *J.A.M.A.*, **277**, 25–31.

Eysenbach, G., Tuische, J. and Diepgen, T.L. (2001). Evaluation of the usefulness of internet searches to identify unpublished clinical trials for systematic reviews. *Med. Inform. Internet Med.*, **26**, 203–218.

Ferreira, P., Ferreira, M., Maher, C., Refshauge, K., Herbert, R. and Latimer, J. (2002). Effect of applying different "levels of evidence" on conclusions of Cochrane reviews of interventions for low back pain. *J. Clin. Epidemiol*, **55**, 1111–1114.

Fransen, M., McConnell, S. and Bell, M. (2002). Therapeutic exercise for people with osteoarthritis of the hip or knee. A systematic review. *J. Rheumatol.*, **29**, 1737–1745.

Ginn, K.A., Herbert, R.D., Khouw, W and Lee, R. (1997). A randomised, controlled clinical trial of a treatment for shoulder pain. *Phys. Ther.*, **77**, 802–811.

Gregoire, G., Derderian, F. and Le Lorier, J. (1995). Selecting the language of the publications included in a meta-analysis: is there a tower of Babel bias? *J. Clin. Epidemiol.*, **48**, 159–163.

Gross, A.R., Aker, P.D., Goldsmith, C.H. and Peloso, P. (2002). Physical medicine modalities for mechanical neck disorders (Cochrane review). In: *The Cochrane Library*, Issue 4, 2002. Oxford: Update Software.

Hedges, L.V. and Olkin, I. (1980). Vote-counting methods in research synthesis. *Psychol. Bull.*, **88**, 359–369.

Helmer, D., Savoie, I., Green, C. and Kazanjian, A. (2001). Evidence-based practice: extending the search to find material for the systematic review. *Bull. Med. Library Assoc.*, **89**, 346–352.

Herbert, R.D. (2000a). How to estimate treatment effects from reports of clinical trials. I: Continuous outcomes. *Aust. J. Physiother.*, **46**, 229–235.

Herbert, R.D. (2000b). How to estimate treatment effects from reports of clinical trials. I: Dichotomous outcomes. *Aust. J. Physiother.*, **46**, 309–313.

Hides, J.A., Jull, G.A. and Richardson, C.A. (2001). Long-term effects of specific stabilizing exercises for first-episode low back pain. *Spine*, **26**, E243–E248.

Hollis, S. and Campbell, F. (1999). What is meant by intention to treat analysis? Survey of published randomised controlled trials. *Br. Med. J.*, **319**, 670–674.

Hoving, J., Koes, B., de Vet, H. et al. (2002). Manual therapy, physical therapy or continued care by a general practitioner for patients with neck pain. A randomised controlled trial. *Ann. Intern. Med.*, **136**, 713–722.

Jadad, A.R., Moore, R.A., Carroll, D. et al. (1986). Assessing the quality of reports of randomised clinical trials: is blinding necessary? *Controlled Clin. Trials*, **7**, 177–188.

Jones, D.R. (1995). Meta-analysis: weighing the evidence. *Statistics Med.*, **14**, 137–149.

Juni, P., Witschi, A., Bloch, R. and Egger, M. (1999). The hazards of scoring the quality of clinical trials in meta-analysis. *J.A.M.A.*, **282**, 1054–1060.

Juni, P., Holenstein, F., Sterne, J., Bartlett, C. and Egger, M. (2002). Direction and impact of language bias in meta-analysis of controlled trials: empirical study. *Int. J. Epidemiol.*, **31**, 115–123.

Khan, K.S., Daya, S. and Jadad, A. (1996). The importance of quality of primary studies in producing unbiased systematic reviews. *Arch. Intern. Med.* **156**, 661–666.

La Mantia, K. and Marks, R. (1995). The efficacy of aerobic exercises for treating osteoarthritis of the knee. *NZ J. Physiother.*, **23**, 23–30.

Loney, P.L. and Stratford, P.W. (1999). The prevalence of low back pain in adults: a methodological review of the literature. *Phys. Ther.* **79**, 384–396.

Maher, C.G., Herbert, R.D., Sherrington, C., Moseley, A.M. and Elkins, M. (2003). Critical appraisal of randomised trials, systematic reviews of randomised trials, and clinical practice guidelines. In: *Grieve's Modern Manual Therapy: The Vertebral Column*, 3rd edn, ed. J. Boyling and G. Jull. Edinburgh: Elsevier.

McManus, R.J., Wilson, S., Delaney, B.C. et al. (1998). Review of the usefulness of contacting other experts when conducting a literature search for systematic reviews. *Br. Med. J.* **317**, 1562–1563.

Moher, D., Jadad, A., Nichol, G., Penman, M., Tugwell, P. and Walsh, S. (1995). Assessing the quality of randomized controlled trials: an annotated bibliography of scales and checklists. *Control. Clin. Trials*, **16**, 62–73.

Moher, D., Fortin, P., Jadad, A.R. et al. (1996). Completeness of reporting of trials published in languages other than English: implications for conduct and reporting of systematic reviews. *Lancet*, **347**, 363–366.

Moher, D., Cook, D.J., Eastwood, S., Olkin, I., Rennie, D. and Stroup, D.F. (1999). Improving the quality of reports of meta-analyses of randomised controlled trials: the QUOROM statement. Quality of reporting of meta-analyses. *Lancet*, **354**, 1896–1900.

Moseley, A.M., Herbert, R.D., Sherrington, C. and Maher, C.G. (2002). Evidence for physiotherapy practice: a survey of the Physiotherapy Evidence Database (PEDro). *Aust. J. Physiother.*, **48**, 43–49.

National Health and Medical Research Council (NHMRC) (1999). *How to Review the Evidence: Systematic Identification and Review of the Scientific Literature*. Canberra: Biotext.

Oxman, A.D. and Guyatt, G.H. (1993). The science of reviewing research. *Ann. NY Acad. Sci.*, **703**, 125–133.

Oxman, A.D., Cook, D.J., Guyatt, G. for the Evidence Based Medicine Working Group (2003). How to use an overview. Available online at: (http://www.cche.net/usersguides/overview.asp) accessed 7 January 2003.

Petticrew, M. (2001). Systematic reviews from astronomy to zoology: myths and misconceptions. *Br. Med. J.*, **322**, 98–101.

Richardson, W.S., Wilson, M.C., Nishikawa, J. and Hayward, R.S. (1995). The well-built clinical question: a key to evidence-based decisions. *ACP J. Club*, **123**, A12–A13.

Sackett, D.L., Straus, S.E., Richardson, W.S., Rosenberg, W. and Haynes, R.B. (2000). *Evidence-Based Medicine: How to Practice and Teach EBM*, 2nd edn. Edinburgh: Churchill Livingstone.

Schulz, K.F. (1995). Subverting randomization in controlled trials. *J.A.M.A.*, **274**, 1456–1458.

Sherrington, C., Herbert, R.D., Maher, C.G. and Moseley, A.M. (2000). PEDro. A database of randomized trials and systematic reviews in physiotherapy. *Manual Ther.*, **5**, 223–226.

Sim, J. and Reid, N. (1999). Statistical inference by confidence intervals: issues of interpretation and utilization. *Phys. Ther.*, **79**, 186–195.

Solomon, D.H., Simel, D.L., Bates, D.W., Katz, J.N. and Schaffer, J.L. (2001). Does this patient have a torn meniscus or ligament of the knee? Value of the physical examination. *J.A.M.A.*, **286**, 1610–1620.

Stern, J.M. and Simes, R.J. (1997). Publication bias: evidence of delayed publication in a cohort study of clinical research projects. *Br. Med. J.*, **315**, 640–645.

Verhagen, A., de Vet, H., de Bie, R., Boers, M. and van den Brandt, P. (2001). The art of quality assessment of RCTs included in systematic reviews. *J. Clin. Epidemiol.*, **54**, 651–654.

Walker, A.M., Martin-Moreno, J.M. and Artalejo, F.R. (1988). Odd man out: a graphical approach to meta-analysis. *Am. J. Public Health*, **78**, 961–966.

Wickstrom, G. and Bendix, T. (2000). The "Hawthorne effect" – what did the original Hawthorne studies actually show? *Scand. J. Work, Environ. Health*, **26**, 363–367.

Chapter 8

Persisting pain: using cognitive-behavioural principles for activity-based pain management

M.K. Nicholas and L. Tonkin

CHAPTER CONTENTS

One of the problems confronting people with persisting spinal pain is the question of activity versus rest. Should they rest (wait for the pain to settle) and only engage in activities which do not aggravate pain (commonly known as 'let pain be your guide')? Or should they try to ignore their pain, having been advised by their doctor and physiotherapist that there is nothing seriously wrong with their back (i.e. there are 'no red flags'), and gradually try to resume normal activities, including exercises?

The weight of current expert opinion, supported by studies like those of Indahl et al. (1995), Lindstrom et al. (1992) and Linton and Andersson (2000), as well as systematic reviews (Waddell and Burton, 1999), is that providing there are no 'red flags' present (indicative of major pathology) people with acute and subacute low back pain, for example, should be encouraged to resume normal activities as soon as possible. The evidence from these studies suggests that those who follow this approach tend to suffer less disability and distress, return to work sooner and use health care services less than those who are treated in more traditional ways that are often more concerned with symptom relief as the focus of treatment.

It is not difficult to imagine that when a patient is experiencing pain which has persisted for more than 6–8 weeks they may be starting to become concerned about what is happening. This concern could well be increased if they feel that no one has been able to give them a clear explanation for the pain or to improve it significantly. They may well fear that by continuing to do things despite the pain they are risking causing further damage or prolonging their condition. Fear of pain may also develop – either because of its possible implications or as a somewhat natural aversion to the experience of pain. This may be compounded if they come to believe that they can't do things when in pain.

At the same time a person in this position is also likely to be getting all sorts of advice on what to do about the pain. This advice may be from doctor, physiotherapist, chiropractor, family and friends, even people at work. It would be surprising if this advice was consistent. Some may be urging further investigations or possible lines of treatment while others may be recommending a 'take-it-easy' approach, with activity avoidance and resting as key strategies. In this setting it is also likely that many people in persisting pain will have their normal household chores taken over by others in an attempt to ease their burden and to enable them to recover. While this help will be well-meaning it could have the unintended consequence of effectively reinforcing disability – both in the pain-sufferer's mind and in the minds of those around them. As a result the person in pain could well become increasingly inactive and passive, while waiting for someone to 'fix' the problem.

We also know that often when people stop doing things which they normally enjoy or which give their life meaning (like working, socializing, playing sport, participating in family activities) their mood is likely to become increasingly despondent and frustrated (Lewinsohn, 1974). In time, many will become quite depressed. When this low mood is coupled with the other aspects of the picture (the fear of pain or reinjury, the failure of treatments to help, belief in inability to do things when in pain and increasing disability) there is a strong risk of the person losing confidence and starting to feel increasingly helpless. As a result, the risk of developing all the common features of chronic disabling pain (depressed mood, inactivity, disturbed sleep, reliance on passive treatments like drugs and withdrawal from most normal activities including work) becomes greatly heightened (Linton, 2000). Curative treatments for those who reach this state are increasingly unlikely.

For those whose low back pain does not settle within 8–12 weeks there is clearly a high risk of their slipping into the chronic disabling pain category (Waddell and Bryn-Jones, 1994). This is particularly true of those who develop the features outlined above. It has become a standard belief of guidelines on acute and subacute low back pain that intervening in this process before the patient gets to this stage will limit their progression to chronic disability (even if their pain cannot be relieved). The few available studies which have examined this proposition have generally reported positive results (Lindstrom et al., 1992; Indahl et al., 1995; Linton and Andersson, 2000), but it is important to note that they were not effective in preventing all patients from developing into chronic cases. A small proportion of cases will, therefore, require further and more intensive interventions (Vlaeyen et al., 1995; Williams et al., 1999; Guzman et al., 2001; Von Korff et al., 2002).

Two main approaches have been described to encourage resumption of ceased activities in patients with persisting spinal pain. Indahl et al. (1995) utilized encouragement to resume normal activities as soon as possible. Lindstrom et al. (1992), on the other hand, utilized a structured exercise programme as a means of restoring confidence and functional capacity. The use of exercises in restoration of function has also been a common feature of most so-called 'work-hardening' or 'work-conditioning' programmes (Teasel and Harth, 1996) aimed at returning injured workers to work. However, both exercises and encouragement to resume normal activities, by themselves, have been shown to have limitations as a means of functional rehabilitation. Malmivaara et al. (1995), for example, demonstrated that simply prescribing exercises is unlikely to be enough to help a person with acute low back pain regain previous levels of functioning. There is also dispute about which exercises people should perform (Maher et al., 1999). In addition, Indahl et al. (1995) reported the failure of 30% to return to work within 6 months. One reason that activity or exercise prescription may not suffice in many cases was outlined by Vlaeyen and Linton's (2000) review which indicated that psychosocial events, like fear of pain or reinjury and catastrophic thinking styles, could become effective obstacles to progress in a simple exercise programme as well as simple encouragement to resume normal activities.

Lindstrom et al. (1992) attempted to address obstacles of this type by employing a programme of graduated exercises, whereby patients were encouraged gradually to resume more normal activities despite their pain, with the exercises being a tool to assist in achieving this goal. Lindstrom et al. mentioned using 'behavioural principles', mainly encouragement and graduated goal-setting, as the basis of their approach. Indahl et al. (1995) also tried to address any fears held by their patients by coupling their encouragement to resume exercises with a thorough musculoskeletal examination followed by attempts to reassure the patients verbally that they were well and could safely become more active. Linton and Andersson (2000) attempted to address these same issues via a series of group cognitive-behavioural therapy sessions with a psychologist to train the patients directly in ways of overcoming fears and managing their pain.

Thus, besides encouraging the resumption of normal activities and exercises, the use of a number of psychological principles or methods derived from these principles can be observed in each of these studies. Similar approaches have been successfully used in more intensive, multidisciplinary programmes with more disabled and distressed patients with chronic pain conditions (Morley et al., 1999; Guzman et al., 2001). However, the degree to which the cognitive and behavioural principles and methods employed have been described (and used) in these studies inevitably has been quite variable. This chapter will attempt to provide a clear account of these principles and methods in ways which might assist physiotherapists, and others, to utilize them to promote activities and exercises in patients with persisting pain conditions.

BASIC PRINCIPLES

So-called 'behavioural' principles were initially generated from laboratory studies of learning (or conditioning) with humans and other animals by researchers like Pavlov and Skinner. They were then systematically applied in clinical settings with people suffering from both mental and physical disabilities (Aylon and Azrin, 1968; Marks, 1975; Fordyce, 1976). During the 1970s and 1980s the developing concepts of cognitions or thought processes, sometimes referred to as 'self-talk' (Meichenbaum, 1975), were increasingly incorporated with the behavioural principles in clinical applications. Some began to refer to these interventions as primarily cognitive therapy (Beck et al., 1979), although behavioural elements were usually involved as well. Others specifically integrated both cognitive and behavioural approaches (Hawton et al., 1989). Currently, this family of therapies is usually referred to under the rubric of 'cognitive-behavioural therapies'.

This chapter will take a similar, integrated cognitive and behavioural approach to clinical applications of the main features of these two strands. It will be assumed that the task to be addressed involves helping people experiencing persisting pain to make changes to the ways in which they behave. This may involve learning new behaviours or skills, or it may involve the resumption of activities which have been ceased or restricted due to pain.

As with any treatment, whether medical, psychological or physical, no patient should be expected to undertake a form of intervention without an adequate explanation of what the treatment involves, its rationale and expected outcomes, and the patient's role in the process. An important element of this process concerns a reformulation or reconceptualization of the patient's problem(s) that will help him or her to make sense of the treatment (Turk and Holzman, 1986). Thus, if a patient believes that all his or her problems are due to their pain and all that is required is a diagnosis of the cause (so, presumably, the right treatment can be administered to resolve the problem), then he or she will take some convincing to accept an exercise or activity programme which will not take this approach and may not resolve the pain. In these cases, the therapist will need to develop ways of explaining the patient's problems that will make the proposed treatment appear reasonable and worth pursuing. This issue will be returned to later.

Also, in common with any treatment, cognitive-behavioural interventions should be devised after an appropriate assessment of the patient's presenting problem(s) by a competent health care provider. Thus, a 'cookbook' or 'one-size-fits-all' approach should have no part in the application of the principles and methods outlined in this chapter – they must be tailored to the individual patient/ client's assessed problems and contributing factors. In a number of cases, this assessment (and/or intervention) will require specialized skills, like those possessed by an appropriately experienced clinical psychologist. In a large proportion of cases, however, this should not be necessary, providing the treating doctor or therapist is able to recognize his or her limits and to seek appropriate skilled assistance at those times.

In these instances, physiotherapists must seek out ways in which to work collaboratively with other providers and the patient/client. This is particularly true when there is evidence that psychosocial factors, like unhelpful fears and beliefs, mood disturbance or interpersonal difficulties, are impeding progress in an activity or exercise-based intervention. In more extreme cases this might require the patient/client to be entered into an intensive multidisciplinary programme (Guzman et al., 2001), but in most cases this should not be necessary. Where medication use is an issue then medical involvement is clearly warranted.

However, regardless of their discipline, for maximal effectiveness all health care providers involved in the delivery of cognitive-behavioural interventions should be familiar with the principles and methods outlined in this chapter.

PEOPLE LEARN MOST EFFECTIVELY BY DOING

Providing information – simply telling someone what to do – is generally a poor method of training or learning. Professor Wilbert Fordyce, the pioneer of behavioural treatments for chronic pain, once made this point very clearly when he said: 'information is to behaviour change as spaghetti is to a brick' (personal communication). The history of the 'back school' approach to back pain is a good example of how information (by itself) on back care is of limited use (Van Tulder et al., 1999). Observing others perform (or model) an activity can aid learning (of an activity or task; Bandura, 1986). By far the most effective method of learning a new behaviour or task is to find a way of getting

the person to perform the desired behaviour, or a version of it, and to reinforce it (Fordyce, 1976).

SHAPING

If the task (i.e. behaviour or exercise) is new to patients, a gradual process called 'shaping' can help them to acquire (or learn) the new behaviour. This involves starting at whatever level the person can manage or whatever version of the behaviour (e.g. an exercise) he or she can manage and then practising the behaviour repeatedly, gradually getting closer and closer to the desired goal behaviour. Thus, a perfect performance is not required or expected initially. Rather, the patient should start with a rough approximation (or whatever he or she can manage) and then gradually refine it with repeated practice until the patient can perform the desired or expected task. This is referred to as shaping successive approximations of the goal activity.

REINFORCEMENT

Many behaviours are maintained by their consequences (or what follows the behaviour; Skinner, 1974). If a behaviour is being maintained, the consequences are referred to as 'reinforcers'. In common language they may be thought of as 'rewards', but this can imply a value judgement. 'Reinforcer' may be seen as more neutral as it is defined by its effect (i.e. maintenance of an activity), rather than *a priori* views. Reinforcers are usually something the person desires or wants to achieve (few people are likely to work for something they don't want). Reinforcers do not have to follow a behaviour every time in order to maintain it, just often enough. So you don't have to feel good or win a prize every time you complete an exercise.

Reinforcers often tend to be very individual things, so what one person values as a reinforcer may not suit another person. For example, some people find praise by others (such as their physiotherapist or a family member) helpful in maintaining their performance of an exercise. Others may prefer to see their achievements recognized in the form of a chart showing how much they have improved since they first started.

Furthermore, reinforcers don't have to be external events (like food or praise from others), they can also be internal, like the satisfaction of having achieved something or having done something you are proud of, like achieving a goal.

Behaviours do not need to be reinforced *individually* to be maintained – it can be enough that the same type of behaviour (or a similar behaviour) has been reinforced, or is reinforced. This effect is known as *generalization,* whereby an effect with one behaviour has spread to other similar behaviours. Thus, if a behaviour from a certain class of behaviours is reinforced, other behaviours in that class may also be maintained even without direct reinforcement themselves. For example, if an exercise performed by a patient is reinforced (praised) by the therapist (or just feels good to do), it is possible that the patient will go on to perform other similar exercises without having to be praised by the therapist in every instance. A similar effect can be seen when people learn rules which apply to a number of behaviours, each of which may not be reinforced specifically. This effect has been conceptualized as 'rule-governed behaviour' (Davey, 1988). The main point here is that each individual response or behaviour does not need to be specifically reinforced in order for it to be maintained.

Contingencies of reinforcement

This refers to the relationship between a behaviour and its reinforcer(s). Simply stated, it tells us what a person has to do in order for that behaviour to be reinforced. As an example, one of our patients decided that one way for her to ensure that she did her exercise routine each morning was to delay herself her usual cup of tea and the newspaper until she had done the exercises. Thus, the tea and newspaper were used by her to reinforce her performance of the exercises.

When deciding on what reinforcers to use it is also important that the patient and therapist also work out what the patient must do (and how often) in order to qualify for the reinforcer. Over time, this contingency can be modified and the patient might, for example, require that he or she gradually does more before qualifying for the reinforcer. This is like 'raising the bar' (or standards) in athletics.

Interestingly, it has been found in learning laboratories that one of the strongest reinforcement contingencies (i.e. one whose effects are hardest to extinguish) is that of intermittent reinforcement. This means that reinforcement is delivered only occasionally. To illustrate this, a common example would be comparing using a pay-phone and a gambling device, like a poker machine. When you try to use a pay-phone and it doesn't work, most people will leave it and try another (as it is expected to work every time). On the other hand, if you try a poker machine and there is no pay-out it is likely you will continue inserting coins in the hope that you might be successful next time. In this way, behaviours that are only reinforced occasionally tend to be more resistant to extinction (maintained longer in the absence of reinforcement) than those that are normally reinforced every time they occur.

Possible clinical applications of this principle would include initially frequently reinforcing, say with praise, a patient's efforts at an exercise, but then gradually reducing the frequency of praise or requiring the patient to do more to 'earn' it.

Consistency

Reinforcement for an activity is most effective when it is consistently applied. That means the same activity or task is reinforced in a consistent manner (rather than a competing or contradictory activity). Thus, in a health care setting, this would mean that not only should the therapist reinforce (praise and encourage) the patient's performance of an exercise, say, but also all other health care providers involved with that patient (doctor, nurse, psychologist, etc.) should do so as well. Ideally, so should the patient and his or her family, employer, etc.

When this doesn't happen, for example, when one health care provider encourages rest or avoidance of any activity which might aggravate pain while another is encouraging more activities, it is not hard to imagine that the patient will become confused – and the outcome less predictable.

When a patient is required, as part of the treatment plan, to play an active role (whether it is exercising, taking tablets or following a diet), all those involved in working with the patient must agree to support the single approach. When they don't, the patient is unlikely to adhere to the plan. The same principle applies when only one health provider is involved – consistency in reinforcement is critical.

Self-reinforcement

People can also learn to reinforce themselves for their achievements. Another way of thinking about this is taking credit for your achievements. A good example of people doing this is when a tennis player or a footballer punches the air in excitement when he or she hits a winner or scores a goal. They are recognizing their achievement. In the long run it can be very helpful for maintenance of a behaviour (such as an exercise) if the person concerned can reinforce him- or herself for their achievements. Some people can have trouble doing this – for example, they may feel they are just 'big-noting' (or excessively self-promoting) themselves. Some people will also feel that their achievement is not that great – they may say that they used to be able to do much better than that. Strictly speaking, this can be true, but does it help and did they have a pain condition when they did it before? These are examples of what can be called 'maladaptive cognitions' or thoughts which can effectively undermine performance. These sorts of thinking styles can result in failure to progress and will usually need to be addressed, but we will return to them shortly.

Selecting reinforcers (and goals)

In order to use reinforcers to promote performance or learning it is important to work out what sorts of things the person is likely to find reinforcing. It can help to devise a sort of menu from which the person can select something according to mood. Some variety can also help to prevent the reinforcers losing their potency (they can become boring or less meaningful with too much repetition). Reinforcers should also be feasible or attainable. Naturally, the person (or patient in a clinical setting) must play an active role in identifying possible reinforcers. The therapist can make suggestions of what others have found useful, but as a guide only. Typical examples would include self-praise, small treats (food, drink, a night off studying, an

outing), keeping a record or chart of progress, and so on.

The same principle applies to setting goals. Goals can also be reinforcers – we get a sense of achievement when we reach them and that can keep us motivated to do more. Of course, goals are normally things we are trying to reach for some purpose and not just an aid to motivation. But as with reinforcers generally, goals should be things that are meaningful to us, things we want. Otherwise we are unlikely to try very hard to achieve them. Ideally, it helps to make goals as clear or specific as possible – then we know what we are seeking and when we get there. So rather than say 'I'd like to be fit' (what is that, and when would we know we'd achieved it?), it can be more useful to define it more precisely, like 'I'd like to be able to use the stairs to my office every day without having to sit down to recover'. If we could do that we would be reasonably fit, but we've defined it in terms of something we can measure our performance against and we will know when we have reached it. By setting a goal precisely it can also help us to work out a way to achieve it. Thus, getting 'fit' could mean anything and doesn't really help us work out how to get there. In contrast, climbing stairs is obvious and we can work out a plan to achieve it (e.g. stop for a rest at the top of each flight to begin with and then at the top of every second flight, and so on).

Timing of reinforcers

Reinforcers are more effective if they follow the behaviour (task or exercise) as soon as possible afterwards. So immediate feedback (after a performance) usually works better than delayed feedback. Of course, reinforcers obtained prior to the expected behaviour are unlikely to be as effective – as anyone who has been paid for something before they have done it will recognize. If people feel that it will be a long time before their efforts bear fruit they can be tempted to give up quite easily. Of course, many things we achieve in life do take a long time (e.g. a university degree can take 4–6 years), but we manage to keep going by achieving small goals (reinforcers) along the way. These can be in the form of feedback from others on how well we are doing (like marks for assignments) or small milestones we set for ourselves.

Long-term reinforcers (goals)

Long-term reinforcers will usually be the goal(s) you are trying to achieve (being able to walk the dog, returning to work/study, resuming sport). Most of these tend to be intrinsically reinforcing in themselves. In the end, no one is likely to work for long at something they don't really want to achieve. Thus, the long-term goal(s) of any exercise programme should be clarified early with the patient. Are they just seeking pain relief, to get fitter, or are they wanting to resume ceased activities? This is a critical point in planning an exercise programme. Of course, as with all reinforcers, these goals should be realistic or attainable (in these situations there is no point in aiming at achieving goals which are very unlikely – the risk of failure is too great). So don't plan on becoming an astronaut at this stage.

None of us needs reminding that few people sustain an exercise programme for long, regardless of whether we have pain or not. If you have persisting pain there may be even less motivation to continue to exercise – unless you have a good reason (i.e. something you really want to achieve and you believe the exercises will help you to achieve that goal).

Short-term reinforcers (also short-term goals)

If the ultimate goal (reinforcer) is likely to take some time to achieve, it can also help to have some more easily accessible reinforcers to maintain motivation (i.e. to keep you at the task). These might be called 'short-term reinforcers' (or short-term goals). They are steps towards the ultimate goal. By achieving them it is more likely the ultimate goal will be achieved.

Patients can be asked to develop a list of short-term reinforcers, like a menu. These might include: keeping a chart of their progress and ticking (checking) it each time a stage is completed; a brief statement to themselves that they've done well; or reminding themselves that they've made more progress towards their ultimate goal. To make it more fun they could also do things like having some snack food that they wouldn't normally have or watching a certain programme on TV that night or calling an old and distant friend whom they haven't seen for some time. Depending on their financial means these might also include things like a night out; buying a new article of clothing or something they've been putting off getting; even a trip or weekend away.

Using reinforcers

It is also important that when a reinforcer is provided, the person reminds him or herself what it is for (e.g. 'this is for completing my exercise programme today'). This helps to strengthen the link between the performance of the task or exercise and the reinforcer. It also signifies success – an important consideration when you are in pain.

Initially, it is usually helpful to make the reinforcers or goals easy to achieve. In other words, success can encourage success. The converse, of course, is that if individuals try to achieve something and repeatedly fail, they are likely to become discouraged and stop trying. In someone who is at risk of developing chronic disabling pain this is not what we want. So when starting something like an exercise programme with someone in pain, it is important that the first goals or tasks are fairly easy to achieve. As the person starts to achieve this goal regularly then the task can be made slightly more difficult (or more repetitions may be required). When that level is regularly achieved then the task can be made more difficult again, thus, making it harder to earn the reinforcers. This has the effect of encouraging effort and improved performance. Completion of a task or an exercise is likely to become a reinforcer in itself, but it can be augmented by an external reinforcer like those mentioned above.

To give a concrete example of how a physiotherapist might apply this principle, you would show patients roughly what you would like them to do, then ask them to do it as best they could. When they do it (and not before – remember you should only reinforce a behaviour *after* it has occurred) then you should praise them very lavishly (within reason). The next time they do it, praise again, no matter how poorly they do it – you are really just praising them for trying. Keep this up (providing they are at least doing something) until you see some progress. When this level is being achieved reliably you should then ask them to do a little more – and only praise them when this is achieved. And so on. Soon they should set their own goals and they should start to reinforce themselves for achieving them. You should explain the use of reinforcers to them and praise them for using them as well. By now you should see that we are also using reinforcers to promote shaping (praising closer and closer approximations of what we are trying to get the patient to do).

Feedback as a reinforcer

Another way of thinking about reinforcers is that they are a form of feedback. They tell you when you have achieved your goal. There is evidence that when patients in chronic pain get feedback on their exercise improvements they tend to achieve higher levels of exercise (Cairns and Pasino, 1977; Fordyce et al., 1979).

Fading out your role as a reinforcer

If we are trying to encourage self-reliance in our patients we need to avoid their becoming dependent on us for encouragement. Instead, they should be encouraging (or reinforcing) themselves and perhaps finding ways of getting it from their own environment (e.g. family). Thus, as your patients are starting to make progress with their exercise programme you should begin to praise them less (letting them know beforehand that this does not imply that you are losing interest in them, just trying to encourage them to take responsibility for looking after their own health). As mentioned earlier in relation to reinforcement contingencies, occasional feedback to the patient is important but it doesn't need to be nearly as frequent as in the initial stages of a programme. You can help to prompt it in the patient by making remarks like: 'You must be very pleased with how well you are doing'.

PACING

Linked to the idea of feedback as a reinforcer is the use of quotas in exercise programmes.

Traditionally, people with persisting back pain have been advised to exercise as long as it is comfortable and stop if their pain increases. The trouble with this approach is that it can result in the person focusing too much on the experience of pain. In turn this can mean that patients start to avoid activities which aggravate their pain. But if most activities aggravate their pain this approach will lead to generalized inactivity – the very thing that we are trying to prevent. There is also evidence that when people with back pain do exercise regularly (i.e. they keep going despite the pain), they can actually end up with less pain (Waling et al., 2000). The trick is to find a way of persisting with the exercises (or whatever activity), gradually doing more, but without significantly aggravating the pain – which can lead to feelings of defeat and cessation of the activity.

Fordyce (1976) pioneered a method of achieving this using the concepts of quotas and pacing. By setting quotas for exercises (e.g. five repetitions of one exercise and, say, seven of another) patients have an external goal to aim for (which can help to take their mind off their pain). Quotas also allow patients to know when they have achieved the short-term goal (i.e. the feedback is immediate – a good reinforcement principle), and they give us a benchmark of what patients can do (allowing for planning the next increment).

Pacing up activities

Pacing up activities, means working at a level (e.g. an exercise quota) that can be achieved and, when that is being achieved reliably, doing a bit more until that is achieved reliably and then doing a bit more, and so on. This is similar to the previously mentioned method of shaping.

Taking regular breaks

Pacing can also involve taking regular breaks in activities. Thus, one could exercise for a period (or number of repetitions) that one can tolerate, then take a break for a few minutes (perhaps doing something else in that time, like relaxing or stretching or standing up and walking about), then resuming the task or exercise for the same tolerance period before stopping again, and so on.

To work out the initial tolerance level we normally ask people to try the activity/task/exercise for as long as they can do it comfortably (but before their pain is really stirred-up). The time/distance/number of repetitions is recorded (e.g. 5 min for sitting, 50 m for walking, etc.) and then repeated at least two to three times and then averaged to give us a reasonable baseline or starting point.

To make the first quota of the exercise even easier to achieve (and remember that the initial goals/reinforcers should be easy to achieve to promote encouragement), it can also help to set the task at a little below the baseline average. For example, Fordyce (1976) suggested using a figure of 20% *below* the baseline average (i.e. 80% of the baseline average). Thus, if the average sitting tolerance at baseline was 5 min, then the starting sitting quota would be 80% of 5 min – that is, 4 min.

Once the quota is set it is important patients work to it and don't stop earlier if their pain is worse that day (so they do it *despite* the extra pain). If this starts to become difficult and they keep stopping short of their quota, then the quota should be reset at a slightly lower level, but not to zero, for the next day. Then the patient should start pacing up again from that lower setting.

The amount by which the quota is raised each time and the timing of the rise is something that is usually negotiated between the patient and the therapist. Patients may be keen to raise the level as fast as possible, but this risks overdoing and unnecessarily aggravating their pain (something we are trying to minimize).

Equally, some patients will be very avoidant and pain-focused. They usually don't want to move up until their pain is relieved (which may not be a realistic option). In both these cases the physiotherapist needs to take a middle line. They should advise the 'overdoer' to keep to a realistic pacing-up of quota levels (say, increasing by only so many repetitions every second day). In the case of the 'underdoer' or 'avoider' they should encourage them to try a small increment, perhaps reminding them of the purpose of the exercises and restating that they will not come to any harm by doing these exercises. It may also be necessary to explore patients' concerns if they are particularly hesitant.

In these cases, however, you should be aware of a possible trap you might fall into, whereby you could end up reinforcing inactivity.

Three points should be made here:

1. Try not to push the patient.
2. Patients must learn to reassure themselves.
3. Shift the focus back on to the task (exercise) and reinforce performance.

Try not to push the patient

If you do, patients may become reliant on you to move them along. But when you are not present they could easily stop. The motivation must come from the patient – they must *want* to achieve their stated goals (which should have been worked out with them already). They should also agree that the exercises are a feasible way for them to achieve these goals (the therapist may have to put time into explaining this clearly).

Patients must learn to reassure themselves

It is appropriate for the physiotherapist to explain to and educate patients about their pain, what it signifies and the prognosis. This will usually entail a degree of reassurance that patients are basically well, that there is nothing seriously (dangerously) wrong with their back (they won't end up in a wheelchair because of this problem).

However, once these issues have been addressed but you find the patient is starting to seek reassurance repeatedly about the same issues, this can be a sign of a problem developing (Salkovskis and Warwick, 1986). Each time you try to allay their concerns they could well say that it makes sense and they are satisfied with your explanation and even feel better about it now. But if they come back worried about the same issue again and again, your repeated attempts to reassure them could be starting to reinforce their worries rather than resolve them – exactly the opposite of what you intended. Remember, while you are taking up time listening to their worries and trying to reassure them, they are not exercising, just talking and getting attention from you for doing it.

Certainly, appropriate explanations, answering questions and reassurance are important initial steps and may be *briefly* repeated from time to time, but patients must learn to do it for themselves as well. Thus, when the same questions you answered last time you saw the patient are raised again, you should try to deflect it back. Get patients to do the work, not just depend on you to do it for them.

Thus you might say something like: 'That sounds like what we discussed last time I saw you; is that right?' (always check with the patient that your perception is accurate). If the answer is 'yes' then you might follow that up with something like: 'Well, what did I say about that the last time?' (in other words, try to get patients to recall your earlier advice – you might also need to remind them that they said they were satisfied with that advice). Of course, if patients think there might be a new angle or aspect to it, you will have to judge if that is so, or decide if it really is basically their original concern. If they say they can't recall what you said last time you could repeat it, but then ask them to repeat it back to you so they *demonstrate* they understood it (i.e. not just *say* they did).

Then you need to point out to them that they should now be able to remind themselves of this advice and the next time they start to worry about it they should be able to deal with it as well as you (or anyone else) could.

In some cases they might say that they have a new symptom (e.g. pain in a different site). In these cases you might be concerned that something new has developed (is it a red flag?). This is what the patient is probably concerned about. However, before getting concerned and recommending further investigations, it is worth checking your original assessment of their symptoms and complaints. It is often the case that they have actually reported this 'new' symptom before, but have been overlooking it lately (or it has been less evident lately). In this case you can point this out. It is relevant to remember that many patients with persisting pain do start to focus more than usual on different sensations in their bodies. If they are already concerned that you or the doctor have overlooked something or that they really do have a serious illness, then their report of a 'new' symptom could easily be a reflection of these beliefs and associated somatic focusing rather than a sign of developing disease or disease flare. Remember that when most of us start an exercise programme we

are activating muscles and joints we haven't used much lately, so some extra aches and pains are always likely. Of course, you must use your clinical judgement in these cases, but your initial assessment notes will often be an important place to start your reassessment of the patient's complaints.

Shift the focus back on to the task (exercise) and reinforce performance

Rather than reinforce talking about fears and concerns (without any evidence of patients doing anything about it themselves), it is important, as soon as possible, to shift your focus and attention back to the exercise programme. Reinforce with praise and attention patients' attempts at that, reminding them of how that will ultimately help them to achieve their goals. At the same time, remind them to reinforce themselves for their performance achievements (despite their fears and pain).

USING ASSOCIATION EFFECTS (REMINDERS)

While reinforcers provide the motivation for continued performance, they don't necessarily tell us *when* a given activity will be reinforced. Many of our actions are strongly influenced by learning *when* (under what circumstances or in what situations) our actions will be reinforced.

For example, when you are driving and you see that the traffic lights change to red, you will usually put your foot on the brake to stop the car. That action is reinforced by successful avoidance of a possible collision with another car (or other obvious consequences). What triggered your stopping was not just the motivation to avoid an accident, but rather the sight of the red light. The red light tells us that stopping is the right thing to do at that time (providing we wish to avoid a collision or a fine). However, if the light had been green, stopping would have been the wrong thing to do. The green light tells us that if we keep moving we will not only get where we want to go, but also we will avoid someone running into our tail.

A moment's reflection will reveal that there are many such examples through our normal day where our behaviour is changed upon a signal or a change in situation. The same applies to our routines through the day. In fact, when we try to change the time or place of when/where we normally do something, we can feel uncomfortable. Take cleaning your teeth – usually we do it in the bathroom, but try doing it in the kitchen and it will somehow feel 'not right', even though logically it should make no difference (the water is the same and the drains go to the same place). The main difference is that we are not used to cleaning our teeth in the kitchen. That is, we don't associate the kitchen with cleaning our teeth. But we do associate the bathroom with that activity, and when we see the bathroom after a meal or before bed we are likely to think about cleaning our teeth.

How could we apply these ideas to an exercise programme for our patients?

We are more likely to practise an exercise programme if we can tie it (associate the exercises) with specific times or places. These might be straight after getting out of bed in the morning or after getting home at the end of the day, or even during tea/coffee breaks through the day, for example. We could also improve our memory of when to exercise by using little reminders (e.g. a note in the diary, on the fridge, or even a sticker on a wristwatch).

If we simply tell patients they should exercise, provide a clear rationale and explanation, as well as description of the exercise, and we apply all the reinforcement principles outlined earlier to encourage them to do it (and to keep doing it), we will probably be successful. After all, most patients seem to manage to get through life without health professionals telling them how to spend every 5 min. Most of them will work out a convenient time to do their exercises and, over time, they will get used to doing them at these times (and maybe even feel 'not right' if they don't do them then).

However, some patients will require help in finding suitable times to do the exercises. If this is a new activity (which is most likely), patients will have to make a change to their normal routine – they will already be doing something (even if only lying down) at these times. They will need to think about how they spend their days and look for possible times that could be suitable. They will also

need to make doing the exercises a higher priority than the activity they will replace (or move the existing activity to another time). This may involve rearranging reinforcers for exercises versus other activities.

It is our experience that those patients who make a specific plan for *when* they will do the exercises (and *commit* themselves to it) before they leave the clinic, are more likely to be successful. It is important that they do not leave the clinic saying that they will think about it and 'see how they go'. If there are conflicting issues it is important that patients identify these beforehand and work out possible solutions. If patients come back for review and say they haven't been doing their exercises as they haven't found a suitable time, it tells you something about their motivation and lifestyle. If they are serious about achieving the goals they seek with the treatment or exercise programme then they will need to make it a higher priority and work out ways of dealing with any obstacles.

Remember to avoid the trap that awaits all health professionals in this situation – *don't do it for them* – patients must take the leading role in sorting these issues out, even if it takes longer than you might. Otherwise, they may never learn to deal with such problems. That doesn't mean the therapist should not offer assistance (e.g. suggesting possibilities, questions or prompts), but as much as possible the therapist should give the expectation that the patient/client is expected to do the work.

OVERCOMING FEAR–AVOIDANCE RESPONSES THROUGH EXPOSURE

A key element in the psychological treatment of a phobia (or strong fear of something) is to arrange for the person with the phobia repeatedly to approach what he or she fears. For example, if a person fears crowds, the treatment would involve getting the person repeatedly to go into somewhere like a crowded shopping centre until it didn't bother him or her. It has been found that this is one of the most effective treatments for a phobia and the effect lasts. However, if the phobia or a version of it recurs, the person now knows how to deal with it. This approach is called exposure training (and sometimes desensitization – making someone less sensitive or less reactive to something they fear; Emmelkamp, 1982).

Naturally, the task of getting someone with a phobia to confront what he or she is afraid of can be quite difficult and stressful for that person (as well as the psychologist). So some preparation is usually required and certain skills may also need to be learnt by patients before they will be ready or prepared to try confronting situations they would much rather avoid. This may involve discussion with patients to reassure them about the safety of the task as well as skills like relaxation techniques and cognitive coping strategies (e.g. reminding themselves that they will be all right, that nothing really bad will happen and that they have coped with these situations before).

It is not difficult to see how such an approach could be applicable for people with persisting pain who are avoiding activities due to fear of aggravating their pain or of causing more damage. Indeed, Vlaeyen and his colleagues in the Netherlands have reported taking just such an approach with good effect in single-case experimental design studies (Vlaeyen et al., 2001, 2002).

Possible steps to take

Identify what might be limiting progress with activities/exercises

Is it fear or anxiety about feeling more pain or causing more damage? Remember, many patients have been told to stop if their pain increases – to let pain be their guide (this could also be the view of the patient's spouse – so his or her views should be sought too). Another possibility is that the patient may have a poor understanding of what the pain might mean – he or she could be imagining rather serious possibilities when, in fact, the reality is much more benign.

Clarify the likely basis of pain (in a reassuring way)

As mentioned earlier, it is important to ensure that the treatment or intervention makes sense to the patient before starting (particularly as it will enhance the patient's adherence to the treatment). This will involve an explanation of the problem being treated in terms that are understandable (i.e. not full of jargon). This should be as factual as possible (given the obvious limits on current knowledge), and explain how the treatment will work. For example, Indahl et al. (1995) advised patients that they should think of low back pain as a sign that the blood circulation in the back muscles was inadequate and this could lead to stiffness and pain. It was also explained that this restricted circulation was often due to inflammation in part of the intervertebral disc which caused a reflex action (tension) in the paraspinal muscles. The patients were also told that pain or the anticipation of pain could also result in guarding of the back and increased muscle tension, which in turn could lead to more pain (via the same restriction in circulation). Regardless of what was thought to be the particular cause of a patient's back pain, all patients were told that their back problems are mainly due to heightened stabilization of the back by lumbar paraspinal muscles (i.e. excessive tension in these muscles holding the back rigid). The logical intervention that followed from Indahl's explanation was to resume ceased activities in as normal a manner as possible.

Vague statements that can easily be misinterpreted, such as 'it is just degeneration', should be avoided. Not only might patients feel that their back is crumbling away, but they would want to know how your treatment will prevent this.

Another example might be where neuropathic mechanisms are thought to be involved. The patient might believe a 'bulging disc and pressure on the nerve' is the cause of their pain and he or she may attribute any flare-up in pain to more damage at the disc, despite previous advice from the surgeon that surgery is not appropriate. An alternative formulation might put this in terms of neural plasticity, such as that there has been a change in the ways their spinal nerves are conducting messages to the brain due to an injury. As a result their nervous system may have become more sensitive and overreacts to sensations, even muscle twitches, which it would have previously ignored. It follows from this that they should try to respond to such increases in pain as calmly as possible, reminding themselves what is probably happening. At the same time, if patients have been avoiding activities as a result of this pain, this could compound their back problems due to disuse as well as altered motor control. Accordingly, the intervention should focus on reactivation through exercises and/or gradual resumption of normal activities.

This explanation should also address the fears or concerns you identified in the first step. If patients have scans which have been interpreted as 'negative' or not showing anything significant, point out (as Indahl et al. (1995) described) that this is actually 'positive' – it means there is nothing seriously wrong with their back – they are OK. They are really no different to most people in the community at their age. Most of us experience back pain sooner or later, but it doesn't last in most cases and it doesn't need to stop us getting on with our lives.

Again, ask patients to repeat back to you what they have understood you to have said, just to ensure that you have explained it clearly enough. Suggest that patients tell their spouse the good news too, especially in cases where the spouse has a poor understanding of the problem.

Encourage resumption of feared activities

This should start at a level patients think they can manage, gradually doing more or extending the task in a paced manner. Remember, continued avoidance of these activities must be reversed.

You might ask what patients would find helpful or reassuring. Reassurance, whether from their doctor or therapist, is unlikely to be enough. Most people gain more confidence by actually doing what they are afraid of, finding that they can do it and discovering that they are OK afterwards. Point this out to them. Think of similar examples that are not to do with pain, for example, learning to drive a car, use a computer, raise a child, travel overseas. No matter how much others tell us about these things, we only start to feel confident about doing them when we have actually done them ourselves.

Monitor and reinforce progress and seek to extend the activities

Remember the sections on reinforcement principles above (especially self-reinforcement). Also, the exercises and initial activities should not be the only goal, just the first step. Patients should be encouraged to extend these (gradually) until they have resumed most normal activities in the various areas of their lives (work, home, socially). It is also useful to remind them to apply these principles (of minimizing avoidance, maintenance of activities and self-confidence, and reinforcement) whenever they find themselves having these sorts of problems in the future.

THOUGHTS/BELIEFS/EXPECTATIONS

All of us are influenced by the ways in which we see (or perceive) the world, those around us and even our own behaviour. These perceptions may or may not be accurate, but they can affect how we feel and behave. Thus, if we believe that a bit of pain in the lower back may suggest we could end up in a wheelchair if we are not careful, then we are likely to be very cautious (guarded) in how we move and what we are prepared to do. This, in turn, is likely to have secondary effects on our gait, exercises and the other activities we are prepared to engage in. Hence, ignoring patients' beliefs and expectations about their pain, what it means and its appropriate treatment could easily risk their non-adherence to an exercise programme. On the other hand, if we inquire about these issues then we may be able to correct any inaccurate views and reassure patients about the best course of action. However, recall the point made earlier – repeated requests for reassurance are a warning sign to you that patients may be at risk of becoming dependent on you and failing to take prime responsibility for managing their pain – see the comments on dealing with this.

It is critical to managing back pain that patients' thoughts and beliefs about their pain be sought and discussed by the treating therapist. We cannot assume that the patient will have a good understanding of their pain and its management, no matter how capable or intelligent the patient may appear.

Possible questions to ask could include things like: 'What is your understanding of what has caused your back pain?' or 'What do you think is going on in your back when you have this pain?' or 'Do you ever wonder that when you do something and your pain gets worse you might have damaged something?'

Such questions should elicit some of their beliefs or expectations which you can then discuss in the light of your assessment and the other information available on their back pain. Of course, this could lead to further concerns being raised and you can then address those too.

Care in checking patients' understanding or perceptions of what you have told them is also critical as it is easy for professionals (of all disciplines) to assume that patients understand health issues as well as they do. When checking a patient's beliefs it is recommended that you should avoid asking for 'yes' or 'no' answers. For example, after having explained something to a patient, if you asked: 'Do you understand?' it is likely that the patient, especially one who is lacking in confidence or feels unassertive, would say 'yes' simply to avoid sounding stupid or dumb. Rather, you should try to get the patient to repeat back to you what you have just said.

This could be put like this: 'Now, just to make sure that I have explained it clearly enough, could you tell me what I said, in your own words?'

This way of checking their comprehension avoids the risk of confronting patients directly and placing the responsibility on them for recalling what you said. Rather, it is the therapist who explicitly takes the responsibility for explaining things clearly. Of course, the patient's response can then be corrected as necessary. Most importantly, the therapist should confirm with patients that they have understood (e.g. 'that's right'). They might also like to write it down if they are having trouble remembering.

Things to avoid

When someone has persisting non-specific back pain, especially in the first few weeks after onset, they can be very susceptible to attending to any information that might indicate there is something seriously wrong with them. Such information could easily give rise to heightened anxiety or apprehension – fears which can easily obstruct advice to exercise. It is critical, therefore, that care is taken in how a therapist responds to patients' account of the onset of the pain, their description of symptoms and their pain behaviours, as well as any reports of imaging. Table 8.1 describes some commonly reported statements by therapists and patients.

It usually helps to prepare for encounters like these if you have practised saying the sorts of things you would like to say in these situations, either alone in front of a mirror or with colleagues. These examples also highlight the importance of checking with patients that they have understood what you told them.

Options to try

If patients are concerned about possible awful things happening to them when they exercise (for example, damaging the spine), ask them to clarify as much as possible exactly what they are

Table 8.1 Common anxiety-inducing responses by therapists

Anxiety-inducing responses by therapist could include statements like	Possible interpretations by patient
'Let pain be your guide'	The pain means I'm doing too much
'If it hurts, stop'	I could be damaging myself
'Be careful'	If I'm not careful, I'll make it worse
'Avoid any activities that aggravate your pain'	They might make matters worse
'These scans indicate a fair bit of degeneration'	I'm falling apart
'These scans show there's a disc bulging'	It must be about to burst
'These scans look pretty terrible'	There must be something terribly wrong
'There is some instability in your spine'	My back could snap in two
'If the exercises hurt, let me know; you must be doing them incorrectly'	The exercises should take my pain away. If they don't, it's my fault

concerned about. Has anyone suggested anything to them (either inadvertently or intentionally), e.g. the possibility of needing surgery, otherwise they might end up in a wheelchair one day? Equally, have they read or heard something (newspapers, TV, or even someone they know) which made them wonder about their back?

If they can't be specific, then ask what is the worst thing they could imagine happening to them if they exercise while in pain.

Once you have this sort of information, you will need to discuss with patients how likely (or unlikely) these things are. Typically, you will try to reassure them that they are very unlikely. However, some patients will still say, 'yes, I know it is unlikely, but it would be terrible if it happened and so I don't want to risk it'. Of course, you can never say that something terrible will never happen, regardless of how unlikely it is. It is also true that some things that happen to people can be very unpleasant and even tragic. So, there is a grain of truth in what these patients say. What are the options for dealing with this situation?

1. Agree with them and say maybe it is better that they just take it easy and see how they go. (OK, but this does raise the risk of avoidance of activities which, in turn, could lead to greater disability and worse outcomes in the long run – in this group who are still seeking help at 8–12 weeks postonset.)

2. Having emphasized that the thing they fear is extremely unlikely (and could just as easily happen to you), explore exactly how terrible it might be. Yes, people do have spinal cord injuries and become quadraplegic, but are their lives over? Look at the Paralympics – many of the competitors there seem to manage quite well, and are often more active than those with no physical impairments.

   In other words, even if the worst thing happened, would it really be so terrible, or would they just have to find a way to manage – as they have done through their lives already when something has gone wrong? Equally, if they spend their lives worrying about what might happen or not doing useful things about their back pain in case something terrible could possibly happen as a result, where might they

end up? Could it be that they might actually be increasing the risk of something awful happening by not resuming normal activities and exercises?

In this way, you will not only be addressing the rarity of the thing they fear, but also getting them to see that what they fear may not be so bad anyway. Even if the worst thing did happen, they would still find a way to manage and to get on with their lives, just as thousands of others have done when seriously injured. Most of us will know of examples of people who have overcome great adversity. Reminding the patient of these people or asking them if they know of anyone like that could be useful (they might still say something like: 'that's all right for them, but I know I couldn't do it' – but you could point out that neither could most of those people before they were injured).

SHORT QUIZ

Now a short quiz – remember that checking whether you've explained things clearly enough is another learning principle.

1. Achieving goals is just a matter of willpower (T/F).
2. If you tell patients to do an exercise, they will usually do just as you expected (T/F).
3. Reinforcers or rewards should be tailored to the individual patient (T/F).
4. If the patient is being encouraged to lie down or rest by one health care provider and to exercise by another, we can be sure they will still do the exercises (T/F).
5. Reinforcers should follow a behaviour that we are trying to encourage a patient to learn (T/F).
6. Reinforcers provide a form of feedback to the patient (T/F).
7. The therapist must motivate patients, otherwise they won't do anything (T/F).
8. Pacing involves a gradual build-up in activity levels and taking regular breaks in activity (T/F).
9. If patients repeatedly seek reassurance from you that they are doing the right thing and that they will be OK, you should give it to them as long as they seek it (T/F).

10. When checking if patients have understood what you have told them, it is best to get them to repeat it back to you (T/F).

11. If a patient with non-specific low back pain reports a new symptom, you should drop everything and re-examine him/her and advise more investigations, especially scans (T/F).

12. If patients are reluctant to do an exercise in case their pain is aggravated, it is best to tell them not to do it until they feel up to it (T/F).

(Note: if you are not confident of your answers, have another look at the chapter.)

REFERENCES

Aylon, T. and Azrin, N. (1968). *The Token Economy*. New York: Appleton Century Crofts.

Bandura, A. (1986). *Social Foundations of Thought and Action: A Social Cognitive Theory*. Englewood Cliffs, NJ: Prentice-Hall.

Beck, A.T., Rush, A.J., Shaw, B.F. and Emery, G. (1979). *Cognitive Therapy of Depression*. New York: Guilford Press.

Cairns, D. and Pasino, J. (1977). Comparison of verbal reinforcement and feedback in the operant treatment of disability due to low back pain. *Pain*, **2**, 301–308.

Davey, G. (1988). Trends in human operant theory. In: *Human Operant Conditioning and Behavior Modification*, ed. G. Davey and C. Cullen, pp. 1–14. Chichester: John Wiley.

Emmelkamp, P.M.G. (1982). *Phobic and Obsessive Compulsive Disorders: Theory, Research and Practice*. New York: Plenum Press.

Fordyce, W.E. (1976). *Behavioural Methods for Chronic Pain and Illness*. St Louis: C.V. Mosby.

Fordyce, W.E., Caldwell, L. and Hongadorom, T. (1979). Effects of performance feedback on exercise tolerance in chronic pain. Unpublished manuscript, University of Washington.

Guzman, J., Esmail, R., Karjaleinan, K., Malmivaara, A., Irvin, E. and Bombardier, C. (2001). Multidisciplinary rehabilitation for chronic low back pain: systematic review. *Br. Med. J.*, **322**, 1511–1515.

Hawton, K., Salkovskis, P.M., Kirk, J. and Clark, D.M. (eds) (1989). *Cognitive Behaviour Therapy for Psychiatric Problems: A Practical Guide*. Oxford: Oxford Medical Publications.

Indahl, A., Velund, L. and Reikeraas, O. (1995). Good prognosis for low back pain when left untampered: a randomized clinical trial. *Spine*, **20**, 473–477.

Lewinsohn, P.M. (1974). A behavioral approach to depression. In: *The Psychology of Depression: Contemporary Theory and Research*, ed. R.J. Friedman and M.M. Katz. Washington, DC: Winston.

Lindstrom, I., Ohland, C., Eek, C., Wallin, L., Peterson, L.E. and Nachemson, A. (1992). Mobility, strength, and fitness after a graded activity program for patients with subacute low back pain. A randomized prospective clinical study with a behavioral therapy approach. *Spine*, **17**, 641–649.

Linton, S.J. (2000). A review of psychological risk factors in back and neck pain. *Spine*, **25**, 1148–1156.

Linton, S.J. and Andersson, T. (2000). Can chronic disability be prevented? A randomized trial of a cognitive-behavioral intervention and two forms of information for spinal pain patients. *Spine*, **25**, 2825–2831.

Maher, C., Latimer, J. and Refshauge, K. (1999). Prescription of activity for low back pain: what works? *Aust. J. Physiother.*, **45**, 121–132.

Malmivaara, A., Hakkinen, U., Aro, T. et al. (1995). The treatment of acute low back pain – bed rest, exercises, or ordinary activity? *N. Engl. J. Med.*, **332**, 351–355.

Marks, I.M. (1975). Behavioural treatment of phobic and obsessive-compulsive disorders: a critical appraisal. In: *Progress in Behavior Modification*, ed. M. Hersen, R.M. Eisler and P.M. Miller, pp. 66–158. New York: Academic Press.

Meichenbaum, D.H. (1975). Self-instructional methods. In: *Helping People Change: A Textbook of Methods*, ed. F.H. Kanfer and A.P. Goldstein. New York: Guilford Press.

Morley, S., Eccleston, C. and Williams, A.C.deC. (1999). Systematic review and meta-analysis of randomised controlled trials of cognitive behaviour therapy for chronic pain in adults, excluding headache. *Pain*, **80**, 1–13.

Salkovskis, P.M. and Warwick, H.M.C. (1986). Morbid preoccupations, health anxiety and reassurance: a cognitive-behavioural approach to hypochondriasis. *Behav. Res. Ther.*, **24**, 597–602.

Skinner, B.F. (1974). *About Behaviorism*. London: Jonathan Cape.

Teasell, R.W. and Harth, M. (1996). Functional restoration: returning patients with chronic low back pain to work – revolution or fad? *Spine*, **21**, 844–847.

Turk, D.C. and Holzman, A.D. (1986). Commonalities among psychological approaches in the treatment of chronic pain: specifying the meta-constructs. In: *Pain Management: A Handbook of Psychological Treatment Approaches*, ed, A.D. Holzman and D.C. Turk, pp. 257–268. New York: Pergamon Press.

Van Tulder, M.W., Esmail, R., Bombardier, C. and Koes, B.W. (1999). Back schools for non-specific low back pain. Cochrane Review. In: the Cochrane Library, issue 3. Oxford: Update Software.

Vlaeyen, J.W.S., Haazen, I., Shuerman, J., Kole-Snijders, A. and Eek, H. (1995). Behavioural rehabilitation of chronic low back pain: comparison of an operant treatment, an operant-cognitive treatment and an operant-respondent treatment. *Br. J. Clin. Psychol.*, **34**, 95–118.

Vlaeyen, J.W.S. and Linton, S.J. (2000). Fear-avoidance and its consequences in chronic musculoskeletal pain: a state of the art. *Pain*, **85**, 317–332.

Vlaeyen, J.W.S., de Jong, J., Geilen, M., Heuts, P.H.T.G. and van Breukelen, G. (2001). Graded exposure in vivo in the treatment of pain-related fear: a replicated single-case experimental design in four patients with chronic low back pain. *Behav. Res. Ther.*, **39**, 151–166.

Vlaeyen, J.W.S., de Jong, J., Geilen, M., Heuts, P.H.T.G. and van Breukelen, G. (2002). The treatment of fear of movement/(re)injury in chronic low back pain: further evidence on the effectiveness of exposure in vivo. *Clin. J. Pain*, **18**, 251–261.

Von Korff, M., Russell, E.G. and Sharpe, M. (2002). Organising care for chronic illness. *Br. Med. J.*, **325**, 92–94.

Waddell, G. and Bryn-Jones, M. (1994). British sickness and invalidity benefit for back incapacities: 1953–54 to 1991–2. Unpublished data prepared for the National Back Pain Association and CSAG, 1993. In: *Report of a CSAG Committee on Back Pain*, ed. M. Rosen. London: HMSO.

Waddell, G. and Burton, K. (1999). Evidence review. In: *Occupational Health Guidelines for the Management of Low Back Pain at Work – Principal Recommendations*, ed. J.T. Carter and L.N. Birrell. London: Faculty of Occupational Medicine.

Waling, K., Sundelin, G., Ahgren, C. and Jarvholm, B. (2000). Perceived pain before and after three exercise programs – a controlled clinical trial of women with work-related trapezius myalgia. *Pain*, **85**, 201–208.

Williams, A.C.deC., Nicholas, M.K., Richardson, P.H., Pither, C.E. and Fernandes, J. (1999). Generalizing from a controlled trial: the effects of patient preference versus randomization on the outcome of inpatient versus outpatient chronic pain management. *Pain*, **83**, 57–65.

Index